Meta-Inflammation and Obesity

Edited by

Asija Začiragić

Department of Human Physiology, Faculty of Medicine,
University of Sarajevo, Sarajevo,
Bosnia and Herzegovina

Meta-inflammation and Obesity

Editor: Asija Začiragić

ISBN (Online): 978-981-14-7965-6

ISBN (Print): 978-981-14-7963-2

ISBN (Paperback): 978-981-14-7964-9

need for a court order if at any point you breach any terms of this License Agreement. In no event will any delay or failure by Bentham Science Publishers in enforcing your compliance with this License Agreement constitute a waiver of any of its rights.

3. You acknowledge that you have read this License Agreement, and agree to be bound by its terms and conditions. To the extent that any other terms and conditions presented on any website of Bentham Science Publishers conflict with, or are inconsistent with, the terms and conditions set out in this License Agreement, you acknowledge that the terms and conditions set out in this License Agreement shall prevail.

Bentham Science Publishers Pte. Ltd.
80 Robinson Road #02-00
Singapore 068898
Singapore
Email: subscriptions@benthamscience.net

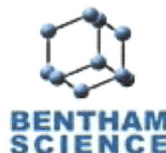

**BENTHAM
SCIENCE**

CONTENTS

PREFACE

With great pleasure, we present you the publication entitled "Meta-inflammation and Obesity". The book is the result of a joint effort and represents a state-of-the-art compilation and overview of current scientific evidence on the role of meta-inflammation in obesity and obesity-related disorders. Obesity embodies a global epidemic with severe and overwhelming health and economic repercussions. The multifaceted physiological mechanisms control the equilibrium of energy intake and expenditure in the body. These complex mechanisms incorporate neuronal activity within structures of the central nervous system with signals coming from the adipose tissue and endocrine glands as well as from the autonomic nervous and gastrointestinal system. A pivotal role in obesity is played by adipokines, which are cytokines produced and secreted from white adipose tissue. Adipokines use autocrine, paracrine, and endocrine mechanisms in the regulation of copious physiological processes. Studies have shown that adipokines are significant players in the regulation of glucose metabolism and tolerance, insulin resistance, inflammation, and oxidative stress, as well as in angiogenesis and atherosclerosis. Moreover, adipokines have a major role in the equilibrium between satiety and appetite as well as in the maintaining energy expenditure and body fat stores. In obesity, visceral adipose tissue is accumulated and undergoes significant morphofunctional changes with numerous pathophysiological consequences. Visceral obesity is characterized by adipocyte dysfunction, which is followed by a disrupted adipokine discharge pattern and the inception of meta-inflammation. The term "meta-inflammation" denotes chronic metabolic and systemic low-grade inflammation that has an important role in the pathogenesis of various metabolic diseases. The majority of authors thus far agree that meta-inflammation could be the linkage between obesity and obesity-related diseases. Bearing in mind that meta-inflammation is a relatively novel concept, it is still widely investigated. The distribution of visceral adipose tissue exhibits a different gender pattern. Physiological and psychosocial alterations between women and men have an impact on the pathophysiology of numerous disorders, and type 2 diabetes mellitus (T2DM) is one of the examples. Obesity represents a major risk factor for T2DM. One of the possible explanations for gender differences in obesity-related T2DM may be meta-inflammation as well as the actions of sex hormones (estrogens and androgens), that have been shown to affect adipose tissue function and metabolism alongside with biological characteristics. Novel evidence points to the significant role of obesity not only in the development of metabolic and cardiovascular diseases but in the pathophysiology of Alzheimer's disease (AD) as well. Studies have shown that meta-inflammation affects brain function together with disturbed insulin signaling and insulin resistance. Based on this notion, certain authors refer to this condition as brain diabetes or diabetes type 3 to denote cognitive decline in AD patients that develops as the consequence of inflammatory and metabolic trajectories. Obesity is followed by changes in the redox state with consequent oxidative stress. Obese patients have been shown to have decreased antioxidant defense and increased levels of reactive oxygen or nitrogen products. Further on, obesity is accompanied by altered brain metabolism. The neuron's synaptic plasticity may be affected by oxidative stress and meta-inflammation, and these processes often result in apoptosis or cell necrosis within the central nervous system with consequent neurodegenerative disorders characterized by brain atrophy, cognitive impairment, and neuroinflammation. Bearing in mind that the aging population worldwide is on the rise, significant scientific efforts are directed towards the unraveling of the basis for human aging. In recent years the term inflammaging has been introduced to indicate the possible role of chronic systemic low-grade inflammation as the cornerstone for human aging. Although the prominence of inflammaging in the aging process is now proven by the evidence from literature, its etiology is not yet fully elucidated. Moreover, future studies should answer the question whether chronic systemic low-grade inflammation is the cause or the consequence of obesity and obesity- and aging-related diseases.

The preface aims to give an insight into the content of our book, and we as the authors sincerely hope that our readers and colleagues will find it interesting and useful in the acquisition of cutting-edge research novelties on the interplay between meta-inflammation and obesity, that carries significant clinical consequences.

Asija Začiragić
Department of Human Physiology, Faculty of Medicine
University of Sarajevo, Sarajevo
Bosnia and Herzegovina

List of Contributors

Almir Fajkić Department of Pathophysiology, University of Sarajevo, Sarajevo, Bosnia and Herzegovina

Amela Dervišević Department of Human Physiology, University of Sarajevo, Sarajevo, Bosnia and Herzegovina

Amina Valjevac Department of Human Physiology, University of Sarajevo, Sarajevo, Bosnia and Herzegovina

Asija Začiragić Department of Human Physiology, University of Sarajevo, Sarajevo, Bosnia and Herzegovina

Lejla Opardija General Hospital Bugojno, Sarajevo, Bosnia and Herzegovina

Nermina Babić Department of Human Physiology, University of Sarajevo, Sarajevo, Bosnia and Herzegovina

Orhan Lepara Department of Human Physiology, University of Sarajevo, Sarajevo, Bosnia and Herzegovina

Selma Spahić Department of Human Physiology, University of Sarajevo, Sarajevo, Bosnia and Herzegovina

CHAPTER 1

Etiology of Obesity

Selma Spahić*

Department of Human Physiology, Faculty of Medicine, University of Sarajevo, Sarajevo, Bosnia and Herzegovina

Abstract: Numerous models have been proposed that try to explain the complex etiology of obesity. Etiology maps have been created to interconnect the various endogenous and exogenous variables that contribute to the pathophysiological pathways that lead to overweight and obesity. No country in the world has solved the problem of overweight and obesity, and the health and economic consequences that are suffered around the world are on the rise since the world population is getting more obese by the day. We aim to reflect on those variables that we see as potential target points for weight loss and to present the best available current data on the overweight and obesity epidemic. The goal of this review chapter is to emphasize the importance of different obesity determinants: host factors, social environment, built environment and behavioral determinants. Obesity is a risk factor for metabolic syndrome, hormonal dysfunction and depression, it lowers lifetime expectancy and reduces the overall health-related quality of life. Searching for a one-size-fits-all solution has been shown ineffective in preventing the escalating obesity rates. Efforts should be directed towards defining targeted, individualized strategies, while creating a network of support that includes healthcare professionals, family members and national regulations. A multi modal interdisciplinary approach and patient-centered care is mandatory to stop the global obesity epidemic.

Keywords: Body weight, Built environment, Behavior, Determinants, Energy imbalance, Inflammation, Metabolically healthy obesity, Microbiome, Obesity, Risk factors.

INTRODUCTION

Obesity is a chronic, non-communicable, adiposity-based, relapsing disease [1]. From data collected around the world during the last century, it is evident that obesity is on the rise. Currently, over 650 million adults (18 years and older) and 340 million children and adolescents are obese. Since 1975, the number of obese people has nearly tripled.

---

* **Corresponding author Selma Spahić:** Department of Human Physiology, Faculty of Medicine, University of Sarajevo. Sarajevo, Bosnia and Herzegovina; Tel: +387 33 226 478, Ext. 529; E-mail: selma.spahic@mf.unsa.ba

Asija Začiragić (Ed.)

In 2016, more than 1.9 billion adults were overweight, which suggests that, following the current trend, obesity prevalence can easily further multiply [2]. Estimates are that by 2030, every fifth citizen of the world will be obese [3]. The world prevalence of overweight and obesity in children under the age of 5 has expanded from approximately 5% in 2000 to 6% in 2010; and 6.3% in 2013. The most prominent rise occurred in Asia and Africa where an increase from 11 to 19% in certain countries in southern Africa, and from 3 to 7% in South-East Asia was observed. Estimates predict that overweight in children under the age of 5 is going to rise to 11% globally by 2025 if current patterns proceed [4]. Obesity is present in both genders and in all age groups regardless of ethnicity, region or socioeconomic status; however, the prevalence is generally greater in the elderly and women [5]. For decades, obesity was considered a behavioral problem, and we are just starting to uncover all the hidden factors that contribute to the complex pathophysiology of weight gain. Looking at current evidence and reviewing the timeline of obesity research, it seems that tackling the obesity epidemic will be a long and demanding task. No country to date managed to reverse its obesity epidemic [6]. A lack of success is understandable considering that appropriate management of obesity demands addressing not only behavior, but multiple dysfunctions (host, environmental and societal). Although they all play a definite role in disease development, it is safe to say that none of them satisfactorily, to a full extent, explains the obesity epidemic [7]. Defining the mechanisms involved in obesity must engage disciplines that analyze the genetic and epigenetic framework, as well as the development stages in host biology that impact disease pathogenesis; the neurological and psychological background of feeding behaviors; metabolic changes due to specific nutrient intake; the effect of physical activity and body composition; environmental availability of healthy foods and the impact of presentation to ecological factors extending from endocrine-disturbing synthetic substances (EDCs) to the social and cultural machinery that drives public opinions and produces regulations and policies [8]. A simplified overview of these determinants and their interplay is proposed in Fig. (**1**), and further explained in the text. Recently, to bring together most of the relevant variables that lead to overweight and obesity and to show their interdependencies, Systems Science [9] was used and etiology maps were generated. Those have been very helpful, although not fully comprehensive, as they present an apprehensible overview of the complexity of obesity and highlight multiple levels where the variables interconnect. The maps are in accordance with the obesity paradigm shift, from obesity being perceived as a problem arousing from a lack of willpower with an easy one-size-fits-all solution that comes down to "eat less, move more"; to one of the biggest health hazards of the 21st century [10, 11].

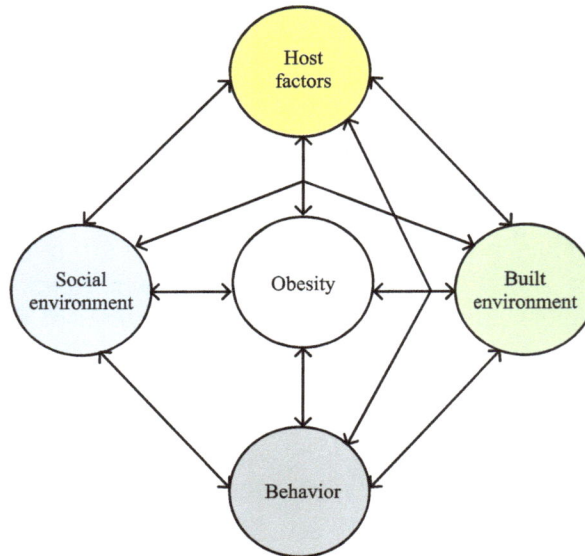

Fig. (1). Obesity determinants.

BODY WEIGHT CLASSIFICATION IN ADULTS

The most commonly used measure of obesity is the Body Mass Index (BMI). Based on the BMI, a healthy weight range for height is easily determined by dividing weight in kilograms with height in meters squared. The BMI is widely accepted as a general marker for obesity, and although the index is not representing a genuine proportion of adiposity, it is easy to use in health screenings and epidemiological reviews. The index is considered a reliable measure in estimating worldwide obesity prevalence. However, due to its limitations, it is not recommended to use only the BMI for individual assessment and nationwide studies, especially for children, elderly and the Asian population [12]. A combination of the BMI with other anthropometric measures such as waist circumference, waist-to-hip ratio and other adiposity estimation methods is advocated. A BMI measure above 25 kg/m^2 classifies for overweight, and a BMI greater or equal to 30 kg/m^2 qualifies as obesity. The BMI is, by itself, a strong predictor of overall mortality both above and below the apparent optimum of about 22.5–25 kg/m^2 [13], even though a BMI from 18.5 to 25 kg/m^2 is considered normal. The degree of obesity is expressed through further categorization of obesity into subclasses for BMI values above 30 kg/m^2. Three subcategories of obesity are defined: class 1 (BMI of 30 to <35 kg/m^2), class 2 (BMI of 35 to <40 kg/m^2), and class 3 (BMI of >40 kg/m^2) [14].

BODY WEIGHT CLASSIFICATION IN CHILDREN

Assessing BMI in children requires adjusting for both biological sex and age with corresponding growth charts; since children are still growing, the children's body composition changes as they age and it varies between girls and boys. The World Health Organization, the Centers for Disease Control and Prevention (CDC) and the International Obesity Task Force (IOTF) proposed their BMI classification systems adopted for the use in children. A comparison of these tools with respect to prevalence approximation tied with demographic factors yielded different estimates and showed inconsistencies [15]. The CDC and IOTF classification systems are a widely used diagnostic tool for overweight and obesity among children and adolescents aged 2-18 years. Percentile classification charts tailored for age and gender form data referenced in national studies from the UK, Hong Kong, the Netherlands, Brazil, Singapore, and the USA are used when conducting epidemiological studies [16]. The ≥85th BMI centile and the ≥95th BMI centile render age- and gender-specific BMI cut-offs that match the cut-offs for adults' overweight and obesity, respectively. These cut-offs are referred to as the International Obesity Task Force (IOTF) body mass index cut-offs. They allow for international associations of obesity prevalence in children, but their use is not recommended for a clinical setting [17].

WEIGHT GAIN AS A CONSEQUENCE OF ENERGY SURPLUS

An increased energy intake, a decreased energy expenditure or a combination of both processes, result in an energy surplus that ultimately leads to the formation of energy reserves in adipocytes. All proposed obesity determinants affect energy intake, energy expenditure or energy storage, thereby affecting energy balance. Two proposed underlying processes related to obesity pathogenesis are prolonged positive energy balance and an increased value of the body weight "set point" [8]. Researches that support the "thrifty gene hypothesis" claim that a positive energy balance was of an evolutionary advantage [18], because food resources were scarce and the body prepared itself for periods of famine and fasting. However, in an obesogenic environment where calorie-dense, processed food is readily available, with a decrease in time spent in physical activities, energy excess occurs easily and is not counterbalanced. Maladaptive eating behaviors, and subsequently weight gain develop seemingly unnoticed. A slight but consistent energy surplus, of merely 100 kcal more per day, results in a gradual yearly weight gain [19]. On the other hand, the body weight "set point" hypothesis, if true would elucidate why weight loss is hard to maintain and why lost weight will probably be regained over time, which represents an important obstacle for successful and sustained obesity management. Accordingly, new treatment approaches attempt to address the processes that reset the guarded body weight level back to a lower, closer to normal value. At which point, the gained weight becomes refractory to change and biologically defended is still not fully understood [8]. Debate still exists, essentially questioning if outside determinants cause biological control malfunction, and if the internal body's 'set point' feedback system is substituted by several 'settling points' that are impacted by energy and nutrient intake which cause new zero-energy balance points. Both proposed models are hypotheses, and fail to fully explain the data from human observational studies, and alternative models based on gene-by-environment interplay are needed to attain a complete understanding of body weight control [20 - 22].

Obesity is now recognized as an adiposity-based chronic disease, and weight gain is only one component of obesity. Many authors agree that most health repercussions of obesity occur because of an induced low-grade systematic inflammation. Once entered the vicious circle of hormonal and metabolic changes complementary to excess adiposity, weight loss becomes very hard to achieve.

DETERMINANTS OF OBESITY

The questions that still remain unanswered are why do some individuals gain weight easier than others, and why do some individuals remain lean in an obesogenic environment? Host risk factors (Fig. **2**) include biological determinants (genetic, epigenetic, perinatal), determinants obtained through long term lifestyle that are not easily modifiable (brain-gut axis, gut microbiome, and viruses) and secondary causes of obesity (neuroendocrine conditions, physical and intellectual disability, medications). Behavior is the key regulating and modifiable factor in obesity prevention and treatment. In order to modulate behavior, a broad understanding of its determinants is needed. A biological foundation that gets expressed in a distinct built and social environment ascertains behavior. Behavioral factors that promote obesity include excessive calorie intake, unhealthy eating patterns, dominantly sedentary lifestyles, insufficient sleep, and inefficient stress management. The biological determinants that underpin the development of obesity include genetic, epigenetic and prenatal factors. Determinants of the built environment or "human-made" determinants include urban planning, the food industry and food availability, utilization of endocrine disruptor chemicals, *etc.* Social determinants embed the effects of socio-economic and political influences, *i.e.,* traditions and customs, opinions towards food and physical activity, ethnicity, presence of supportive policies, culture, inequalities and stigmatization into the obesity etiology framework [23]. Altogether, the energy balance of the body is regulated within the brain that serves as an integration center for inputs from peripheral receptors, hormones, mediators and neurotransmitters as signals for hunger and satiation. The coordination of the signals received is planned to involve a minimum of 2 parallel systems: the metabolic homeostatic system and the brain reward system [24]. Therefore, is important to note that eating patterns are also changed in response to psychological stress and various external cues [25]. The metabolic homeostasis is primarily controlled by hypothalamic and brainstem neuronal circuits. The hedonic pathway of the consumed food involves the mesolimbic brain area and the cortex. Combinations of several groups of risk factors contribute to the process of gaining excess weight to developing unhealthy obesity. The process is usually polygenic and long.

BIOLOGICAL DETERMINANTS

Results from twins, family and adoption studies led to the recognition of causative gene-phenotype interactions in monogenic forms of obesity. However, hereditary factors cannot be considered the primary origin of the global obesity epidemic since the genome is not inclined to change within a few years. Advances in epigenetic studies extended the contemporary understanding of the pandemic of obesity [26]. Epigenetic alterations—DNA methylation, histone tails, and miRNAs modifications—involved in the evolution of obesity are increasingly apparent. There is evidence that the embryo-fetal and perinatal period play a fundamental role in the development and the programming of proper functioning in all human organs and tissues [27]. Hereditary determinants of obesity broadly can be grouped into monogenic causes, syndromic causes and polygenic causes. Monogenic causes are induced by a single gene mutation, principally found in the leptin-melanocortin pathway.

So far, there are eight well-recognized monogenic obesity genes: leptin (LEP), leptin receptor (LEPR), brain-derived neurotrophic factor (BDNF), neurotrophic tyrosine kinase receptor type 2 (NTRK2), prohormone convertase 1 (PCSK1), melanocortin 4 receptor (MC4R), proopiomelanocortin (POMC) and single-minded homologue 1 (SIM1). Severe early-onset obesity and overeating can be explained with single-gene mutations in these eight genes in up to 10% of severely obese children. Single gene mutations commonly result in leptin and leptin receptor deficiency, POMC deficiency, Prohormone convertase deficiency, Melanocortin Receptor 4 deficiency, SIM 1 insufficiency, BDNF and TrkB insufficiency. Syndromic obesity is linked with different phenotypes such as neurodevelopmental anomalies, and other organ and/or system malformations. Syndromic obesity is associated with Prader–Willi syndrome, Bardet–Biedl syndromes, Alstrom–Hallgren syndrome, Beckwith–Wiedemann syndrome, Carpenter syndrome and Cohen syndrome [28]. Polygenic obesity is induced by a large number of genes, with a cumulative augmentation, where the effect of gene dysfunction is magnified within an obesogenic environment. Maternal-fetal stress, poor nutrition of the mother and various intoxications during pregnancy can conflict proper programming of cells, tissues, and organs. The roots of obesity may be fastened in utero. Intrauterine conditioning of the fetus and the plasticity during gestational growth is critical for adapting the fetus to its foreseen environment. Multiple animal and human studies have shown that obesity in pregnancy affects control of appetite and metabolism, immunity, growth, insulin signaling and inflammation [29]. An increased susceptibility to obesity may be predefined in patients born *via* Caesarean section and in patients whose mothers used antibiotics during pregnancy, because of an alteration in the natural maternal-offspring microbiota transfer. This contributes to anomalous microbial colonization of the infant's gut [30].

THE BRAIN-GUT AXIS

The Brain-gut axis is comprised of neuronal pathways in the central nervous system (CNS), enteric nervous system (ENS) and the autonomic nervous system (ANS) and neuroendocrine and immunological systems, including also the gut microbiome, which will be discussed below [31]. These axis components allow the brain and the gut to correspond with each other. Neurohumoral communication within the axis is established *via* local, paracrine and/or endocrine secretion. It is formed through sensory information being translated into neural, hormonal and immunological signals, which are relayed bidirectional from the CNS to the gut. The axis modulates appetite, energy balance and food consumption, which are centrally regulated in response to homeostatic and non-homoeostatic inputs. The arcuate nucleus of the hypothalamus integrates signals in the homeostatic system and regulates satiety and hunger *via* relaying inputs to higher cortical centers that stimulate the ANS, gastric function, and hormone secretion accordingly [32]. After a meal, due to the presence of nutrients in the gut, a variety of gut-derived peptides are produced from enteroendocrine cells including glucagon-like peptide 1 (GLP1), cholecystokinin (CCK), pancreatic polypeptide (PP), peptide YY3−36 (PYY), and oxyntomodulin, thereby signaling changes in the nutritional status to inform the brain. Gut to brain signaling occurs *via* afferent nerves, and direct secretion into the blood. Microbiota-derived metabolites, for example, short-chain fatty acids can modify gut hormone secretion, due to binding to receptors on enteroendocrine cells, and thus affect appetite and satiety. Obese patients have decreased satiation, higher fasting gastric volume, quickened gastric emptying, lower levels of CCK and GLP-1, higher levels of acyl-ghrelin, and increased levels of adipocyte secreted leptin, commonly accompanied with leptin resistance. A proposed subclassification of obesity in relation to the main abnormality in the brain-gut axis is based on a principal component analysis of characteristics from obesity patients. Based on the findings, the suggested traits that can differentiate between obesity subphenotypes are: abnormal satiety, abnormal gastric motor function and motility, and affect [33]. Whether brain-gut axis alterations that are coupled with excessive food consumption are a cause or an effect of obesity is still uncertain [34].

THE MICROBIOME

The gut microbiota is comprised of 10-100 trillion microorganisms that produce bioactive metabolites in a diet-dependent manner, including short-chain fatty acids and conjugated fatty acids impacting body weight through its effects on energy metabolism and systemic inflammation. Obesity-associated microbiota alter host energy harvesting, insulin resistance, inflammation, and fat deposition. Increased plasma levels of lipopolysaccharide, an endotoxin in the cell wall of Gram-negative bacteria, cause metabolic endotoxaemia, inducing a strong immune system response and contributing to the obesity-related low-grade inflammation. Dietary fat is crucial in this process because it increases intestinal lipopolysaccharide absorption through incorporation into chylomicrons. Moreover, impaired intestinal barrier integrity might also contribute to this metabolic endotoxaemia. The industrialized microbiota has an increased capacity to degrade the intestinal mucus layer [35]. Gut bacteria are therefore becoming increasingly recognized as the key regulators of host physiology and pathophysiology. Microbiota-derived metabolites have peripheral effects and also regulate metabolism, adiposity, homoeostasis, and energy balance as well as central appetite and food reward signaling. Alterations in the composition of the human gut microbiota especially early in life, are linked with metabolic disorders such as obesity, diabetes, and eating disorders, as well as stress-related neuropsychiatric disorders, including depression and anxiety, which are also characterized by changes in eating behavior. Growing evidence suggests that the success of bariatric surgery is due to its effects on the microbiota [36]. Gut bacteria can directly affect the CNS *via* modulation of endocrine signaling pathways of the microbiota–gut–brain axis such as GLP-1 and peptide YY signaling, or activation of reward pathways that together have crucial roles in obesity. Alterations in diet can profoundly affect the composition of gut bacteria at multiple levels of the gastrointestinal tract, and obesity itself may affect the composition of gut bacteria. Although the gut microbiota is a contributing and potential causal factor for obesity and metabolic syndrome, the exact mechanisms underlying this relationship are unclear. Further investigations are needed to elucidate the intricate gut-microbiota–host relationship and the potential of gut-microbiota-targeted strategies, such as dietary interventions including prebiotics, probiotics and fecal microbiota transplantation, as promising metabolic therapies that can help patients to maintain a healthy weight throughout life.

VIRUSES

Research into the origins of the obesity pandemic has encouraged the theory that distinct infectious agents might play a causal role in etiology of obesity, but this hypothesis is frequently omitted. Animal models infected with certain viral strains can develop obesity. Primarily adenoviruses Ad36 and Ad37 emerged as pathogens associated with adipogenesis. An Ad36 infection is linked to adipocyte proliferation and a body weight increase as reported in various preclinical models [37]. Obese individuals have significantly higher antibody titers to Ad36 than lean individuals. In a study of 502 US participants, where individuals have been screened for Ad36 prevalence, the virus was significantly more prevalent in the obese than in the lean (30% *vs*. 11%) [38]. These findings raise the question of whether susceptibility to infections contributes to the development of obesity. Extensive research and more human studies are required to explore this hypothesis and confirm a definitive causation. If enough strong evidence emerges, proving this causation, current approaches to obesity treatment and prevention would be profoundly impacted.

NEUROENDOCRINE CONDITIONS CAUSING SECONDARY OBESITY

Secondary obesity is caused by several neuroendocrine diseases. Patients need to be evaluated for potential hormone balance dysfunctions. Common disorders like hypothyroidism and polycystic ovarian syndrome, and other rather rare disorders like Cushing's syndrome, central hypothyroidism, hypothalamic disorders, and combined hormone deficiencies lead to obesity *via* various processes that align with the mechanisms of the primary endocrine condition [39].

PHYSICAL AND INTELLECTUAL DISABILITY

People with physical and intellectual disabilities comprise a vulnerable group since evidence shows that they are more prone to developing obesity than the general population. They may experience difficulties in weight control because creating and sustaining a healthy lifestyle is laborious. The possible obstacles that people with disabilities may face are numerous [40]. Difficulties with chewing or swallowing food, or experiencing food taste or texture, with a concomitant lack of healthy food decisions impact energy intake and digestion. Their prescribed medications may impact energy balance and have weight-related side effects. Physical restrictions due to disability reduce a person's ability to exercise additionally to physical activity barriers experienced by the general population like motivation and time. There are fewer possibilities for sports participation and/or they are inaccessible. Pain and a general energy deficiency further limit their participation in physical activity. The management of obesity occurring within this vulnerable group is specifically troublesome considering that they are at risk for the same weight-related complications and comorbidities as the general population, while additionally being at increased risk for chronic conditions linked with their disability. The co-occurrence of disability and weight gain forms vicious cycles and poses added health burdens, restricting patient functionality and independence, and reducing health-related quality of life [41]. More health-promotion programs targeting appropriate exercise regimes for people with disabilities are needed.

PRESCRIPTION DRUGS

It seems that the increased utilization of prescription drugs that lead to weight gain as a side-effect, at least partially contributes to the overweight and obesity pandemic. Classes of pharmaceuticals including antihyperglycemics, antidepressants, antipsychotics [42], corticosteroids, and antihypertensives contain medications that were associated with significant weight gain.

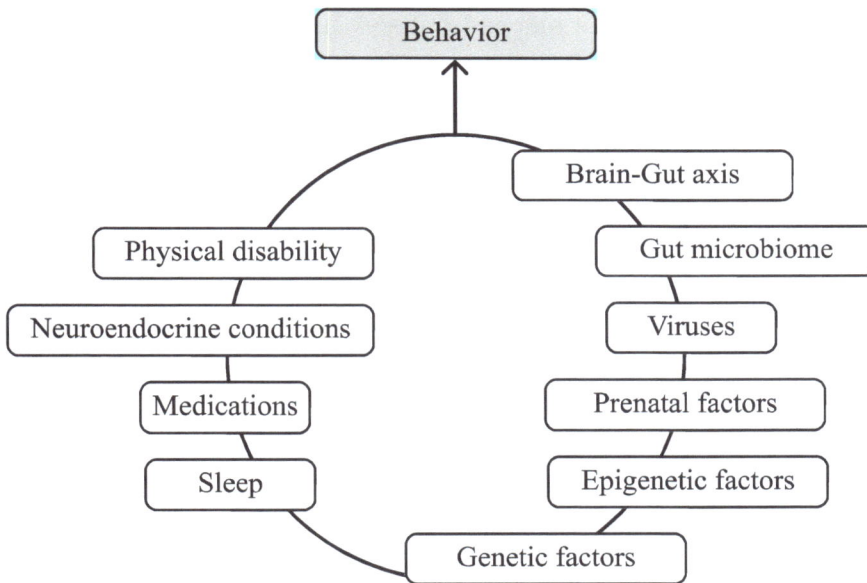

Fig. (2). Host risk factors.

Furthermore, diabetes, hypertension, and depression are well-known complications of obesity, and prescribing certain medications to treat these comorbidities worsens obesity, hence, a vicious circle is formed. Medication-induced gain of weight is often agonizing for the patient as well as for health care providers [43]. Reviewing prescribed medications is imperative in the evaluation of the obese patient because it can reveal the cause of the patients' weight being refractory to weight loss, or the cause of inability to achieve weight loss maintenance [44]. When possible changing medication with a weight-neutral or even weight-reducing alternative is preferable in overweight or obese patients. When alternative pharmaceuticals are not available, or therapy change is impossible, adjunctive treatment, changes in dosing, changes in medication delivery or lifestyle modifications should be discussed with the patient.

BUILT ENVIRONMENT RISK FACTORS

Built environment factors favoring obesity development include the abundance and commercialization of processed calorie-dense food, the utilization of endocrine disruptor chemicals (EDCs), the increasingly sedentary employment settings with a concomitant decrease of occupational physical activity, the absence of bicycle lanes, scarcity of pedestrian zones for walking, *etc* [45]. Various components of the built environment have been asserted as independent predictors of obesity. Neighborhoods either have or do not have parks and recreational spaces. The stores, supermarkets, theatres, restaurants, and workplaces can be located outside walking distances, inquiring more frequent use of motorized transportation (car, train, bus, taxi) [46]. The United States department of agriculture has mapped out so-called "food deserts" defined as a low-income area with limited access to healthy and nutritious food [47].

Current perspectives imply that BMI tends to lower values in regions where the intake of fruits and vegetables is higher. When investigating obesity risk, a reliable correlation between distances from home to healthy food sources is not easily made. It seems that access to healthier foods is rather associated with economics than with distance from home. Neighborhood characteristics analysis has the potential to contribute to customized obesity prevention programs. Connections between neighborhood-built environment characteristics and obesity have been extensively reported. Healthy People 2020 includes goals for supporting physical activity through neighborhood-built environment inter-ventions [48].

Readily available ultra-processed food often has decreased micronutrient content, little fiber and is stripped of most microorganisms, becoming nearly sterile [49]. Low-cost foods are generally, high in salt content and supplemented with sugars and fats. These inexpensive foods also have a high reward value and are promptly available. It has been hinted that the intake of such foods relieves the stress of daily life in some individuals. Numerous studies link exposure to EDCs to a variety of outcomes of potential relevance to obesity, including stimulation of adipogenesis and changes of insulin secretion, insulin sensitivity, and liver metabolism. Low-level exposure to EDCs is common and widespread in communities. Especially dangerous is maternal exposure to ECDs that can be transmitted to the fetus, where even if present in low levels, a higher susceptibility to obesity is imposed when compared to adult exposure. The Endocrine Society Scientific Statement recently provided a comprehensive review of this topic [50].

SOCIO-CULTURAL ENVIRONMENT RISK FACTORS

The neighborhood social environment is less profoundly studied. The social context, including sociodemographic composition and residential social processes, is potent in shaping obesity risk [51]. The relationships between individuals reflect on social cohesion and collective efficacy. Social norms, social capital, neighborhood safety, and segregation need to be assessed when investigating the social environment and its impacts on individual and public health. Socio-economic status (SES)-encouraged dietary changes and their contribution to obesity prevalence rise have been studied extensively. However, because of confounding variables the real influence of SES on obesity prevalence needs to be further investigated with different approaches like geolocalization and mapping approaches that can track the social, racial, and residential segregation patterns in neighborhoods. Overall, most observations link an increase in obesity risk among lower-income groups to insufficient healthy food budgets [52]. In future linking SES to obesity risk must include the examination of the effect on the energy homeostasis system, and not solely diet, physical activity, and behavior. Obesity among both adults and children has been linked to a lack of neighborhood safety [53]. The social environment is significant for habit formation. The results of a recent study, where a natural experiment was performed to examine whether obesity is more likely to be acquired when individuals are exposed to communities with high obesity rates, indicate that obesity has features of a social contagion [54]. Expressing opinions *via* online interactions has created a new body of evidence for psychological and sociological research. The stored databases are the hallmark for resourcing public opinions and beliefs nowadays [55]. Weight-related stigmatization within the personal environment on a global scale threatens the mental health of obese patients. Because of idealized body images, body dissatisfaction is common, as well as are eating disorders and a negligence of regular physical activities. The mental health of the youth need special public health programs to shift the perceived body image away from its appearance and towards its functionality. UK Youth Parliament's 'Make Your Mark' ballot showed that one million young adults pointed out body image as a one of the primary causes of their life problems [56]. The general public and health professionals stigmatize those who suffer from obesity, and this needs to be urgently addressed [43]. Nutrition is not sufficiently thought in schools, and universities. There is a lack of knowledge about the means of prevention, the burden of the disease and treatment. It seems that in order to build empathy, reduce prejudice, attain and establish social justice, simply spreading information will be insufficient [57]. A conceptual model of the above mentioned is proposed in Fig.(**3**).

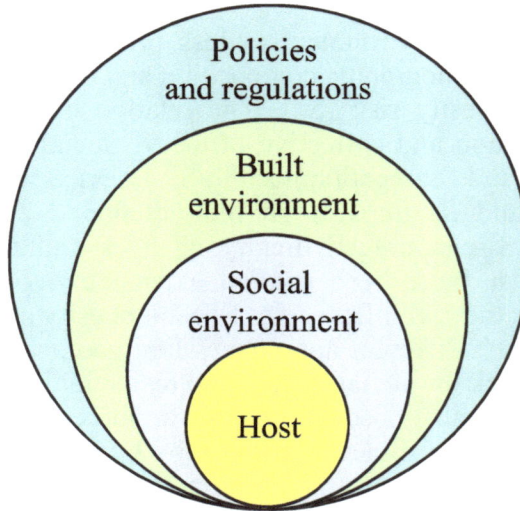

Fig. (3). Obesity model.

BEHAVIORAL RISK FACTORS

Despite being influenced by environmental factors individual decisions are precipitating the obesity disease development. An unhealthy diet, reduced physical activity, insufficient sleep [58], inadequate stress management and smoking cessation are self-inflicted and therefore modifiable risk factors for obesity and cardio-metabolic dysfunctions. The general population does not have a sustained, healthy dietary pattern. Essential nutrients and wholefoods including fruit and vegetables are consumed less when compared to unhealthy and processed foods, and sugar- sweetened beverages (SSBs) [59]. Evidence consolidated a positive association of SSBs consumption with obesity indices in adults and children; therefore a reduction of SSBs consumption through public health policies is advisable [60]. Engagement in physical activity is the most variable element of daily energy expenditure. Estimates are that in the past 50 years occupational physical activity reductions resulted in a decrease in total daily energy expenditure by 100 cal/day [8]. Scientific evidence points out that sleep disruption and circadian misalignment contribute to metabolic physiology dysregulations. Sufficient sleep is of key importance for a healthy metabolic function. However, many people do not sustain a habit of getting enough sleep, by cutting sleeping hours in order to participate in shift work, social activities, or other activities. These behaviors create a predisposition for poor metabolic health, by favoring excess caloric consumption in response to reduced sleep, food intake at times when the internal metabolic physiology systems are not prepared, reduced energy expenditure and disordered glucose metabolism [61]. Physiological stress, if not handled correctly, through efficient stress management methods, has the potential to drive maladaptive eating behaviors and mental health problems. 38 Stress induces cortisol secretion, together with other stress-induced physiological responses, both food intake and energy expenditure are modified, thereby making weight control more difficult to achieve [62].

Luckily, a substantial reduction in cigarette smoking rates was observed in the past decades [63]. Numerous health benefits accompany smoking cessation. Nevertheless, at least partially due to nicotine withdrawal and loss of the pharmacological effect of nicotine to suppress food consumption, smoking cessation is linked to a 3–5 kg average weight gain. The possible mechanisms of weight gain include a positive energy balance due to increased energy intake, reduced energy expenditure and resting metabolic rate, and an increase in lipoprotein lipase activity. Therefore, body weight monitoring and promotion of lifestyle changes need to be part of smoking cessation plans. Nicotine replacement and bupropion may help prevent weight gain in this vulnerable group. However, obesity remains a problem among both current smokers and people who never smoked [64].

COMPLICATIONS AND COMORBIDITIES OF OVERWEIGHT AND OBESITY

In the general population, obesity relates to more deaths than underweight [2]. The risk of death rises by 20%-40% in overweight people and is two-to-three times higher in obese people when compared to normal-weight individuals, as shown in a prospective cohort study of 527,265 U.S. citizens age 50 to 71 years, where the BMI was correlated to all-cause risk of death [65]. The Lancet published a report by the Prospective Studies Collaboration (PSC) that included 57 prospective studies with approximately 900 000 subjects, whose findings were analyzed to evaluate the correlation linking total and disease-specific mortality with the BMI values. The study proved that total mortality associated with a BMI value above 30 kg/m^2 is increased in both women and men in all age groups from 35 to 89 years. Increased mortality in subjects with a high BMI was principally caused by ischemic heart disease, diabetes, stroke, and liver disease [13].

The crosstalk between the multiple cell types that compose adipose tissue and the investigation into their function, led to the understanding that adipose tissue does not only serve as a storage organ, but rather has a dynamic metabolic and homeostatic, endocrine response in the regulatory pathways of body composition, hunger and satiety, and inflammatory modulation. Adipocytes and their precursors, immune cells, vascular cells, and neuronal cells constitute adipose tissue [66]. Some obese individuals are prone to developing comorbidities while others express metabolic health despite abundant weight. This observation resulted in two distinct phenotype formulations, metabolically healthy obesity and metabolically unhealthy obesity, based on the presence of complications in patients with an increased BMI. The separation of these two profiles seems justified when calculating the risk for disease progression and deciding on treatment modalities. Impairments in adipocyte amount, distribution and function are the drives of obesity-related health risks. Obesity complications occur mainly due to two processes. Firstly, the amount of stored fat inflicts mechanical complications coming from physical forces exerted on the patient (fat mass disease) [1]. The most commonly described complications resulting from this process are osteoarthritis, gastroesophageal reflux disease, and obstructive sleep apnea [67]. Secondarily, the processes of adiposopathy (sick fat disease) inflict immunological and metabolic/endocrine consequences on the patient through meta-inflammation [1].

The adipocytes adapt to excess energy through hypertrophy and hyperplasia *i.e.* adipogenesis where new adipocytes are formed from progenitor and stem cells [68]. Excess energy is stored as glycogen or through the metabolic formation of fat. The increase in fat tissue consequently requires a bigger blood pool, therefore the formation of new blood vessels *via* angiogenesis is also crucial. In physiological circumstances, adipokines signal the regulatory mechanisms involved in these processes, and a molecular exchange with other organ systems is established, protecting the organism from a lipid overflow. Adipose tissue has a limited storage capacity, and cannot expand indefinitely through tissue remodeling. Excess energy is stored partially in subcutaneous adipose tissue, and partially in visceral adipose tissue. In terms of metabolic health, visceral adiposity imposes a bigger threat than subcutaneous adipose tissue. When a capacity maximum is reached, the process of adipocyte apoptosis becomes a key regulator of macrophage activation. Involved are two major classes of macrophages, the classically activated pro-inflammatory M1 class, and the anti-inflammatory M2 class [69]. Activation of pro-inflammatory macrophages is linked with insulin resistance and meta-inflammation. Metabolic obesity-related diseases originate from impairments in fatty acid storage and release as well as under- and overproduction of adipokines. A fatty acids "leak" causes ectopic fat deposition, and a lipid overflow. In obesity, fat is stored in the liver, the pancreas, inside of muscle cells, around the heart and kidney and there is a general body fat distribution dysfunction. These ectopic fat depots disturb the physiological functions of the affected organs.

Individuals who recruit new subcutaneous adipocytes to store excess energy instead of accumulating ectopic fat manage to preserve a relatively healthy metabolic status [14]. The above-mentioned processes imply that more fat does not necessarily mean more metabolic disease. Current guidelines that distinguish between metabolically healthy and metabolically unhealthy obesity [70] yield inconsistencies in management approach [71]. This is partially due to the on-going debate that metabolically healthy obesity only serves as a prologue to metabolically unhealthy obesity, and must not be considered as a stable disease phenotype [72]. More research into adipose tissue inflammation and metabolic inflexibility will provide a better understanding of current dilemmas.

Nevertheless, multiple hormonal signals interpreted by the central nervous system influence appetite, and asking a patient to resist increased appetite through willpower and discipline seems inadequate from this standing point. Certain behaviors are modifiable, whereas others are not [73]. There is evidence that metabolic signaling, glucotoxicity, lipotoxicity, leptin and insulin resistance accompanied by oxidative stress lead to neuroinflammation and cognitive impairment [74]. Another set of complications arose from the socio-environmental frame of obesity. Namely, additional to already faulty homeostatic regulation and impaired hypothalamic signaling, stigmatization and peer-pressures lead to various psychiatric diseases such as depression, anxiety, eating disorders and a higher risk of self-harm and suicide [75].

Cancer incidence is also higher in obese patients. There is an increased risk of predominantly colon, rectum and prostate cancer in men, and breast, endometrium and gallbladder cancer in women [14].

Due to the role of adipose tissue in the hormonal conversion of steroid hormones, adiposity dysfunction is linked with Polycystic Ovarian Syndrome and infertility [76]. Pregnant obese women have an increased risk of gestational diabetes and hypertensive disorders like preeclampsia. Instrumentally assisted births and cesarean sections are conducted more often. There is an increased risk of preterm birth, macrosomia, congenital abnormalities, fetal defects, and perinatal mortality. Compared with healthy weight women, infections of subsequent surgical wounds are more likely to befall obese women. Obese mothers have lower breastfeeding initiation rates, and breastfeeding is ceased earlier when matched with healthy-weight mothers [14].

Obesity imposes an increasing threat to healthcare systems, with huge financial implications due to obesity-related medical costs. If the world population continues to gain weight, institutions that provide health care need to be adjusted for oversized patients. Larger doors, beds, chairs, emergency wagons, imaging machines, and costumed equipment are needed to perform successful and unrestricted ICU interventions. Critical care management for the morbidly obese patient is implicated by patient size and comorbidities on multiple levels [77].

CONCLUDING REMARKS

The question that is often overlooked is, how do the patients feel about their disease? It is well known that the foundation of every successful treatment involves primarily patient compliance. Host behavior underpins treatment efficacy, but as explained in detail, the behavior is not only a function of host willpower. Accepting that obesity is a disease is the first step to successful treatment. Patients, as well as healthcare providers, need to look beyond outdated beliefs. As A. Huxley famously said: "Facts do not cease to exist because they are ignored. "

CONSENT FOR PUBLICATION

Not applicable.

CONFLICT OF INTEREST

The authors confirm that this chapter content has no conflict of interest.

ACKNOWLEDGEMENTS

The authors would like to express their sincere thanks to the editor and anonymous reviewers for their time and valuable suggestions.

REFERENCES

[1]   Frühbeck G, Busetto L, Dicker D, *et al.* The ABCD of obesity: An EASO position statement on a diagnostic term with clinical and scientific implications. Obes Facts 2019; 12(2): 131-6.
        [http://dx.doi.org/10.1159/000497124] [PMID: 30844811]

[2]   Obesity and overweight [Internet]. Who.int. 2019 [cited 4 October 2019]. Available from: https://www.who.int/news-room/fact-sheets/detail/obesity-and-overweight

[3]   Kelly T, Yang W, Chen CS, Reynolds K, He J. Global burden of obesity in 2005 and projections to 2030. Int J Obes 2008; 32(9): 1431-7.
        [http://dx.doi.org/10.1038/ijo.2008.102] [PMID: 18607383]

[4]   2019.https://www.who.int/end-childhood-obesity/facts/en/

[5]   Chooi YC, Ding C, Magkos F. The epidemiology of obesity. Metabolism 2019; 92: 6-10.
        [http://dx.doi.org/10.1016/j.metabol.2018.09.005] [PMID: 30253139]

[6]   Roberto CA, Swinburn B, Hawkes C, *et al.* Patchy progress on obesity prevention: emerging examples, entrenched barriers, and new thinking. Lancet 2015; 385(9985): 2400-9.
        [http://dx.doi.org/10.1016/S0140-6736(14)61744-X] [PMID: 25703111]

[7]   Niccolai E, Boem F, Russo E, Amedei A. The Gut-Brain axis in the neuropsychological disease model of obesity: A classical movie revised by the emerging director "microbiome". Nutrients 2019; 11(1): 156.
        [http://dx.doi.org/10.3390/nu11010156] [PMID: 30642052]

[8] Schwartz MW, Seeley RJ, Zeltser LM, *et al.* Obesity pathogenesis: An endocrine society scientific statement. Endocr Rev 2017; 38(4): 267-96.
[http://dx.doi.org/10.1210/er.2017-00111] [PMID: 28898979]

[9] Wang Y, Xue H, Liu S. Applications of systems science in biomedical research regarding obesity and noncommunicable chronic diseases: opportunities, promise, and challenges. Adv Nutr 2015; 6(1): 88-95.
[http://dx.doi.org/10.3945/an.114.007203] [PMID: 25593147]

[10] Vandenbroeck IP, Goossens J, Clemens M. Foresight Tackling Obesities: Future Choices—Building the Obesity System Map. Government Office for Science, UK Government's Foresight Programme. 2018. Available from: https://www.gov.uk/government/publications/reducing-obesity-obesity-system-map

[11] Finegood DT, Merth TD, Rutter H. Implications of the foresight obesity system map for solutions to childhood obesity. Obesity (Silver Spring) 2010; 18(1s) (Suppl. 1): S13-6.
[http://dx.doi.org/10.1038/oby.2009.426] [PMID: 20107455]

[12] Expert Consultation WHO. Appropriate body-mass index for Asian populations and its implications for policy and intervention strategies. Lancet 2004; 363(9403): 157-63.
[http://dx.doi.org/10.1016/S0140-6736(03)15268-3] [PMID: 14726171]

[13] Whitlock G, Lewington S, Sherliker P, *et al.* Prospective Studies Collaboration. Body-mass index and cause-specific mortality in 900 000 adults: collaborative analyses of 57 prospective studies. Lancet 2009; 373(9669): 1083-96.
[http://dx.doi.org/10.1016/S0140-6736(09)60318-4] [PMID: 19299006]

[14] Bray GA, Heisel WE, Afshin A, *et al.* The science of obesity management: An endocrine society scientific statement. Endocr Rev 2018; 39(2): 79-132.
[http://dx.doi.org/10.1210/er.2017-00253] [PMID: 29518206]

[15] Gonzalez-Casanova I, Sarmiento OL, Gazmararian JA, *et al.* Comparing three body mass index classification systems to assess overweight and obesity in children and adolescents. Rev Panam Salud Publica 2013; 33(5): 349-55.
[http://dx.doi.org/10.1590/S1020-49892013000500006] [PMID: 23764666]

[16] Reilly JJ, Kelly J, Wilson DC. Accuracy of simple clinical and epidemiological definitions of childhood obesity: systematic review and evidence appraisal. Obes Rev 2010; 11(9): 645-55.
[http://dx.doi.org/10.1111/j.1467-789X.2009.00709.x] [PMID: 20059704]

[17] Cole TJ, Bellizzi MC, Flegal KM, Dietz WH. Establishing a standard definition for child overweight and obesity worldwide: international survey. BMJ 2000; 320(7244): 1240-3.
[http://dx.doi.org/10.1136/bmj.320.7244.1240] [PMID: 10797032]

[18] Neel JV. Diabetes mellitus: a "thrifty" genotype rendered detrimental by "progress"? Am J Hum Genet 1962; 14: 353-62.
[PMID: 13937884]

[19] Selassie M, Sinha AC. The epidemiology and aetiology of obesity: A global challenge. Best Pract Res Clin Anaesthesiol 2011; 25(1): 1-9.
[http://dx.doi.org/10.1016/j.bpa.2011.01.002] [PMID: 21516909]

[20] Müller MJ, Bosy-Westphal A, Heymsfield SB. Is there evidence for a set point that regulates human body weight? F1000 Med Rep 2010; 2: 59.
[http://dx.doi.org/10.3410/M2-59] [PMID: 21173874]

[21] Müller MJ, Geisler C, Heymsfield SB, Bosy-Westphal A. Recent advances in understanding body weight homeostasis in humans. F1000 Res 2018; 7: 1025.
[http://dx.doi.org/10.12688/f1000research.14151.1] [PMID: 30026913]

[22] Speakman JR, Levitsky DA, Allison DB, *et al.* Set points, settling points and some alternative models: theoretical options to understand how genes and environments combine to regulate body adiposity. Dis

Model Mech 2011; 4(6): 733-45.
[http://dx.doi.org/10.1242/dmm.008698] [PMID: 22065844]

[23]   González-Muniesa P, Mártinez-González MA, Hu FB, *et al.* Obesity. Nat Rev Dis Primers 2017; 3(1): 17034.
[http://dx.doi.org/10.1038/nrdp.2017.34] [PMID: 28617414]

[24]   Kenny PJ. Reward mechanisms in obesity: new insights and future directions. Neuron 2011; 69(4): 664-79.
[http://dx.doi.org/10.1016/j.neuron.2011.02.016] [PMID: 21338878]

[25]   Brewer JA, Ruf A, Beccia AL, *et al.* Can mindfulness address maladaptive eating behaviors? why traditional diet plans fail and how new mechanistic insights may lead to novel interventions. Front Psychol 2018; 9: 1418.
[http://dx.doi.org/10.3389/fpsyg.2018.01418] [PMID: 30250438]

[26]   Lopomo A, Burgio E, Migliore L. Epigenetics of obesity. Prog Mol Biol Transl Sci 2016; 140: 151-84.
[http://dx.doi.org/10.1016/bs.pmbts.2016.02.002] [PMID: 27288829]

[27]   van Dijk SJ, Molloy PL, Varinli H, Morrison JL, Muhlhausler BS. Members of EpiSCOPE. Epigenetics and human obesity. Int J Obes 2015; 39(1): 85-97.
[http://dx.doi.org/10.1038/ijo.2014.34] [PMID: 24566855]

[28]   Kaur Y, de Souza RJ, Gibson WT, Meyre D. A systematic review of genetic syndromes with obesity. Obes Rev 2017; 18(6): 603-34.
[http://dx.doi.org/10.1111/obr.12531] [PMID: 28346723]

[29]   Stubert J, Reister F, Hartmann S, Janni W. The risks associated with obesity in pregnancy. Deutsches Aerzteblatt Online 2018.
[http://dx.doi.org/10.3238/arztebl.2018.0276]

[30]   Liu Y, Qin S, Song Y, *et al.* The perturbation of infant gut microbiota caused by cesarean delivery is partially restored by exclusive breastfeeding. Front Microbiol 2019; 10: 598.
[http://dx.doi.org/10.3389/fmicb.2019.00598] [PMID: 30972048]

[31]   Bliss ES, Whiteside E. The gut-brain axis, the human gut microbiota and their integration in the development of obesity. Front Physiol 2018; 9: 900.
[http://dx.doi.org/10.3389/fphys.2018.00900] [PMID: 30050464]

[32]   Agustí A, García-Pardo MP, López-Almela I, *et al.* Interplay between the gut-brain axis, obesity and cognitive function. Front Neurosci 2018; 12: 155.
[http://dx.doi.org/10.3389/fnins.2018.00155] [PMID: 29615850]

[33]   Camilleri M, Acosta A. Gastrointestinal traits: Individualizing therapy for obesity with drugs and devices. Gastrointest Endosc 2016; 83(1): 48-56.
[http://dx.doi.org/10.1016/j.gie.2015.08.007] [PMID: 26271184]

[34]   Lean ME, Malkova D. Altered gut and adipose tissue hormones in overweight and obese individuals: cause or consequence? Int J Obes 2016; 40(4): 622-32.
[http://dx.doi.org/10.1038/ijo.2015.220] [PMID: 26499438]

[35]   Sonnenburg ED, Sonnenburg JL. The ancestral and industrialized gut microbiota and implications for human health. Nat Rev Microbiol 2019; 17(6): 383-90.
[http://dx.doi.org/10.1038/s41579-019-0191-8] [PMID: 31089293]

[36]   Torres-Fuentes C, Schellekens H, Dinan TG, Cryan JF. The microbiota-gut-brain axis in obesity. Lancet Gastroenterol Hepatol 2017; 2(10): 747-56.
[http://dx.doi.org/10.1016/S2468-1253(17)30147-4] [PMID: 28844808]

[37]   Dhurandhar NV. Is obesity caused by an adenovirus? Expert Rev Anti Infect Ther 2012; 10(5): 521-4.
[http://dx.doi.org/10.1586/eri.12.41] [PMID: 22702313]

[38]   Ponterio E, Gnessi L. Adenovirus 36 and obesity: An overview. Viruses 2015; 7(7): 3719-40.

[http://dx.doi.org/10.3390/v7072787] [PMID: 26184280]

[39]   Weaver JU. Classical endocrine diseases causing obesity. Front Horm Res 2008; 36: 212-28.
        [http://dx.doi.org/10.1159/000115367] [PMID: 18230905]

[40]   Liou TH, Pi-Sunyer FX, Laferrère B. Physical disability and obesity. Nutr Rev 2005; 63(10): 321-31.
        [http://dx.doi.org/10.1111/j.1753-4887.2005.tb00110.x] [PMID: 16295145]

[41]   Froehlich-Grobe K, Lollar D. Obesity and disability: time to act. Am J Prev Med 2011; 41(5): 541-5.
        [http://dx.doi.org/10.1016/j.amepre.2011.07.015] [PMID: 22011427]

[42]   Igel L. Antipsychotic medication-induced weight gain. Obes Manag 2018; 61-7.

[43]   Medici V, McClave SA, Miller KR. Common medications which lead to unintended alterations in
        weight gain or organ lipotoxicity. Curr Gastroenterol Rep 2016; 18(1): 2.
        [http://dx.doi.org/10.1007/s11894-015-0479-4] [PMID: 26700070]

[44]   Wharton S, Raiber L, Serodio KJ, Lee J, Christensen RA. Medications that cause weight gain and
        alternatives in Canada: a narrative review. Diabetes Metab Syndr Obes 2018; 11: 427-38.
        [http://dx.doi.org/10.2147/DMSO.S171365] [PMID: 30174450]

[45]   Sallis JF, Floyd MF, Rodríguez DA, Saelens BE. Role of built environments in physical activity,
        obesity, and cardiovascular disease. Circulation 2012; 125(5): 729-37.
        [http://dx.doi.org/10.1161/CIRCULATIONAHA.110.969022] [PMID: 22311885]

[46]   Suglia SF, Shelton RC, Hsiao A, Wang YC, Rundle A, Link BG. Why the Neighborhood Social
        Environment Is Critical in Obesity Prevention. J Urban Health 2016; 93(1): 206-12.
        [http://dx.doi.org/10.1007/s11524-015-0017-6] [PMID: 26780582]

[47]   USDA ERS - Food Access Research Atlas [Internet]. Ers.usda.gov. 2020 [cited 16 April 2020].
        Available from: https://www.ers.usda.gov/data/fooddesert/

[48]   Physical Activity: Built Environment Approaches Combining Transportation System Interventions
        with Land Use and Environmental Design | Healthy People 2020 [Internet]. Healthypeople.gov. 2020
        [cited 6 August 2020]. Available from: https://www.healthypeople.gov/2020/tools-resources/evidenc-
        -based-resource/physical-activity-built-environment-approaches

[49]   Miclotte L, Van de Wiele T. Food processing, gut microbiota and the globesity problem. Crit Rev
        Food Sci Nutr 2019; 1-14.
        [http://dx.doi.org/10.1080/10408398.2019.1596878] [PMID: 30945554]

[50]   Gore AC, Chappell VA, Fenton SE, *et al.* EDC-2: The Endocrine Society's Second Scientific
        Statement on Endocrine-Disrupting Chemicals. Endocr Rev 2015; 36(6): E1-E150.
        [http://dx.doi.org/10.1210/er.2015-1010] [PMID: 26544531]

[51]   Carrillo-Álvarez E, Kawachi I, Riera-Romaní J. Neighbourhood social capital and obesity: a
        systematic review of the literature. Obes Rev 2019; 20(1): 119-41.
        [http://dx.doi.org/10.1111/obr.12760] [PMID: 30306717]

[52]   Cummins S, Macintyre S. Food environments and obesity--neighbourhood or nation? Int J Epidemiol
        2006; 35(1): 100-4.
        [http://dx.doi.org/10.1093/ije/dyi276] [PMID: 16338945]

[53]   Borrell LN, Graham L, Joseph SP. Associations of Neighborhood Safety and Neighborhood Support
        with Overweight and Obesity in US Children and Adolescents. Ethn Dis 2016; 26(4): 469-76.
        [http://dx.doi.org/10.18865/ed.26.4.469] [PMID: 27773973]

[54]   Datar A, Nicosia N. Assessing Social Contagion in Body Mass Index, Overweight, and Obesity Using
        a Natural Experiment. JAMA Pediatr 2018; 172(3): 239-46.
        [http://dx.doi.org/10.1001/jamapediatrics.2017.4882] [PMID: 29356816]

[55]   Chou WY, Prestin A, Kunath S. Obesity in social media: a mixed methods analysis. Transl Behav Med
        2014; 4(3): 314-23.
        [http://dx.doi.org/10.1007/s13142-014-0256-1] [PMID: 25264470]

[56]   Bray I, Slater A, Lewis-Smith H, Bird E, Sabey A. Promoting positive body image and tackling overweight/obesity in children and adolescents: A combined health psychology and public health approach. Prev Med 2018; 116: 219-21.
[http://dx.doi.org/10.1016/j.ypmed.2018.08.011] [PMID: 30144484]

[57]   Frederick DA, Saguy AC, Gruys K. Culture, health, and bigotry: How exposure to cultural accounts of fatness shape attitudes about health risk, health policies, and weight-based prejudice. Soc Sci Med 2016; 165: 271-9.
[http://dx.doi.org/10.1016/j.socscimed.2015.12.031] [PMID: 26776492]

[58]   Spaeth A. Insufficient sleep and obesity. Sleep Health 2019; 189-201.

[59]   Peeters A. Obesity and the future of food policies that promote healthy diets. Nat Rev Endocrinol 2018; 14(7): 430-7.
[http://dx.doi.org/10.1038/s41574-018-0026-0] [PMID: 29799023]

[60]   Luger M, Lafontan M, Bes-Rastrollo M, Winzer E, Yumuk V, Farpour-Lambert N. Sugar-Sweetened Beverages and Weight Gain in Children and Adults: A Systematic Review from 2013 to 2015 and a Comparison with Previous Studies. Obes Facts 2017; 10(6): 674-93.
[http://dx.doi.org/10.1159/000484566] [PMID: 29237159]

[61]   McHill AW, Wright KP Jr. Role of sleep and circadian disruption on energy expenditure and in metabolic predisposition to human obesity and metabolic disease. Obes Rev 2017; 18 (Suppl. 1): 15-24.
[http://dx.doi.org/10.1111/obr.12503] [PMID: 28164449]

[62]   Hewagalamulage SD, Lee TK, Clarke IJ, Henry BA. Stress, cortisol, and obesity: a role for cortisol responsiveness in identifying individuals prone to obesity. Domest Anim Endocrinol 2016; 56 (Suppl.): S112-20.
[http://dx.doi.org/10.1016/j.domaniend.2016.03.004] [PMID: 27345309]

[63]   Ritchie H, Roser M. Smoking [Internet]. Our World in Data. 2020. Available from: https://ourworldindata.org/smoking

[64]   Karam J, McFarlane S. Secondary causes of obesity. Therapy 2007; 4(5): 641-50.
[http://dx.doi.org/10.2217/14750708.4.5.641]

[65]   Adams KF, Schatzkin A, Harris TB, *et al.* Overweight, obesity, and mortality in a large prospective cohort of persons 50 to 71 years old. N Engl J Med 2006; 355(8): 763-78.
[http://dx.doi.org/10.1056/NEJMoa055643] [PMID: 16926275]

[66]   Seijkens T, Kusters P, Chatzigeorgiou A, Chavakis T, Lutgens E. Immune cell crosstalk in obesity: a key role for costimulation? Diabetes 2014; 63(12): 3982-91.
[http://dx.doi.org/10.2337/db14-0272] [PMID: 25414012]

[67]   Daniel S, Soleymani T, Garvey WT. A complications-based clinical staging of obesity to guide treatment modality and intensity. Curr Opin Endocrinol Diabetes Obes 2013; 20(5): 377-88.
[http://dx.doi.org/10.1097/01.med.0000433067.01671.f5] [PMID: 23974764]

[68]   Oñate B, Vilahur G, Camino-López S, *et al.* Stem cells isolated from adipose tissue of obese patients show changes in their transcriptomic profile that indicate loss in stemcellness and increased commitment to an adipocyte-like phenotype. BMC Genomics 2013; 14(1): 625.
[http://dx.doi.org/10.1186/1471-2164-14-625] [PMID: 24040759]

[69]   Atri C, Guerfali FZ, Laouini D. Role of Human Macrophage Polarization in Inflammation during Infectious Diseases. Int J Mol Sci 2018; 19(6): 1801.
[http://dx.doi.org/10.3390/ijms19061801] [PMID: 29921749]

[70]   Mongraw-Chaffin M, Foster MC, Anderson CAM, *et al.* Metabolically Healthy Obesity, Transition to Metabolic Syndrome, and Cardiovascular Risk. J Am Coll Cardiol 2018; 71(17): 1857-65.
[http://dx.doi.org/10.1016/j.jacc.2018.02.055] [PMID: 29699611]

[71] Muñoz-Garach A, Cornejo-Pareja I, Tinahones FJ. Does Metabolically Healthy Obesity Exist? Nutrients 2016; 8(6): 320.
[http://dx.doi.org/10.3390/nu8060320] [PMID: 27258304]

[72] Jung CH, Lee WJ, Song KH. Metabolically healthy obesity: a friend or foe? Korean J Intern Med (Korean Assoc Intern Med) 2017; 32(4): 611-21.
[http://dx.doi.org/10.3904/kjim.2016.259] [PMID: 28602062]

[73] Perry B, Wang Y. Appetite regulation and weight control: the role of gut hormones. Nutr Diabetes 2012; 2(1): e26-6.
[http://dx.doi.org/10.1038/nutd.2011.21] [PMID: 23154682]

[74] Guillemot-Legris O, Muccioli GG. Obesity-Induced Neuroinflammation: Beyond the Hypothalamus. Trends Neurosci 2017; 40(4): 237-53.
[http://dx.doi.org/10.1016/j.tins.2017.02.005] [PMID: 28318543]

[75] Ouakinin SRS, Barreira DP, Gois CJ. Depression and Obesity: Integrating the Role of Stress, Neuroendocrine Dysfunction and Inflammatory Pathways. Front Endocrinol (Lausanne) 2018; 9: 431.
[http://dx.doi.org/10.3389/fendo.2018.00431] [PMID: 30108549]

[76] Silvestris E, de Pergola G, Rosania R, Loverro G. Obesity as disruptor of the female fertility. Reprod Biol Endocrinol 2018; 16(1): 22.
[http://dx.doi.org/10.1186/s12958-018-0336-z] [PMID: 29523133]

[77] Bajwa SJ, Sehgal V, Bajwa SK. Clinical and critical care concerns in severely ill obese patient. Indian J Endocrinol Metab 2012; 16(5): 740-8.
[http://dx.doi.org/10.4103/2230-8210.100667] [PMID: 23087857]

CHAPTER 2

The Endocrine Function of Adipose Tissue

Amina Valjevac[*]

Department of Human Physiology, Faculty of Medicine University of Sarajevo; Čekaluša 90, 71000 Sarajevo; Bosnia and Herzegovina

Abstract: White adipose tissue secretes adipokines that regulate numerous biological processes by autocrine, paracrine, and endocrine mechanisms. Adipokines are essential in the balance between appetite and satiety, regulation of body fat stores and energy expenditure, glucose tolerance, insulin release and sensitivity, cell growth, inflammation, oxidative stress, angiogenesis, and atherosclerosis. Cytokines are secreted directly from adipocytes, but also from other stromal cells in the adipose depot and primarily play a role in immune regulation. Among adipokines, leptin, resistin, and visfatin were described as markers that are positively related to body weight, fat mass, insulin resistance, and exhibit pro-inflammatory properties. Opposite to the pro-inflammatory cytokines, adipose tissue can secrete a series of anti-inflammatory adipokines, including adiponectin, apelin, vaspin, and omentin, which play crucial protective roles in inflammation states, insulin resistance, and atherosclerosis. In obese person dysregulation of adipokines secretion, in addition to upregulated inflammatory response, contributes to obesity-induced insulin resistance and systemic low-grade inflammation. Brown adipose tissue (BAT) might also have a secretory role, secreting "brownkines" that act in a paracrine or autocrine manner. Most of these factors promote hypertrophy and hyperplasia of BAT, vascularization, innervation and blood flow, processes that are all associated with BAT recruitment when thermogenic activity is enhanced.

Keywords: Adiponectin, Apelin, Adipsin, Brown adipose tissue, Inflammation, Leptin, Omentin, Resistin, Visfatin, Vaspin, White adipose tissue.

INTRODUCTION

There are two forms of adipose tissue in humans, white adipose tissue (WAT), historically recognized as energy storage for triglycerides, and brown adipose tissue (BAT) needed for thermogenesis.

WAT is widely distributed across the body. WAT is found in subcutaneous adipose tissue (SAT) and intra-abdominal region known as visceral adipose tissue

[*] **Corresponding author Amina Valjevac:** Department of Human Physiology, Faculty of Medicine, University of Sarajevo, Sarajevo, Bosnia and Herzegovina; Tel: +387 33 226 478, Ext. 526; E-mail: amina.valjevac@mf.unsa.ba

Asija Začiragić (Ed.)

(VAT). The human SAT primarily occurs in the belly, hip, while VAT is located mostly in the omentum, mesenterium, and perirenal area [1]. In addition to its traditional role as a reservoir of energy, WAT is now recognized as an endocrine organ [2]. WAT secretes several hormones, which are called adipokines, as they are derived from adipocytes. Adipokines have endocrine actions and affect cells expressing receptors. Adipokines possess pleiotropic activity triggering intracellular signaling pathways, which modulate human metabolism [3]. Acting as orexigenic and anorexigenic hormones in the nucleus arcuatus in the hypothalamic region, adipokines play a crucial role in energy metabolism through the communication of the organism's nutrient status. Adipokines are currently known to be important players in inflammation and immunity since most are increased in obesity and lead to the 'low-grade inflammatory disease' as observed in obese subjects. The most extensively researched are leptin and adiponectin, but resistin, visfatin, vaspin, apelin, omentin, and adipsin have gained research interest lately [4]. Importantly, accumulating evidence showed that adipose tissue holds a large number of immune cells, such as macrophages, eosinophils, T and B cells, which control immune homeostasis and inflammation, thereby influencing the metabolism of adipose tissue and the entire body [5].

LEPTIN

Leptin is a 16-kDa sized hormone encoded by the OB gene on human chromosome 7q31.3a. Human leptin is a protein consisting of 167 amino acids, produced mainly in the white adipose tissue adipocytes. Leptin is also released by BAT cells, placenta, ovaries, skeletal muscles, gastric glands, mammary glands, bone marrow, pituitary, and liver [6].

It is well recorded that the serum leptin concentration is positively correlated with the fat mass and the body mass index (BMI) [7]. Moreover, the percentage of body fat postmenopausal women may be the strongest predictor of serum leptin [8].

The main physiological function of leptin is to control food intake and energy expenditure through its interaction with various neuropeptides in the hypothalamus. The leptin's site of action is located in the arcuate nucleus of the hypothalamus, where it acts on two types of neurons. Leptin directly stimulates neurons to secrete proopiomelanocortin (POMC), a protein that is subsequently cleaved into, among others, αmelanocyte-stimulating hormone (α-MSH), an anorexigenic peptide that lowers food intake. Leptin also stimulates POMC neurons, which activate cocaine- and amphetamine-regulated transcript (CART) and subsequently suppresses the appetite. In conjunction with the stimulation of POMC neurons, leptin reduces appetite by inhibiting AgRP/NPY neurons that coexpress the orexigenic neuropeptides agouti-related peptide (AgRP) and neuropeptide Y (NPY) [9].

Leptin levels follow a circadian pattern, with peak levels during the night and lowest levels in the afternoon. Circulating concentration of leptin during the night can be up to 75.6 percent greater than in the afternoon. The pulsatile properties of leptin secretion in obese and lean individuals are similar, although obese subjects have higher pulsatile amplitudes [10]. It has been shown that women have greater leptin concentrations compared to age- and BMI-matched men [6]. Leptin exhibits dimorphism, with levels higher in women than in men. The amplitude of leptin pulses in females is 2-3 times higher than in men and the leptin mRNA levels in subcutaneous adipose tissue are substantially higher in females than in males [11]. Furthermore, the rate of leptin secretion in the SAT in males is 66% that of female's as shown by *in vitro* study [12]. This suggests that the secretion of leptin is under the influence of estrogen. Some authors suggest that the difference in leptin secretion is not due to the high estrogen levels in females, but rather due to higher circulating androgens levels in men. Studies have suggested that androgens have a rather suppressive effect on leptin production and reduce leptin secretion [13, 14]. However, the influence of circulating androgens is not supported by other studies [15].

Leptin exerts its effects by binding with six different receptor isoforms, secretory (ObRe), long (ObRb) and short (ObRa, ObRc, ObRd, ObRf) forms. Secretory leptin receptor (ObRe) is found in plasma, binds leptin and carries it to the brain. ObRb form, found in several hypothalamic nuclei, has active intracellular signaling domains, which, when activated, decreases food intake [6].

Besides its role in appetite suppression and energy expenditure promotion, leptin, under normal physiological conditions, increases the sympathetic activity, facilitates glucose utilization, and improves insulin sensitivity [16]. Leptin can acutely suppress insulin secretion but it increases long-term β cell survival and function [17] (Fig. **1**). By activating the sympathetic nervous system, leptin increases energy expenditure but also increases systemic blood pressure [18]. High circulating leptin levels have been reported in obese individuals with increased renal sympathetic tone [19]. Moreover, leptin increases fatty acid uptake and oxidation in the skeletal muscle and liver, promotes angiogenesis and atherosclerosis acting as a growth factor for endothelial cells [20] (Fig. **2**). Contrary to the leptin's positive effects in the muscle where it sensitizes insulin receptors, leptin has rather negative effects in type 2 diabetes development by enhancement of inflammatory processes especially in obese subjects. It has been shown that leptin favours cell propagation towards pro-inflammatory Th1 cells, while suppressing anti-inflammatory Th2 cells [21]. Leptin also stimulates IL-6 and TNFα release from B cells favouring inflammation [22]. Taken together, these studies confirm associations between leptin, immunity, and inflammation, providing evidence that high leptin levels could intensify chronic inflammation (Fig. **2**).

ADIPONECTIN

Adiponectin is a 30 kDa protein, primarily expressed in white adipose tissue [23], but its expression has been demonstrated in various tissues such as brown adipose tissue [24], skeletal muscle [25], liver [26], cardiac myocytes [27], bone-forming cells [28], placenta [29] and cerebrospinal fluid [30].

Plasma adiponectin concentrations range from 0.5-30 μg/mL accounting for up to 0.01% of total plasma proteins in humans [23]. The major determinant of plasma adiponectin concentration is body fat mass. Increased body fat mass impairs adiponectin synthesis and secretion due to obesity-associated low-grade inflammation and oxidative stress in adipose tissue [31].

The monomer of adiponectin (about 30 kDa), is a protein containing four different domains (an aminoterminal signal sequence, a variable region, a collagen domain and a carboxyterminal globular domain) and corresponds to the 'full-length' form of the hormone [32].

Single monomers of adiponectin can combine to form trimeric complexes, which can further polymerize through their collagenous domains into hexameric forms (or low molecular weight forms (LMW)) or high molecular weight (HMW) complexes containing 12 – 18 molecules corresponding to the circulating forms of adiponectin in the plasma [33].

Predominant forms of adiponectin in plasma are low molecular weight (LMW) hexamer (180-kDa) and high molecular weight (HMW) multimer (360 kDa). A globular adiponectin (gAd) form also circulates in human plasma and represents a proteolytic cleavage of adiponectin [34]. Circulating adiponectin has a half-life of 75 minutes and is cleared from plasma by the hepatocytes, while HMW adiponectin has the slowest clearance rate with relatively stable serum levels [35].

Numerous physiological processes are regulated by adiponectin. Adiponectin released from adipose tissue travels to distant cells that express adiponectin's receptors, representing its endocrine effects. In addition, adiponectin released from other tissues act locally, which represents its autocrine or paracrine effect [36].

Adiponectin regulates glucose and fatty acid metabolism in skeletal muscle [36]. *In vitro* studies suggest that adiponectin can increase glucose uptake and increase fatty acid uptake, both basally and postprandially [36] (Fig. **1**). Adiponectin improves energy homeostasis by regulating glucose and fatty acid metabolism, sensitizes insulin receptors in hepatocytes and decreases TNFα levels. Decreased adiponectin levels have been associated with steatosis, hepatomegaly, a pro-inflammatory process in the liver [31, 36].

Many studies have established positive associations between circulating adiponectin and cardiovascular health, but the underlying mechanisms are now clearly defined. It has been proven that adiponectin has cardioprotective properties promoting cardiac energy metabolism, hypertrophy, fibrosis, and apoptosis. In addition, the benefits of adiponectin's actions on the cardiovascular system are attributed to its anti-inflammatory, vasodilatory, and anti-atherosclerotic effects [36].

Adiponectin's diverse actions in these tissues are mediated by its receptors. Three adiponectin receptors, AdipoR1, AdipoR2 and T-cadherin, have been identified. AdipoR1 and AdipoR2, belong to the seven-transmembrane-spanning receptor family but are not coupled to G-protein. The expression of both receptors is inversely regulated by insulin both in physiological and pathophysiological conditions such as fasting/refeeding, insulin deficiency and hyperinsulinemia and correlates with adiponectin sensitivity [32]. AdipoR1 is found on many cells, among which cardiomyocytes and myocytes in skeletal muscles contain numerous AdipoR1 receptors which, when activated trigger AMP-activated kinase (AMPK) pathways. AdipoR2 is found mostly on hepatocytes and activates peroxisome proliferator-activated receptor (PPAR)-α pathways [37]. T-cadherin mostly expressed on vascular endothelial cells and smooth muscle, is a receptor for hexameric and HMW adiponectin [38]. The activation of AdipoR1 and AdipoR2 results in increased hepatic and skeletal muscle fatty acid oxidation, increased skeletal muscle lactate production, reduced hepatic gluconeogenesis, increased cellular glucose uptake and inhibition of inflammation and oxidative stress [34] (Fig. **2**). Activation of T-cadherin is protective in vascular endothelial cells against oxidative stress-induced apoptosis and is strongly expressed in areas affected by atherosclerosis [38].

The concentrations of adiponectin in plasma are relatively constant during the day, exhibiting slight fluctuation (20%), with levels slightly decreasing during the night [39, 40]. It is still not clear whether adiponectin levels oscillation could be affected by meal or body composition. In obese subjects, adiponectin has been reported to increase after a meal to levels which are four-fold higher, but similar findings could not be detected in lean subjects [41]. Other studies reported no change in adiponectin concentrations over the course of a day, neither in lean or overweight/obese subjects, despite significant post-prandial increases in blood glucose and insulin [40].

Although a negative correlation between serum insulin and adiponectin levels has been confirmed in human subjects, *in vivo* and *in vitro* studies showed inconsistent results on the effects of insulin on adiponectin secretion [42]. It is still not clear whether short-term caloric restriction affects adiponectin concentration, while long-term caloric restriction associated with significant weight loss increases adiponectin concentrations [43].

Women have significantly higher circulating adiponectin concentrations than men, despite featuring a higher body fat content [42]. This is attributed primarily to the inhibitory effect of the androgen testosterone on adiponectin secretion. In particular, adiponectin secretion has been found to be reduced in visceral fat compared with subcutaneous fat, thus accounting (together with the involvement of sex steroids), for the relatively higher degree of insulin resistance in males compared with female counterparts [44].

Glucocorticoids and growth hormones regulate the level of circulating adiponectin by inhibiting its expression and secretion in human adipocytes [45, 46].

RESISTIN

Resistin was named upon demonstration that it can reduce insulin sensitivity in a rat model [47] (Fig. **1**). In humans, resistin is produced and secreted from monocytes and macrophages rather than adipocytes [48]. Increased adiposity favours resistin release in both genetic and diet-induced obese mouse models due to accumulation and activation of inflammatory cells in hypertrophic adipose tissue [49]. This implies that resistin plays a role in immune/inflammatory responses resembling the effects of TNFα [50] (Fig. **2**). Resistin's role in glucose homeostasis was shown in mice models where exogenous injections of resistin reduced insulin sensitivity and induce glucose intolerance [51]. Furthermore, obese resistin-deficient mice have improved fasting glucose levels compared to obese resistin- sufficient mice [52]. Although resistin receptors have not been established in humans, it is suggested that toll-like receptor 4 (TLR4) might be resistin-specific receptors [53]. Adipose tissues immune cells are responsible for the secretion of resistin, suggesting that resistin, by activating TLR4-downstream effects, has a role in inflammatory processes. In support of this, recent studies demonstrate human resistin to be a cytokine that activates adenylyl cyclase-associated protein 1 (CAP1) and induces low-grade inflammation [54].

VISFATIN

Visfatin, known as the cytokine PBEF (pre-B-cell colony enhancing factor), is an extracellular form of the enzyme Nampt (nicotinamide phosphor ribosyl transferase), an essential enzyme in the NAD biosynthetic pathway starting from nicotinamide [55]. Therefore, any NAD+ dependent process is probably regulated by visfatin, including cell adhesion, redox potential, oxidative stress, aging and longevity [56]. Visfatin is expressed in multiple tissues, although adipose tissue is the most important visfatin source [57]. Visfatin secretion from visceral fat tissue is higher than the subcutaneous adipose tissue [57]. Plasma visfatin levels have been reported to be higher in obese compared to normal weight subjects [57 - 60], possibly due to activated macrophages, whose infiltration in adipose tissue is prominently increased in obesity. In addition, visfatin levels from leukocytes are also higher in obese compared to lean subjects [61]. Visfatin has been implicated in decreased glucose uptake, insulin secretion and increased insulin resistance [62] (Fig. **1**), osteoarthritis and osteoporosis [63]. Growing scientific evidence suggests that visfatin can stimulate vascular inflammation by activating endothelial cells, vascular smooth muscle cells, monocytes and macrophages [64]. Visfatin is shown to promote the synthesis of pro-inflammatory cytokines, such as tumor necrosis factor-α (TNF-α) and IL-8 by activating monocytes [65]. Exogenous administration of visfatin enhances the expression of a pro-inflammatory enzyme, inducible nitric oxide synthase (iNOS), contributing to dysregulated NO production and subsequent peroxynitrite formation [66]. Visfatin has also been shown to activate the endothelial cells, promoting upregulation of cell adhesion molecules and cytokines, both implicated in leukocyte recruitment and adhesion of monocytes to endothelial cells [67, 68] (Fig. **2**).

VASPIN

Vaspin is predominantly secreted by visceral fat. Vaspin belongs to the serine protease inhibitor family that exhibits approximately 40% homology with α1-antitrypsin [69]. Its levels are increased in obese patients and associated with increased BMI and waist-to-hip ratio (WHR) [70]. Central administration of vaspin in rats reduces appetite and body weight [71], while intraperitoneal administration failed to exert the same effects on body weight in rats on high-fat diet [69]. Studies have shown that vaspin can improve glucose tolerance and insulin sensitivity in obese rats by lowering blood glucose and insulin plasma levels [69, 72] (Fig. **1**).

Vaspin downregulates inflammatory response [73, 74]. It has been shown that vaspin protects vascular endothelial cells by inhibiting NF-κB/protein kinase C theta and expression of intercellular adhesion molecule-1 induced by TNF-α and IL-6 in smooth muscle cells of vessels [75, 76] (Fig. **2**).

APELIN

Apelin is mostly produced by adipocytes but also by neurons, cardiomyocytes, and endothelial cells and exerts its effects by binding to APJ G-protein coupled receptor expressed in many cells and tissues [77]. Apelin has been shown to play a role in glucose, energy and fluid homeostasis [78 - 80], stimulation of angiogenesis and cardiac function [81, 82].

It has been suggested that apelin might reverse insulin resistance and postpone diabetes mellitus progression by regulating insulin response to hyperglycaemia [83] (Fig. **1**). However, obese and insulin-resistant subjects have increased apelin levels [84]. Intracerebral administration of apelin in rats causes a decrease in food intake [85] and increased water intake [86]. Apelin has also been shown to decrease inflammation inhibiting cytokine activation such as TNF-α, IL-1, MCP-1, MIP-1α, IL-6 [86]. In conclusion, apelin's beneficial effects on the regulation of food and fluid balance, insulin secretion and inflammation make this adipokine a promising target for subjects with overweight/obesity and prediabetes.

ADIPSIN

Adipsin is produced mostly by sessile macrophages and adipocytes. Its levels rise in subjects with obesity in whom it activates the complement alternative pathway and stimulates the accrual of triglycerides in adipocytes [87]. Recently its role in glucose homeostasis has been proposed in a study which showed that administration of adipsin in db/db mice decreases fasting plasma glucose, improves glucose clearance and regulates glucose-mediated insulin release [88]. These results suggest its role in the protection of β-cell function and regulation of basal and postprandial insulin secretion (Fig. **1**). But the data on the association and interplay between adipsin and type 2 diabetes mellitus is not adequately defined. Zhou *et al*. [89] recently showed that serum adipsin was significantly lower in patients with impaired glucose tolerance and type 2 diabetes mellitus compared to healthy individuals and negatively associated with fasting plasma glucose and HbA1c levels. Additionally, data from this study suggest that adipsin might independently regulate insulin levels, especially first-phase insulin secretion and β-cell function.

OMENTIN

Omentin is predominantly secreted from visceral adipose tissue [90]. Plasma omentin levels are significantly higher in normal weight subjects compared to overweight and obese [91]. Omentin seems to exert beneficial effects on glucose homeostasis and insulin release (Fig. **1**). In vitro study has shown that omentin could also decrease inflammatory response by suppressing cytokine releases such as IL-6 and TNFα and at the same time, play a role in hindering insulin resistance [92] (Figs. **1** and **2**).

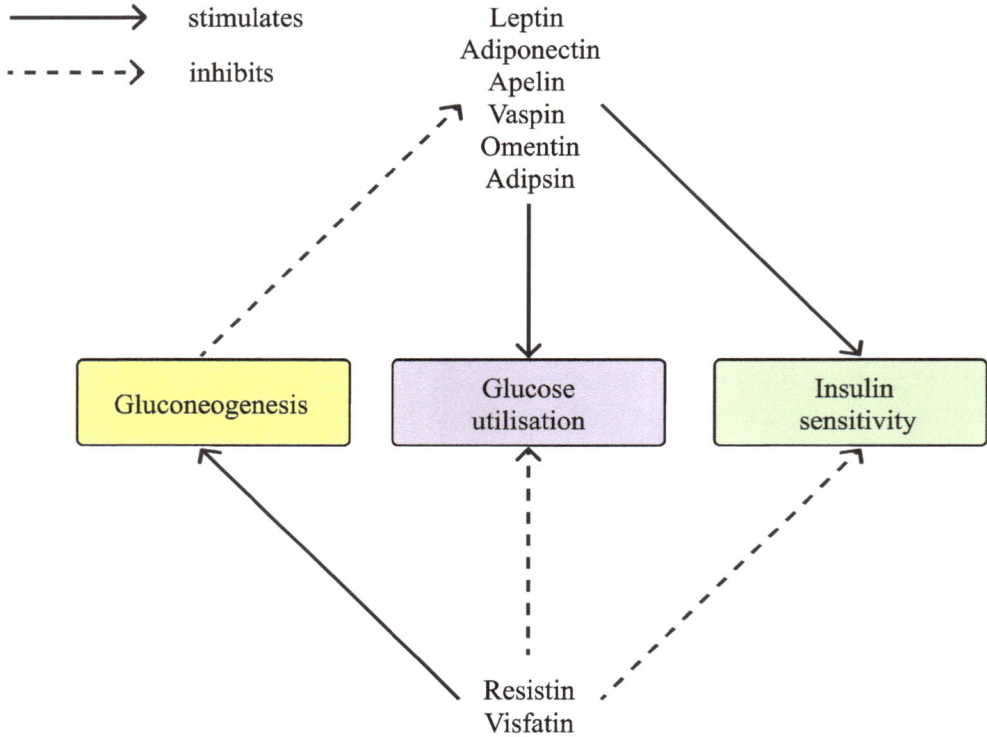

Fig. (1). The role of adipokines in glucose homeostasis.

ADIPOKINES AND INFLAMMATION

In addition to adipocytes, fibroblasts and endothelial cells which are predominant components of WAT, extensive collection of immune cells such as macrophages, neutrophils, eosinophils, mast cells, T and B cells can also be found in adipose tissue. Expansion of WAT in obese persons results in adipocyte expansion followed by dysregulation of adipokines secretion and infiltration of inflammatory cells [93]. Dysregulation of adipokines secretion in obesity is characterized by increased secretion of pro-inflammatory adipokines such as leptin, resistin, and visfatin which are all positively associated with obesity, insulin resistance, and inflammation (Fig. **2**). Best described so far is leptin, which regulates vast metabolic functions including immunological and inflammatory processes. Another important adipokine that is upregulated in obesity is resistin, which exhibits pro-inflammatory properties associated with low-grade chronic inflammatory metabolic diseases including insulin resistance, diabetes, obesity, and cardiovascular disease. Visfatin, produced mainly by VAT, is a multifunctional protein, acting as a cytokine, hormone, and enzyme. In addition to dysregulation of adipokines secretion in obese persons, activation of T cells is a hallmark of expanding WAT. Activated T-cells such as CD4+ helper T (Th) cells and CD8+ cytotoxic T lymphocytes (CTLs), are considered to mediate obesity-induced WAT inflammation [94]. Upregulation of proinflammatory cytokines such as tumor necrosis factor (TNF)-α and interleukin (IL)-6 are also mediators of systemic low-grade inflammation and insulin resistance in obesity [95, 96].

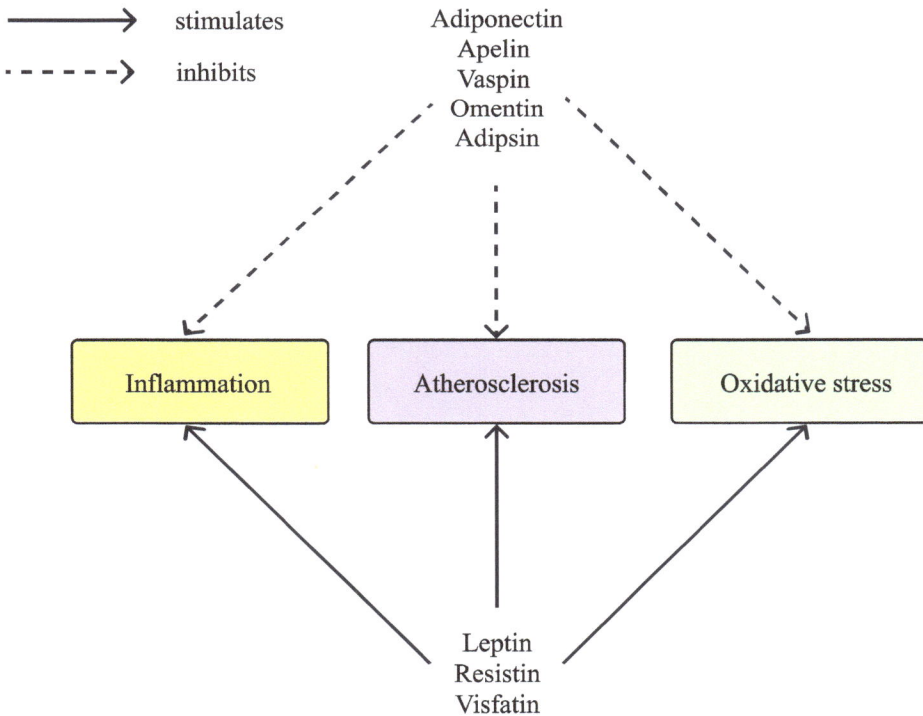

Fig. (2). The role of adipokines in inflammation, oxidative stress and atherosclerosis.

WAT has the ability to secrete a range of anti-inflammatory adipokines, including adiponectin and omentin, which play important protective roles in inflammatory conditions. However, in obese person, the level of these protective adipokines are diminished and the pro-inflammatory adipokines predominate. Adiponectin possesses anti-inflammatory, anti-atherogenic, and insulin-sensitizing properties.

Omentin and vaspin secreted by the stromal cells, exert also anti-inflammatory and anti-atherogenic effects. Omentin stimulates endothelial nitric oxide synthesis, vaspin inhibits nuclear factor-kappa B (NF-kB), and thus both play important role in protecting vascular endothelial cells and regulating blood pressure through relaxation of smooth cells in the vessels [97]. In addition, eosinophils and T regulatory cells (Treg), the main resident T cell population, secrete anti-inflammatory cytokines (IL-10 and IL-4) and protective adiponectin that polarize adipose tissue macrophages towards an anti-inflammatory phenotype [93].

BROWN ADIPOSE TISSUE AND BROWNKINES

Brown adipose tissue (BAT), in contrast to WAT, has uncoupling protein-1 (UCP1) which is crucial for fatty acid oxidation and heat production (thermogenesis) [98]. BAT utilizes energy from macronutrients such as fatty acids and glucose to induce nonshivering thermogenesis. This thermogenic capacity of BAT has been well described in small mammals and infants in whom it assists in maintaining the temperature of the internal environment of the body [99]. It was previously thought that BAT is mostly found in infants, but current evidence has proven that adult humans, although to a lesser extent, also have BAT, usually situated in the supraclavicular, paravertebral, and cervical regions [100]. Accumulating data suggests that BAT activity is inversely related to age, body mass index (BMI) and diabetes in adults, suggesting that BAT activation could serve as an important target in treating metabolic diseases such as diabetes and obesity [100].

In addition to the classic brown adipocytes, usually found in specific brown fat depots, it has been reported previously that brown adipocytes can often exist in white adipose depots in reaction to sustained cold exposure or b-adrenergic stimulation [98]. This phenomenon has recently been termed "browning" or "beiging." These cells possess a high thermogenic capacity and thus significantly contribute to energy expenditure in various *in vivo* models [101]. In addition to cold and b-adrenergic stimulation, multiple genetic factors have recently been identified to regulate the browning of WAT, highlighting the transcriptional complexity underlying this process [99].

Protective effects of BAT in the development of a chronic metabolic disease have conventionally been attributed to its capacity to employ glucose and lipids for thermogenesis. Nevertheless, as the new evidence emerges, it seems that BAT might protect against chronic metabolic diseases by secreting metabolically active mediators, so-called 'brownkines'. These BAT-derived molecules can act locally in BAT, where they stimulate hypertrophy and hyperplasia, neovascularization, all of which are required during increased needs for thermogenesis. But, animal models have suggested that brownkines such as fibroblast growth factor 21, IL-6 and neuregulin 4 might have an endocrine role affecting distant and vast cells exerting systemic effects [102].

FACTOR FIBROBLAST GROWTH FACTOR 21 (FGF21)

FGF21 is mainly produced by the liver. However, when BAT is activated by cold exposure, brown adipocytes express and release high amounts of FGF21 contributing to systemic FGF21 levels [103]. FGF21 promotes glucose use in adipose tissues and improves glycaemia and lipidaemia [104]. Administration of an FGF21 to rodents has been shown to induce thermogenesis, improved glucose homeostasis, lipid profile, and weight loss [105]. However, in humans, FGF21 is absurdly increased in insulin-resistant states such as obesity or type 2 diabetes; suggesting that humans could either be prone to develop resistance to FGF21 effects or that other mechanisms counter fight above mentioned effects [106].

NEUREGULIN 4

Neuroregulin 4 (Nrg4) has been implicated in the development of several malignancies and has been associated with high-grade tumors, suggesting its potential roles in cancer initiation and progression. However, recent studies demonstrated that Nrg4 is also highly expressed in BAT and could exert its metabolic effect on the liver where Nrg4 has been shown to inhibit lipogenesis and liver steatosis, while downplaying insulin resistance [107]. It has also been shown in animal models on high-fat diet, that overexpression of Nrg4 reduces fat mass and obesity, increases energy expenditure through activation of fatty acid oxidation and provoking protective adipokine secretion [108]. In contrast, animals depleted of Nrg4 developed metabolic disorders such as obesity, dyslipidemia, hepatic steatosis, hyperglycemia, hyperinsulinemia and insulin resistance [107].

RETINOL BINDING PROTEIN 4

Retinol binding protein 4 is another browkine secreted from BAT during noradrenergic stimulation which might favour the transport of retinoids released after lipolysis [109].

IL-6

Noradrenergic stimulation of BAT leads to increased secretion of IL6. This observation might seem inconsistent with the role of IL6 as a proinflammatory cytokine but IL-6 is now known to be released by skeletal muscle in response to exercise and to promote insulin sensitivity [110]. In adipose tissue, IL6 mediated signalling promotes macrophage activation by sensitizing these cells to the action of IL4, which in this context is concomitant with an enhancement of insulin sensitivity [111].

ANGIOPOIETIN-LIKE 8

Angiopoietin-like 8 (Angptl8) is synthesized in BAT when BAT is exposed to cold although the implication of enhanced release is currently unclear [112]. Lipoprotein lipase activity can be suppressed by Angptl8, which serves as a regulatory mechanism since BAT exposure to cold increases lipoprotein lipase activity [113]. Increased BAT activity, in conditions such as cold exposure, regulates glucose homeostasis and insulin sensitivity which could lead to speculation that diabetes protective effects might be mediated by Angptl8 [112].

CONCLUDING REMARKS

White adipose tissue is an active endocrine organ consisting of adipocytes, fibroblasts, endothelial cells and a broad array of immune cells. Adipokines released from adipocytes modulate human metabolism affecting inflammation, insulin secretion and sensitivity, oxidative stress and atherosclerosis. In obese persons, positive energy balance results in adipocyte expansion, infiltration of inflammatory cells and enhanced cytokines secretion. In addition, dysregulation of adipokines secretion where proinflammatory adipokines such as leptin, resistin, and visfatin are upregulated, while the anti-inflammatory adipokines, such as adiponectin, apelin, vaspin and omentin are downregulated, plays a crucial role in systemic low-grade inflammation, obesity-induced insulin resistance and immune system dysfunction. The ability of brown adipose tissue to protect against chronic metabolic disease has been attributed to its capacity to utilize glucose and lipids for thermogenesis, but recent studies suggest that secreted brownkines such as fibroblast growth factor 21, neuregulin 4 and IL-6 can contribute to the improvement of glycaemia and lipidaemia by inhibiting hepatic lipogenesis and obesity-associated insulin resistance. Although many effects of adipokines and brownkines have been elucidated in recent times, the detail of their integration is a missing link which should be further investigated with the ultimate goal to better understand obesity-induced inflammatory diseases for the development of novel therapeutic approaches.

CONSENT FOR PUBLICATION

Not applicable.

CONFLICT OF INTEREST

The authors confirm that this chapter content has no conflict of interest.

ACKNOWLEDGEMENTS

The authors would like to express their sincere thanks to the editor and anonymous reviewers for their time and valuable suggestions.

REFERENCES

[1]   Tchkonia T, Thomou T, Zhu Y, *et al.* Mechanisms and metabolic implications of regional differences among fat depots. Cell Metab 2013; 17(5): 644-56.
[http://dx.doi.org/10.1016/j.cmet.2013.03.008] [PMID: 23583168]

[2]   Coelho M, Oliveira T, Fernandes R. Biochemistry of adipose tissue: an endocrine organ. Arch Med Sci 2013; 9(2): 191-200.
[http://dx.doi.org/10.5114/aoms.2013.33181] [PMID: 23671428]

[3]   Kiess W, Petzold S, Töpfer M, *et al.* Adipocytes and adipose tissue. Best Pract Res Clin Endocrinol Metab 2008; 22(1): 135-53.
[http://dx.doi.org/10.1016/j.beem.2007.10.002] [PMID: 18279785]

[4]   Galic S, Oakhill JS, Steinberg GR. Adipose tissue as an endocrine organ. Mol Cell Endocrinol 2010; 316(2): 129-39.
[http://dx.doi.org/10.1016/j.mce.2009.08.018] [PMID: 19723556]

[5]   Wang Q, Wu H. T cells in adipose tissue: Critical players in immunometabolism. Front Immunol 2018; 9: 2509.
[http://dx.doi.org/10.3389/fimmu.2018.02509] [PMID: 30459770]

[6]   Mantzoros CS, Moschos SJ. Leptin: in search of role(s) in human physiology and pathophysiology. Clin Endocrinol (Oxf) 1998; 49(5): 551-67.
[http://dx.doi.org/10.1046/j.1365-2265.1998.00571.x] [PMID: 10197068]

[7]   Hadji P, Hars O, Bock K, *et al.* The influence of menopause and body mass index on serum leptin concentrations. Eur J Endocrinol 2000; 143(1): 55-60.
[http://dx.doi.org/10.1530/eje.0.1430055] [PMID: 10870031]

[8]   Mahabir S, Baer D, Johnson LL, *et al.* Body Mass Index, percent body fat, and regional body fat distribution in relation to leptin concentrations in healthy, non-smoking postmenopausal women in a feeding study. Nutr J 2007; 6: 3.
[http://dx.doi.org/10.1186/1475-2891-6-3] [PMID: 17229323]

[9]   Dardeno TA, Chou SH, Moon HS, Chamberland JP, Fiorenza CG, Mantzoros CS. Leptin in human physiology and therapeutics. Front Neuroendocrinol 2010; 31(3): 377-93.
[http://dx.doi.org/10.1016/j.yfrne.2010.06.002] [PMID: 20600241]

[10]   Sinha MK, Ohannesian JP, Heiman ML, *et al.* Nocturnal rise of leptin in lean, obese, and non-insuli--dependent diabetes mellitus subjects. J Clin Invest 1996; 97(5): 7-1344.

[11]   Havel PJ, Kasim-Karakas S, Dubuc GR, Mueller W, Phinney SD. Gender differences in plasma leptin concentrations. Nat Med 1996; 2(9): 949-50.
[http://dx.doi.org/10.1038/nm0996-949b] [PMID: 8782440]

[12]   Di Carlo C, Tommaselli GA, Nappi C. Effects of sex steroid hormones and menopause on serum leptin concentrations. Gynecol Endocrinol 2002; 16(6): 479-91.
[http://dx.doi.org/10.1080/gye.16.6.479.491] [PMID: 12626035]

[13]   Rosenbaum M, Nicolson M, Hirsch J, *et al.* Effects of gender, body composition, and menopause on

plasma concentrations of leptin. J Clin Endocrinol Metab 1996; 81(9): 3424-7.
[PMID: 8784109]

[14]   Petzel M. Action of leptin on bone and its relationship to menopause. Biomed Pap Med Fac Univ Palacky Olomouc Czech Repub 2007; 151(2): 195-9.
[http://dx.doi.org/10.5507/bp.2007.034] [PMID: 18345251]

[15]   Bednarek-Tupikowska G, Filus A, Kuliczkowska-Płaksej J, Tupikowski K, Bohdanowicz-Pawlak A, Milewicz A. Serum leptin concentrations in pre- and postmenopausal women on sex hormone therapy. Gynecol Endocrinol 2006; 22(4): 207-12.
[http://dx.doi.org/10.1080/09513590600702774] [PMID: 16723307]

[16]   Dong M, Ren J. What fans the fire: insights into mechanisms of leptin in metabolic syndrome-associated heart diseases. Curr Pharm Des 2014; 20(4): 652-8.
[http://dx.doi.org/10.2174/13816128200414021316093] [PMID: 23688014]

[17]   Wauters M, Considine RV, Yudkin JS, Peiffer F, De Leeuw I, Van Gaal LF. Leptin levels in type 2 diabetes: associations with measures of insulin resistance and insulin secretion. Horm Metab Res 2003; 35(2): 92-6.
[http://dx.doi.org/10.1055/s-2003-39054] [PMID: 12734788]

[18]   Carlyle M, Jones OB, Kuo JJ, Hall JE. Chronic cardiovascular and renal actions of leptin: role of adrenergic activity. Hypertension 2002; 39(2 Pt 2): 496-501.
[http://dx.doi.org/10.1161/hy0202.104398] [PMID: 11882597]

[19]   Eikelis N, Schlaich M, Aggarwal A, Kaye D, Esler M. Interactions between leptin and the human sympathetic nervous system. Hypertension 2003; 41(5): 1072-9.
[http://dx.doi.org/10.1161/01.HYP.0000066289.17754.49] [PMID: 12668587]

[20]   Ghantous CM, Azrak Z, Hanache S, Abou-Kheir W, Zeidan A. Differential role of leptin and adiponectin in cardiovascular system. Int J Endocrinol 2015; 2015: 534320.
[http://dx.doi.org/10.1155/2015/534320] [PMID: 26064110]

[21]   Lord GM, Matarese G, Howard JK, Baker RJ, Bloom SR, Lechler RI. Leptin modulates the T-cell immune response and reverses starvation-induced immunosuppression. Nature 1998; 394(6696): 897-901.
[http://dx.doi.org/10.1038/29795] [PMID: 9732873]

[22]   Agrawal S, Gollapudi S, Su H, Gupta S. Leptin activates human B cells to secrete TNF-α, IL-6, and IL-10 *via* JAK2/STAT3 and p38MAPK/ERK1/2 signaling pathway. J Clin Immunol 2011; 31(3): 472-8.
[http://dx.doi.org/10.1007/s10875-010-9507-1] [PMID: 21243519]

[23]   Scherer PE, Williams S, Fogliano M, Baldini G, Lodish HF. A novel serum protein similar to C1q, produced exclusively in adipocytes. J Biol Chem 1995; 270(45): 26746-9.
[http://dx.doi.org/10.1074/jbc.270.45.26746] [PMID: 7592907]

[24]   Viengchareun S, Zennaro MC, Pascual-Le Tallec L, Lombes M. Brown adipocytes are novel sites of expression and regulation of adiponectin and resistin. FEBS Lett 2002; 532(3): 345-50.
[http://dx.doi.org/10.1016/S0014-5793(02)03697-9] [PMID: 12482590]

[25]   Delaigle AM, Jonas JC, Bauche IB, Cornu O, Brichard SM. Induction of adiponectin in skeletal muscle by inflammatory cytokines: *in vivo* and *in vitro* studies. Endocrinology 2004; 145(12): 5589-97.
[http://dx.doi.org/10.1210/en.2004-0503] [PMID: 15319349]

[26]   Yoda-Murakami M, Taniguchi M, Takahashi K, *et al.* Change in expression of GBP28/adiponectin in carbon tetrachloride-administrated mouse liver. Biochem Biophys Res Commun 2001; 285(2): 372-7.
[http://dx.doi.org/10.1006/bbrc.2001.5134] [PMID: 11444852]

[27]   Piñeiro R, Iglesias MJ, Gallego R, *et al.* Adiponectin is synthesized and secreted by human and murine cardiomyocytes. FEBS Lett 2005; 579(23): 5163-9.

[http://dx.doi.org/10.1016/j.febslet.2005.07.098] [PMID: 16140297]

[28] Berner HS, Lyngstadaas SP, Spahr A, *et al.* Adiponectin and its receptors are expressed in bone-forming cells. Bone 2004; 35(4): 842-9.
[http://dx.doi.org/10.1016/j.bone.2004.06.008] [PMID: 15454091]

[29] Caminos JE, Nogueiras R, Gallego R, *et al.* Expression and regulation of adiponectin and receptor in human and rat placenta. J Clin Endocrinol Metab 2005; 90(7): 4276-86.
[http://dx.doi.org/10.1210/jc.2004-0930] [PMID: 15855268]

[30] Neumeier M, Weigert J, Buettner R, *et al.* Detection of adiponectin in cerebrospinal fluid in humans. Am J Physiol Endocrinol Metab 2007; 293(4): E965-9.
[http://dx.doi.org/10.1152/ajpendo.00119.2007] [PMID: 17623750]

[31] Katsuki A, Suematsu M, Gabazza EC, *et al.* Increased oxidative stress is associated with decreased circulating levels of adiponectin in Japanese metabolically obese, normal-weight men with normal glucose tolerance. Diabetes Res Clin Pract 2006; 73(3): 310-4.
[http://dx.doi.org/10.1016/j.diabres.2006.02.014] [PMID: 16631275]

[32] Chiarugi P, Fiaschi T. Adiponectin in health and diseases: from metabolic syndrome to tissue regeneration. Expert Opin Ther Targets 2010; 14(2): 193-206.
[http://dx.doi.org/10.1517/14728220903530712] [PMID: 20017651]

[33] Wang Y, Lam KS, Yau MH, Xu A. Post-translational modifications of adiponectin: mechanisms and functional implications. Biochem J 2008; 409(3): 623-33.
[http://dx.doi.org/10.1042/BJ20071492] [PMID: 18177270]

[34] Robinson K, Prins J, Venkatesh B. Clinical review: adiponectin biology and its role in inflammation and critical illness. Crit Care 2011; 15(2): 221.
[http://dx.doi.org/10.1186/cc10021]

[35] Halberg N, Schraw TD, Wang ZV, *et al.* Systemic fate of the adipocyte-derived factor adiponectin. Diabetes 2009; 58(9): 1961-70.
[http://dx.doi.org/10.2337/db08-1750] [PMID: 19581422]

[36] Dadson K, Liu Y, Sweeney G. Adiponectin action: a combination of endocrine and autocrine/paracrine effects. Front Endocrinol (Lausanne) 2011; 2: 62.
[http://dx.doi.org/10.3389/fendo.2011.00062] [PMID: 22649379]

[37] Yamauchi T, Nio Y, Maki T, *et al.* Targeted disruption of AdipoR1 and AdipoR2 causes abrogation of adiponectin binding and metabolic actions. Nat Med 2007; 13(3): 332-9.
[http://dx.doi.org/10.1038/nm1557] [PMID: 17268472]

[38] Hug C, Wang J, Ahmad NS, Bogan JS, Tsao TS, Lodish HF. T-cadherin is a receptor for hexameric and high-molecular-weight forms of Acrp30/adiponectin. Proc Natl Acad Sci USA 2004; 101(28): 10308-13.
[http://dx.doi.org/10.1073/pnas.0403382101] [PMID: 15210937]

[39] Gavrila A, Peng CK, Chan JL, Mietus JE, Goldberger AL, Mantzoros CS. Diurnal and ultradian dynamics of serum adiponectin in healthy men: comparison with leptin, circulating soluble leptin receptor, and cortisol patterns. J Clin Endocrinol Metab 2003; 88(6): 2838-43.
[http://dx.doi.org/10.1210/jc.2002-021721] [PMID: 12788897]

[40] Swarbrick MM, Havel PJ. Physiological, pharmacological, and nutritional regulation of circulating adiponectin concentrations in humans. Metab Syndr Relat Disord 2008; 6(2): 87-102.
[http://dx.doi.org/10.1089/met.2007.0029] [PMID: 18510434]

[41] English PJ, Coughlin SR, Hayden K, Malik IA, Wilding JP. Plasma adiponectin increases postprandially in obese, but not in lean, subjects. Obes Res 2003; 11(7): 839-44.
[http://dx.doi.org/10.1038/oby.2003.115] [PMID: 12855752]

[42] Cnop M, Havel PJ, Utzschneider KM, *et al.* Relationship of adiponectin to body fat distribution, insulin sensitivity and plasma lipoproteins: evidence for independent roles of age and sex.

Diabetologia 2003; 46(4): 459-69.
[http://dx.doi.org/10.1007/s00125-003-1074-z] [PMID: 12687327]

[43] Imbeault P. Environmental influences on adiponectin levels in humans. Appl Physiol Nutr Metab 2007; 32(3): 505-11.
[http://dx.doi.org/10.1139/H07-017] [PMID: 17510690]

[44] Böttner A, Kratzsch J, Müller G, *et al.* Gender differences of adiponectin levels develop during the progression of puberty and are related to serum androgen levels. J Clin Endocrinol Metab 2004; 89(8): 4053-61.
[http://dx.doi.org/10.1210/jc.2004-0303] [PMID: 15292348]

[45] Degawa-Yamauchi M, Moss KA, Bovenkerk JE, *et al.* Regulation of adiponectin expression in human adipocytes: effects of adiposity, glucocorticoids, and tumor necrosis factor alpha. Obes Res 2005; 13(4): 662-9.
[http://dx.doi.org/10.1038/oby.2005.74] [PMID: 15897474]

[46] Fukuda I, Hizuka N, Ishikawa Y, *et al.* Serum adiponectin levels in adult growth hormone deficiency and acromegaly. Growth Horm IGF Res 2004; 14(6): 449-54.
[http://dx.doi.org/10.1016/j.ghir.2004.06.005] [PMID: 15519253]

[47] Steppan CM, Brown EJ, Wright CM, *et al.* A family of tissue-specific resistin-like molecules. Proc Natl Acad Sci USA 2001; 98(2): 502-6.
[http://dx.doi.org/10.1073/pnas.98.2.502] [PMID: 11209052]

[48] Patel L, Buckels AC, Kinghorn IJ, *et al.* Resistin is expressed in human macrophages and directly regulated by PPAR gamma activators. Biochem Biophys Res Commun 2003; 300(2): 472-6.
[http://dx.doi.org/10.1016/S0006-291X(02)02841-3] [PMID: 12504108]

[49] Rajala MW, Qi Y, Patel HR, *et al.* Regulation of resistin expression and circulating levels in obesity, diabetes, and fasting. Diabetes 2004; 53(7): 1671-9.
[http://dx.doi.org/10.2337/diabetes.53.7.1671] [PMID: 15220189]

[50] Savage DB, Sewter CP, Klenk ES, *et al.* Resistin / Fizz3 expression in relation to obesity and peroxisome proliferator-activated receptor-gamma action in humans. Diabetes 2001; 50(10): 2199-202.
[http://dx.doi.org/10.2337/diabetes.50.10.2199] [PMID: 11574398]

[51] Steppan CM, Bailey ST, Bhat S, *et al.* The hormone resistin links obesity to diabetes. Nature 2001; 409(6818): 307-12.
[http://dx.doi.org/10.1038/35053000] [PMID: 11201732]

[52] Qi Y, Nie Z, Lee YS, *et al.* Loss of resistin improves glucose homeostasis in leptin deficiency. Diabetes 2006; 55(11): 3083-90.
[http://dx.doi.org/10.2337/db05-0615] [PMID: 17065346]

[53] Tarkowski A, Bjersing J, Shestakov A, Bokarewa MI. Resistin competes with lipopolysaccharide for binding to toll-like receptor 4. J Cell Mol Med 2010; 14(6B): 1419-31.
[http://dx.doi.org/10.1111/j.1582-4934.2009.00899.x] [PMID: 19754671]

[54] Lee S, Lee HC, Kwon YW, *et al.* Adenylyl cyclase-associated protein 1 is a receptor for human resistin and mediates inflammatory actions of human monocytes. Cell Metab 2014; 19(3): 484-97.
[http://dx.doi.org/10.1016/j.cmet.2014.01.013] [PMID: 24606903]

[55] Luk T, Malam Z, Marshall JC. Pre-B cell colony-enhancing factor (PBEF)/visfatin: a novel mediator of innate immunity. J Leukoc Biol 2008; 83(4): 804-16.
[http://dx.doi.org/10.1189/jlb.0807581] [PMID: 18252866]

[56] Imai S, Guarente L. NAD+ and sirtuins in aging and disease. Trends Cell Biol 2014; 24(8): 464-71.
[http://dx.doi.org/10.1016/j.tcb.2014.04.002] [PMID: 24786309]

[57] Fukuhara A, Matsuda M, Nishizawa M, *et al.* Visfatin: a protein secreted by visceral fat that mimics the effects of insulin. Science 2005; 307(5708): 426-30.

[http://dx.doi.org/10.1126/science.1097243] [PMID: 15604363]

[58]   Karbaschian Z, Hosseinzadeh-Attar MJ, Giahi L, *et al*. Portal and systemic levels of visfatin in morbidly obese subjects undergoing bariatric surgery. Endocrine 2013; 44(1): 114-8.
       [http://dx.doi.org/10.1007/s12020-012-9821-x] [PMID: 23104149]

[59]   Auguet T, Terra X, Porras JA, *et al*. Plasma visfatin levels and gene expression in morbidly obese women with associated fatty liver disease. Clin Biochem 2013; 46(3): 202-8.
       [http://dx.doi.org/10.1016/j.clinbiochem.2012.11.006] [PMID: 23174488]

[60]   Li RZ, Ma Xn, Hu XF, *et al*. Elevated visfatin levels in obese children are related to proinflammatory factors. J Pediatr Endocrinol Metab 2013; 26(1-2): 111-8.
       [PMID: 23327785]

[61]   Friebe D, Neef M, Kratzsch J, *et al*. Leucocytes are a major source of circulating nicotinamide phosphoribosyltransferase (NAMPT)/pre-B cell colony (PBEF)/visfatin linking obesity and inflammation in humans. Diabetologia 2011; 54(5): 1200-11.
       [http://dx.doi.org/10.1007/s00125-010-2042-z] [PMID: 21298414]

[62]   Chang YH, Chang DM, Lin KC, Shin SJ, Lee YJ. Visfatin in overweight/obesity, type 2 diabetes mellitus, insulin resistance, metabolic syndrome and cardiovascular diseases: a meta-analysis and systemic review. Diabetes Metab Res Rev 2011; 27(6): 515-27.
       [http://dx.doi.org/10.1002/dmrr.1201] [PMID: 21484978]

[63]   Franco-Trepat E, Guillán-Fresco M, Alonso-Pérez A, *et al*. Visfatin Connection: Present and Future in Osteoarthritis and Osteoporosis. J Clin Med 2019; 8(8): 1178.
       [http://dx.doi.org/10.3390/jcm8081178] [PMID: 31394795]

[64]   Romacho T, Sánchez-Ferrer CF, Peiró C. Visfatin/Nampt: An Adipokine with Cardiovascular Impact Mediators of Inflammation 2013; 2013: 15.
       [PMID: 946427]

[65]   Dahl TB, Yndestad A, Skjelland M, *et al*. Increased expression of visfatin in macrophages of human unstable carotid and coronary atherosclerosis: possible role in inflammation and plaque destabilization. Circulation 2007; 115(8): 972-80.
       [http://dx.doi.org/10.1161/CIRCULATIONAHA.106.665893] [PMID: 17283255]

[66]   Romacho T, Azcutia V, Vázquez-Bella M, *et al*. Extracellular PBEF/NAMPT/visfatin activates pro-inflammatory signalling in human vascular smooth muscle cells through nicotinamide phosphoribosyltransferase activity. Diabetologia 2009; 52(11): 2455-63.
       [http://dx.doi.org/10.1007/s00125-009-1509-2] [PMID: 19727662]

[67]   Kim SR, Bae YH, Bae SK, *et al*. Visfatin enhances ICAM-1 and VCAM-1 expression through ROS-dependent NF-kappaB activation in endothelial cells. Biochim Biophys Acta 2008; 1783(5): 886-95.
       [http://dx.doi.org/10.1016/j.bbamcr.2008.01.004] [PMID: 18241674]

[68]   Liu SW, Qiao SB, Yuan JS, Liu DQ. Visfatin stimulates production of monocyte chemotactic protein-1 and interleukin-6 in human vein umbilical endothelial cells. Horm Metab Res 2009; 41(4): 281-6.
       [http://dx.doi.org/10.1055/s-0028-1102914] [PMID: 19009499]

[69]   Liu S, Duan R, Wu Y, *et al*. Effects of Vaspin on Insulin Resistance in Rats and Underlying Mechanisms. Sci Rep 2018; 8(1): 13542.
       [http://dx.doi.org/10.1038/s41598-018-31923-3] [PMID: 30202052]

[70]   Feng R, Li Y, Wang C, *et al*. Higher vaspin levels in subjects with obesity and type 2 diabetes mellitus: a meta-analysis. Diabetes Res Clin Pract 2014; 106(1): 88-94.
       [http://dx.doi.org/10.1016/j.diabres.2014.07.026] [PMID: 25151227]

[71]   Klöting N, Kovacs P, Kern M, *et al*. Central vaspin administration acutely reduces food intake and has sustained blood glucose-lowering effects. Diabetologia 2011; 54(7): 1819-23.
       [http://dx.doi.org/10.1007/s00125-011-2137-1] [PMID: 21465327]

[72]   Wada J. Vaspin: a novel serpin with insulin-sensitizing effects. Expert Opin Investig Drugs 2008;

17(3): 327-33.
[http://dx.doi.org/10.1517/13543784.17.3.327] [PMID: 18321232]

[73]   Qi D, Wang D, Zhang C, *et al.* Vaspin protects against LPS-induced ARDS by inhibiting
        inflammation, apoptosis and reactive oxygen species generation in pulmonary endothelial cells via the
        Akt/GSK-3β pathway. Int J Mol Med 2017; 40(6): 1803-17.
        [http://dx.doi.org/10.3892/ijmm.2017.3176] [PMID: 29039444]

[74]   Kameshima S, Sakamoto Y, Okada M, Yamawaki H. Vaspin prevents elevation of blood pressure
        through inhibition of peripheral vascular remodelling in spontaneously hypertensive rats. Acta Physiol
        (Oxf) 2016; 217(2): 120-9.
        [http://dx.doi.org/10.1111/apha.12636] [PMID: 26640237]

[75]   Phalitakul S, Okada M, Hara Y, Yamawaki H. Vaspin prevents TNF-α-induced intracellular adhesion
        molecule-1 *via* inhibiting reactive oxygen species-dependent NF-κB and PKCθ activation in cultured
        rat vascular smooth muscle cells. Pharmacol Res 2011; 64(5): 493-500.
        [http://dx.doi.org/10.1016/j.phrs.2011.06.001] [PMID: 21683791]

[76]   Liu S, Dong Y, Wang T, *et al.* Vaspin inhibited proinflammatory cytokine induced activation of
        nuclear factor-kappa B and its downstream molecules in human endothelial EA.hy926 cells. Diabetes
        Res Clin Pract 2014; 103(3): 482-8.
        [http://dx.doi.org/10.1016/j.diabres.2013.12.002] [PMID: 24418398]

[77]   Than A, Tee WT, Chen P. Apelin secretion and expression of apelin receptors in 3T3-L1 adipocytes
        are differentially regulated by angiotensin type 1 and type 2 receptors. Mol Cell Endocrinol 2012;
        351(2): 296-305.
        [http://dx.doi.org/10.1016/j.mce.2012.01.005] [PMID: 22249006]

[78]   Sorhede Winzell M, Magnusson C, Ahren B. The apj receptor is expressed in pancreatic islets and its
        ligand, apelin, inhibits insulin secretion in mice. 2005.
        [http://dx.doi.org/10.1016/j.regpep.2005.05.004]

[79]   O'Carroll AM, Selby TL, Palkovits M, Lolait SJ. Distribution of mRNA encoding B78/apj, the rat
        homologue of the human APJ receptor, and its endogenous ligand apelin in brain and peripheral
        tissues. Biochim Biophys Acta 2000; 1492: 72-80. 73.

[80]   Taheri S, Murphy K, Cohen M, *et al.* The effects of centrally administered apelin-13 on food intake,
        water intake and pituitary hormone release in rats. Biochem Biophys Res Commun 2002; 291(5):
        1208-12.
        [http://dx.doi.org/10.1006/bbrc.2002.6575] [PMID: 11883945]

[81]   Cox CM, D'Agostino SL, Miller MK, Heimark RL, Krieg PA. Apelin, the ligand for the endothelial
        G-protein-coupled receptor, APJ, is a potent angiogenic factor required for normal vascular
        development of the frog embryo. Dev Biol 2006; 296(1): 177-89.
        [http://dx.doi.org/10.1016/j.ydbio.2006.04.452] [PMID: 16750822]

[82]   Ashley EA, Powers J, Chen M, *et al.* The endogenous peptide apelin potently improves cardiac
        contractility and reduces cardiac loading *in vivo.* Cardiovasc Res 2005; 65(1): 73-82.
        [http://dx.doi.org/10.1016/j.cardiores.2004.08.018] [PMID: 15621035]

[83]   Dray C, Knauf C, Daviaud D, *et al.* Apelin stimulates glucose utilization in normal and obese insulin-
        resistant mice. Cell Metab 2008; 8(5): 437-45.
        [http://dx.doi.org/10.1016/j.cmet.2008.10.003] [PMID: 19046574]

[84]   Castan-Laurell I, Dray C, Knauf C, Kunduzova O, Valet P. Apelin, a promising target for type 2
        diabetes treatment? Trends Endocrinol Metab 2012; 23(5): 234-41.
        [http://dx.doi.org/10.1016/j.tem.2012.02.005] [PMID: 22445464]

[85]   Sunter D, Hewson AK, Dickson SL. Intracerebroventricular injection of apelin-13 reduces food intake
        in the rat. 2003.
        [http://dx.doi.org/10.1016/S0304-3940(03)00351-3]

[86]   Lv SY, Yang YJ, Qin YJ, *et al.* Central apelin-13 inhibits food intake via the CRF receptor in mice. Peptides 2012; 33: 8-132. 78.

[87]   Giralt M, Cereijo R, Villarroya F. Adipokines and the Endocrine Role of Adipose Tissues. Handb Exp Pharmacol 2016; 233: 265-82.
[http://dx.doi.org/10.1007/164_2015_6] [PMID: 25903415]

[88]   Lo JC, Ljubicic S, Leibiger B, *et al.* Adipsin is an adipokine that improves β cell function in diabetes. Cell 2014; 158(1): 41-53.
[http://dx.doi.org/10.1016/j.cell.2014.06.005] [PMID: 24995977]

[89]   Zhou Q, Ge Q, Ding Y, *et al.* Relationship between serum adipsin and the first phase of glucose-stimulated insulin secretion in individuals with different glucose tolerance. J Diabetes Investig 2018; 9(5): 1128-34.
[http://dx.doi.org/10.1111/jdi.12819] [PMID: 29432659]

[90]   Booth A, Magnuson A, Fouts J, Foster MT. Adipose tissue: an endocrine organ playing a role in metabolic regulation. Horm Mol Biol Clin Investig 2016; 26(1): 25-42.
[http://dx.doi.org/10.1515/hmbci-2015-0073] [PMID: 26910750]

[91]   de Souza Batista CM, Yang RZ, Lee MJ, *et al.* Omentin plasma levels and gene expression are decreased in obesity. Diabetes 2007; 56(6): 1655-61.
[http://dx.doi.org/10.2337/db06-1506] [PMID: 17329619]

[92]   Pan HY, Guo L, Li Q. Changes of serum omentin-1 levels in normal subjects and in patients with impaired glucose regulation and with newly diagnosed and untreated type 2 diabetes. Diabetes Res Clin Pract 2010; 88(1): 29-33.
[http://dx.doi.org/10.1016/j.diabres.2010.01.013] [PMID: 20129687]

[93]   Huh JY, Park YJ, Ham M, Kim JB. Crosstalk between adipocytes and immune cells in adipose tissue inflammation and metabolic dysregulation in obesity. Mol Cells 2014; 37(5): 365-71.
[http://dx.doi.org/10.14348/molcells.2014.0074] [PMID: 24781408]

[94]   Khan IM, Dai Perrard XY, Perrard JL, *et al.* Attenuated adipose tissue and skeletal muscle inflammation in obese mice with combined CD4+ and CD8+ T cell deficiency. Atherosclerosis 2014; 233(2): 419-28.
[http://dx.doi.org/10.1016/j.atherosclerosis.2014.01.011] [PMID: 24530773]

[95]   Hotamisligil GS, Arner P, Caro JF, Atkinson RL, Spiegelman BM. Increased adipose tissue expression of tumor necrosis factor-alpha in human obesity and insulin resistance. J Clin Invest 1995; 95(5): 2409-15.
[http://dx.doi.org/10.1172/JCI117936] [PMID: 7738205]

[96]   Rotter V, Nagaev I, Smith U. Interleukin-6 (IL-6) induces insulin resistance in 3T3-L1 adipocytes and is, like IL-8 and tumor necrosis factor-alpha, overexpressed in human fat cells from insulin-resistant subjects. J Biol Chem 2003; 278(46): 45777-84.
[http://dx.doi.org/10.1074/jbc.M301977200] [PMID: 12952969]

[97]   Liu S, Li X, Wu Y, *et al.* Effects of vaspin on pancreatic β cell secretion via PI3K/Akt and NF-κB signaling pathways. PLoS One 2017; 12(12): e0189722.
[http://dx.doi.org/10.1371/journal.pone.0189722] [PMID: 29240812]

[98]   Fenzl A, Kiefer FW. Brown adipose tissue and thermogenesis. Horm Mol Biol Clin Investig 2014; 19(1): 25-37.
[http://dx.doi.org/10.1515/hmbci-2014-0022] [PMID: 25390014]

[99]   Cannon B, Nedergaard J. Brown adipose tissue: function and physiological significance. Physiol Rev 2004; 84(1): 277-359.
[http://dx.doi.org/10.1152/physrev.00015.2003] [PMID: 14715917]

[100]   van Marken Lichtenbelt WD, Vanhommerig JW, Smulders NM, *et al.* Cold-activated brown adipose tissue in healthy men. N Engl J Med 2009; 360(15): 1500-8.

[http://dx.doi.org/10.1056/NEJMoa0808718] [PMID: 19357405]

[101] Wu J, Cohen P, Spiegelman BM. Adaptive thermogenesis in adipocytes: is beige the new brown? Genes Dev 2013; 27(3): 234-50.
[http://dx.doi.org/10.1101/gad.211649.112] [PMID: 23388824]

[102] Villarroya F, Cereijo R, Villarroya J, Giralt M. Brown adipose tissue as a secretory organ. Nat Rev Endocrinol 2017; 13(1): 26-35.
[http://dx.doi.org/10.1038/nrendo.2016.136] [PMID: 27616452]

[103] Cuevas-Ramos D, Mehta R, Aguilar-Salinas CA. Fibroblast Growth Factor 21 and Browning of White Adipose Tissue. Front Physiol 2019; 10: 37.
[http://dx.doi.org/10.3389/fphys.2019.00037] [PMID: 30804796]

[104] Cuevas-Ramos D, Aguilar-Salinas CA, Gómez-Pérez FJ. Metabolic actions of fibroblast growth factor 21. Curr Opin Pediatr 2012; 24(4): 523-9. a
[http://dx.doi.org/10.1097/MOP.0b013e3283557d22] [PMID: 22732636]

[105] Véniant MM, Hale C, Helmering J, *et al.* FGF21 promotes metabolic homeostasis *via* white adipose and leptin in mice. PLoS One 2012; 7(7): e40164.
[http://dx.doi.org/10.1371/journal.pone.0040164] [PMID: 22792234]

[106] Cuevas-Ramos D, Almeda-Valdes P, Gómez-Pérez FJ, *et al.* Daily physical activity, fasting glucose, uric acid, and body mass index are independent factors associated with serum fibroblast growth factor 21 levels. Eur J Endocrinol 2010; 163(3): 469-77.
[http://dx.doi.org/10.1530/EJE-10-0454] [PMID: 20566587]

[107] Wang GX, Zhao XY, Meng ZX, *et al.* The brown fat-enriched secreted factor Nrg4 preserves metabolic homeostasis through attenuation of hepatic lipogenesis. Nat Med 2014; 20(12): 1436-43.
[http://dx.doi.org/10.1038/nm.3713] [PMID: 25401691]

[108] Chen Z, Wang GX, Ma SL, *et al.* Nrg4 promotes fuel oxidation and a healthy adipokine profile to ameliorate diet-induced metabolic disorders. Mol Metab 2017; 6(8): 863-72.
[http://dx.doi.org/10.1016/j.molmet.2017.03.016] [PMID: 28752050]

[109] Rosell M, Hondares E, Iwamoto S, *et al.* Peroxisome proliferator-activated receptors-α and -γ, and cAMP-mediated pathways, control retinol-binding protein-4 gene expression in brown adipose tissue. Endocrinology 2012; 153(3): 1162-73.
[http://dx.doi.org/10.1210/en.2011-1367] [PMID: 22253419]

[110] Abdullahi A, Chen P, Stanojcic M, Sadri AR, Coburn N, Jeschke MG. IL-6 signal from the bone marrow is required for the browning of white adipose tissue post burn injury. Shock 2017; 47(1): 33-9.
[http://dx.doi.org/10.1097/SHK.0000000000000749] [PMID: 27648696]

[111] Kaisanlahti A, Glumoff T. Browning of white fat: agents and implications for beige adipose tissue to type 2 diabetes. J Physiol Biochem 2019; 75(1): 1-10.
[http://dx.doi.org/10.1007/s13105-018-0658-5] [PMID: 30506389]

[112] Luo M, Peng D. ANGPTL8: An Important Regulator in Metabolic Disorders. Front Endocrinol (Lausanne) 2018; 9: 169.
[http://dx.doi.org/10.3389/fendo.2018.00169] [PMID: 29719529]

[113] Zhang R. Lipasin, a novel nutritionally-regulated liver-enriched factor that regulates serum triglyceride levels. Biochem Biophys Res Commun 2012; 424(4): 786-92.
[http://dx.doi.org/10.1016/j.bbrc.2012.07.038] [PMID: 22809513]

CHAPTER 3

Neuropeptides and Adipokines in The Control of Food Intake

Amina Valjevac[*]

Department of Human Physiology, Faculty of Medicine University of Sarajevo; Čekaluša 90, 71000 Sarajevo; Bosnia and Herzegovina

Abstract: The balance of energy intake and expenditure in the body is maintained by the complex physiological mechanisms that integrate neuronal activity in various central nervous system structures with signals coming from the gastrointestinal system, adipose tissue, endocrine glands, and the autonomic nervous system. The arcuate nucleus (ARC) in the ventral hypothalamus is considered to be the most important integrational centre in the hypothalamus. Very porous hematoencephalic barrier around arcuate nuclei allows numerous hormones, nutrients and cytokines from the periphery to reach the nuclei and inform ARC of the amount of food consumed and energy stored during the preceding hours, weeks, months and years. Information about short-term fluctuations in the amount of food consumed is carried by hormones released from the gastrointestinal tract (ghrelin, cholecystokinin, peptide YY, glucagon-like peptide) and pancreas (insulin, amylin, pancreatic polypeptide), while information about the amount of food consumed and energy stored during the preceding weeks or months is carried by hormones released from adipose tissue (leptin and adiponectin). ARC, when informed, secrete anorexigenic (alpha-melanocyte stimulating hormone) or orexigenic neurotransmitters (neuropeptide Y, agouti-related protein, melanin-concentrating hormone), which modulate the activity of second order hypothalamic nuclei such as the paraventricular, ventromedial and dorsomedial nuclei, as well as the lateral hypothalamus and thereby control eating behaviour and energy expenditure. In this chapter, the interaction of peripheral hormones with anorexigenic/orexigenic neurons and its effects on food intake are discussed.

Keywords: Adipokines, Anorexogenic, Arcuate nucleus, Gastrointestinal hormones, Neuropeptides, Orexigenic, Pancreatic hormones.

INTRODUCTION

Applying the first law of thermodynamics in weight management considers the balance between calories consumed and calories burned through metabolic processes, waste heat, physical activity, *etc.* When the energy intake and expendi-

---

[*] **Corresponding author Amina Valjevac:** Department of Human Physiology, Faculty of Medicine, University of Sarajevo, Sarajevo, Bosnia and Herzegovina; Tel: +387 33 226 478, ext. 526; E-mail: amina.valjevac@mf.unsa.ba

Asija Začiragić (Ed.)

-ture are balanced there is no change in the body mass, and if the energy intake is higher than its expenditure, the excess energy will be converted and stored as fat [1, 2]. Balance of energy intake and expenditure in the body is maintained by the complex physiological mechanisms that integrate neuronal activity in various central nervous system structures with signals coming from the gastrointestinal system, adipose tissue, endocrine glands, and the autonomic nervous system.

In order to understand the physiological mechanism that regulate food intake, one needs to distinguish two intervening terms: satiation and satiety. Satiation refers to the size of meals consumed, whereas satiety refers to the post-meal period and reflects events occurring in the intervals between eating episodes. Physiological mechanisms involved in the control of food intake can be understood with reference to processes that cause people to begin eating; maintain eating and then bring it to an end, called short term regulation of food intake, and processes that inhibit eating for a given period of time until previously stored energy is used, called long-term regulation of food intake [3].

Gastrointestinal system plays a key role in the short-term regulation of food intake by synthesizing and secreting peptides. The hormones of the gastrointestinal tract mainly involve mechanisms that reduce further food intake, rather than mechanisms that initiate food intake. Peptides such as cholecystokinin, PPY, and glucagon-like peptide, are secreted postprandially and inform the hypothalamus about the presence of nutrients in the digestive tract [4]. Their main role is to control the optimum amount of food consumed during a given meal and prevent overeating. However, a gut hormone, ghrelin, secreted immediately before a meal and usually at times when a person is habituated to eat, initiates food intake.

Adipose tissue and pancreas are involved in the long-term regulation of food intake and energy balance by secreting hormones which bind to their receptors in the hypothalamus. Extensive research of insulin and leptin signalling within the hypothalamus has provided evidence for their role in inhibiting food intake and increasing energy expenditure [5]. So, what are the key signals that the central nervous system uses to control satiation and satiety, and therefore the behaviour of eating?

THE ROLE OF HYPOTHALAMUS

Hypothalamus, a small structure in diencephalon, has a central role in the regulation of food intake. Information about available energy are integrated within several hypothalamic areas involved in food intake: arcuate, lateral, ventromedial, paraventricular and dorsomedial nuclei [6]. Maintenance of body weight requires integration of signals from periphery and other parts of the central nervous system.

The arcuate nucleus (ARC) in the ventral hypothalamus is considered to be the most important integrational centre in hypothalamus. Very porous hematoencephalic barrier around arcuate nuclei allows numerous hormones, nutrients and cytokines from the periphery to reach the nuclei, bind to the receptors and inform ARC of the amount of food consumed and energy stored during the preceding hours, weeks, months and years [7]. Information about short-term fluctuations in the amount of food consumed is carried by hormones released from the gastrointestinal tract (ghrelin, cholecystokinin, PYY, glucagon-like peptide) and pancreas (insulin, amylin, pancreatic polypeptide) [4]. Information about the amount of food consumed and energy stored during the preceding weeks, months and years is carried by hormones released from adipose tissue (adipokines such as leptin and adiponectin) [5]. The first order neurons in the ARC have extensive projections with second order neurons in other hypothalamic nuclei, such as the paraventricular, ventromedial and dorsomedial nuclei, as well as the lateral hypothalamus. ARC when informed, secrete neuropeptides that modulate activity of second order hypothalamic nuclei and thereby control eating behaviour and energy expenditure.

There are two functionally different types of neurons found in the arcuate nuclei which regulate food intake. Activation of anorexigenic neurons leads to a decrease in food intake and increased energy expenditure, while activation of orexigenic neurons results in increased food intake and decreased energy expenditure [6]. Anorexigenic group of neurons within the arcuate nucleus are proopiomelanocortin (POMC) and cocaine- and amphetamine-regulated transcript (CART) neurons [8]. POMC neurons secrete alpha-melanocyte stimulating hormone (α-MSH) which can bind to several types of MCH receptors and cause a decrease in food intake. Therefore, the activation of POMC neurons in the ARC inhibits food intake, while ablation of arcuate POMC neurons results in increased food consumption and body weight. Orexigenic group of neurons within the arcuate nucleus synthetize agouti-related protein (AgRP) and neuropeptide Y (NPY). Studies have shown that AgRP/NPY neurons increase food intake by releasing several orexigenic neurotransmitters: neuropeptide Y, agouti-related protein and melanin-concentrating hormone (MCH) [9]. AgRP/NPY neurons modulate and control the activity of POMC/CART neurons, while reciprocal links from POMC/CART neurons to AgRP/NYP are insignificant (Fig. **1**).

Paraventricular nuclei in the hypothalamus (PVH) integrate information from POMC/CART and AgRP/NPY neurons. Damage of paraventricular nuclei causes gluttony, while damage of dorsomedial nuclei usually causes satiety [10].

Under conditions with prolonged energy intake, hormones from pancreas and adipose tissue bind to their receptors within the ARC and promote the firing of

POMC neurons. POMC neurons project to the paraventricular nucleus (PVN) to decrease food intake and to increase energy expenditure [11]. In the fasted state, AgRP/NPY neurons are activated and send inhibitory signals to reduce firing of POMC neurons. Additionally, AgRP/NYP neurons send numerous links to other areas of hypothalamus including paraventricular nucleus, dorsomedial nuclei and the lateral area of hypothalamus (the feeding centre) thus modulating the activity of various hypothalamus parts and participating in the control of food intake [12]. Stimulation of lateral nuclei of hypothalamus, by orexigenic neurons and neuropeptides, cause excessive food intake and the area is called the feeding centre, whereas stimulation of the ventromedial area, leads to the feeling of satiety and discontinuation of food intake; hence the name the satiety centre [13]. Alternating activation and inhibition of the feeding and satiety centres are at the core of the dual centre hypothesis of the food intake control.

ANOREXOGENIC NEUROTRANSMITTERS

Alpha-melanocyte stimulating hormone (α-MSH) is a hormone cleaved from POMC prepropeptide in addition to melanocyte stimulating hormones (β-, and γ-MSH), adrenocorticotropic hormone (ACTH), β-endorphin, lipotropin (β- and γ-LPH), and met-enkephalin [14]. Alpha-melanocyte stimulating hormone binds to a family of melanocortin receptors: MC1 to MC5. The MC4 receptor is widely expressed throughout the brain, while the MC3 receptor is mostly found in the hypothalamus [15]. Due to the lack of MC3 receptor specific ligands, the role of MC3 receptor in maintaining metabolic homeostasis is still not clear. When administered intracerebrally, α-MSH, causes a decrease in food intake by binding to MC4 receptors in the PVH [16]. The deletion of the gene encoding MC4 receptor results in hyperphagia, increased food consumption, and profound obesity [17]. Mutation or deletion of the MC4 receptor is associated with obesity, hyperphagia, and hyperinsulinaemia suggesting that activation of the MC4 receptor regulates food intake and body fat mass [15] (Fig. **1**).

In addition, α-MSH has a potent protective and anti-inflammatory activity by binding to centrally expressed melanocortin receptors, and blocks proinflammatory mechanisms exerting anti-inflammatory, immunosuppressive, antipyretic, and antimicrobial activities [18].

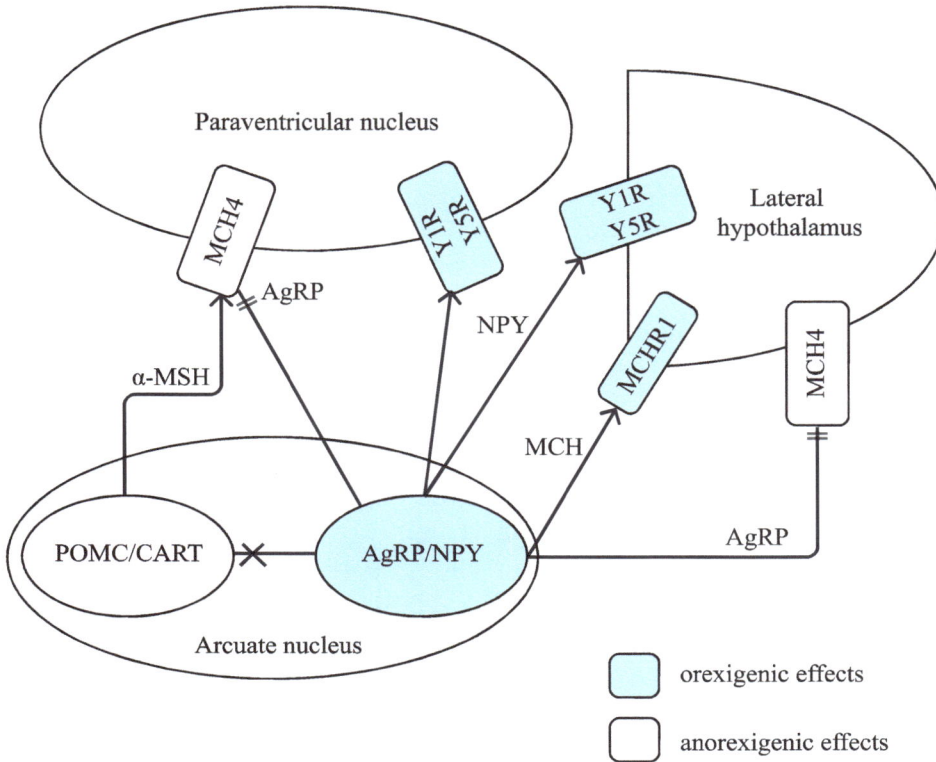

Fig. (1). Orexi- and anorexigenic neurotransmitters in regulation of food intake.
POMC/CART-proopiomelanocortin/cocaine- and amphetamine-regulated transcript neurons; AgRP/NPY-agouti related peptide/neuropeptide Y neurons; αMSH-alpha-melanocyte stimulating hormone; AgRP-agouti related peptide; MCH4-melanocortin receptor type 4; NPY-neuropeptide Y; Y1R-neuropeptide Y receptor type 1; Y5R-neuropeptide Y receptor type 5; MCH-melanin concentrating hormone; MCHR1-melanin concentrating hormone receptor type 1.

OREXIGENIC NEUROTRANSMITTERS

Neuropeptide Y (NPY) belongs to a family of gut–brain peptides including peptide YY (PYY) and PP. NPY is expressed in vast areas of the brain including hippocampus, amygdala, and hypothalamus with the highest expression within the ARC [19]. NPY is the strongest neuroendocrine orexigenic peptide which controls feeding, mobility, energy expenditure, and body temperature [20]. Intracerebral administration of NPY in rats induces hyperphagia, reduced energy expenditure and fatty acid storage in the liver and adipose tissues [21]. Moreover, it has been shown that NPY also plays a role in cardiovascular, immune and musculoskeletal system, as well as stress response and anxiety [22]. Although, PYY and PP have not been detected in the central nervous system, both are involved in food intake since they are predominantly secreted from the intestines and pancreas postprandially and transported to the ARC inhibiting food intake.

NPY binds with equal affinity to all of the five different G protein– coupled receptors: Y1, Y2, Y4, Y5, and Y6, yet different receptors mediate different processes and diseases including food intake, obesity, hypertension, metabolic disorders and atherosclerosis [23]. Moreover, NPY exhibits different and sometimes opposing effects. It has been reported that the activation of Y1 and Y5 can induce feeding, whereas the increased expression of Y2 and Y4 can exert anorexigenic effects [24] (Fig. 1).

In humans, the Y1 receptor is expressed in the colon, heart, adrenal gland, kidney as well as caudate, putamen and arcuate nucleus [23]. The most prominent and significant effects of the Y1R is the regulation of energy homeostasis and initiation of feeding and these effects often require the involvement of the Y5 receptor [25]. In agreement with this, recent studies showed that the Y5 receptor can regulate energy homeostasis, anticonvulsant effects and anxiety [20, 23]. The Y2R is mainly expressed in the hippocampus, thalamus, hypothalamus and some parts of the peripheral nervous system. The most important role of the Y2R is regulation of circadian feeding behaviour, energy homeostasis, and bone formation [23]. In humans, Y2R exerts anorexigenic effects since postprandial secretion of PYY mainly acts by binding to ARC Y2R, inhibiting further meal intake [26]. Also, Y4 receptors bind PP postprandially, which inhibits further food intake by activating α-MSH signalling [27].

Additionally, NPY overexpression can lead to different feeding behaviour depending on the hypothalamic area. NPY overexpression in the lateral hypothalamus causes increase in meal size, while in the paraventricular nucleus, it causes an increase in meal frequency [28, 29].

Also, NPY has been shown to modulate immune cell trafficking, T helper cell differentiation, cytokine secretion, natural killer cell activity, phagocytosis, and the production of reactive oxygen species [30]. Therefore, NPY has a potential role as a therapeutic target in neurodegenerative and neuroimmune diseases, but the NPY receptor mediating the effects in the brain tissue still needs to be identified [31].

Agouti-related protein (AgRP) is mostly expressed in the arcuate nuclei [32]. Agouti-related protein secreting nerve fibres project into the paraventricular nuclei and into the lateral nuclei of the hypothalamus [33]. The primary role of AgRP is the stimulation of food intake. These effects are achieved primarily by antagonising alpha-MSH effects through binding and inhibiting MCR3 and MCR4 receptors [7] (Fig. 1). Both AgRP and NPY are mostly secreted during fasting [34]. They exhibit a circadian rhythm and their levels are significantly higher immediately before meals. It has been shown that intracerebral administration of AgRP leads to an increase in food intake, but with significantly longer lasting effects in comparison to those observed after the administration of neuropeptide Y [35].

Melanin concentrating hormone (MCH) is a neuropeptide expressed in many parts of the central nervous system, especially around the lateral hypothalamus near the feeding center [36]. MCH neurons send their projections broadly across the brain, and MCHR1 is also widely expressed in the brain [37]. Its primary role in humans is to increase food intake [38] by binding to MCHR1 or MCHR2 receptors, whereas rodents express only MCHR1 [39].

In animal models, it has been observed that single intravenous administration of MCH results in increased food intake lasting for about 6 hours, but that the effects of MCH on the amount of food consumed are far smaller in comparison to those after the intravenous administration of NPY [35]. MCH-overexpressing mice exhibit increased food intake and develop mild obesity, while MCH-deficient mice exhibit decreased food intake, lean phenotypes and increased energy expenditure [36]. Furthermore, MCHR1-deficient mice exhibit a lean phenotype and are resistance to high-fat diet-induced obesity [40].

GASTROINTESTINAL HORMONES

Ghrelin, is the only gastrointestinal hormone known to date that promotes food intake and obesity. Ghrelin is predominantly synthesized and secreted from gastric oxyntic cells, but to a lesser extent from the intestines, pancreas, kidneys, lungs and ovaries [41]. Ghrelin level rises several hours before each meal, and reaches its peak just before the meal, then drops within the first hour after eating [42]. Ghrelin is an endogenous ligand for growth hormone (GH) secretagogue receptors (GHS-R) expressed on NPY/AgRP neurons in arcuate nuclei and releases NPY and AgRP favouring food intake, body weight gain, and diabetic hyperphagia [43, 44] (Fig. **2**). Intracerebral injection of ghrelin can rapidly stimulate increased food intake and the effect can persist for 8h, but usually ceases after 24 h [45, 46].

Prolonged administration of ghrelin not only leads to increased food intake but also slows down lipid metabolism and catabolism. Specifically, ghrelin promotes lipogenesis and suppresses lipolysis. Therefore, it believed that ghrelin is also involved in the long-term regulation of energy balance, which sets it apart from other gut peptides which, even after long-term administration, participate only in short-term regulation. It is important to note that ghrelin is the only known hormone that stimulates food intake whether administered centrally or peripherally, whereas most other hypothalamic peptides exhibit this effect only by central administration [47].

Ghrelin has been reported to be lower in obese compared to normal weight subjects [48]. However, postprandial ghrelin levels are higher in obese compared to lean individuals suggesting that obese individuals are experiencing hunger even after meal consumption [49]. The same post meal ghrelin has also been documented in obese children. Therefore, the ghrelinergic system has gained significant attention as a therapeutic objective for reducing the appetite in obesity or stimulating the appetite in anorexia, malnutrition and cachexia [50].

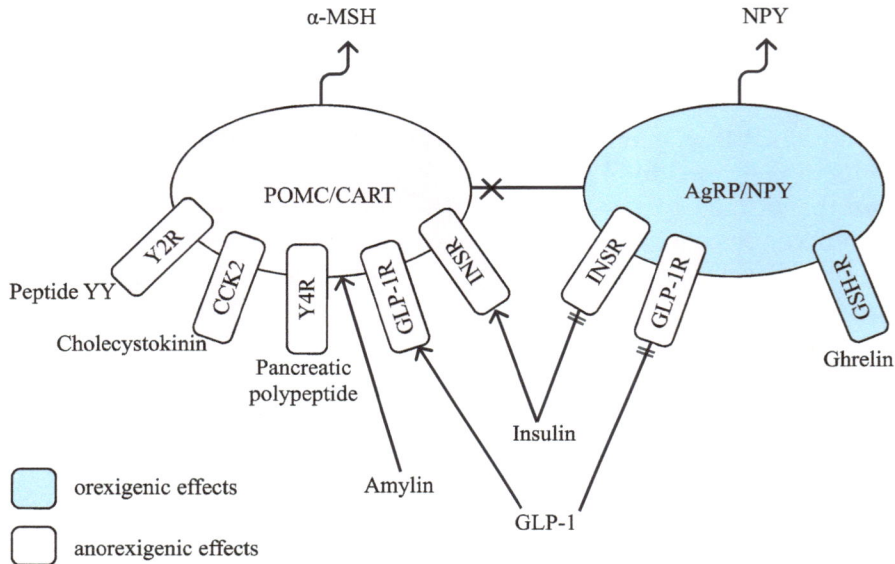

Fig. (2). Interaction between gastrointestinal/pancreatic hormones and neurons in arcuate nucleus. POMC/CART-proopiomelanocortin/cocaine- and amphetamine-regulated transcript neurons; AgRP/NPY-agouti related peptide/neuropeptide Y neurons; αMSH-alpha-melanocyte stimulating hormone; NPY-neuropeptide Y; Y2R-neuropeptide Y receptor type 2; Y4R-neuropeptide Y receptor type 4; CCK2-cholecystokinin receptor type 2; GLP-1R-glucagon-like peptide-1 receptor; INSR-insulin receptor; GHS--ghrelin receptor; GLP-1-glucagon-like peptide-1.

Cholecystokinin is the most researched satiety signal which is secreted in 2 forms, CCK-33 and CCK-8, from I cells within the duodenal and jejunal mucosa [51]. It is also synthesized in the central nervous system, primarily in the form of CCK-8 [52]. Cholecystokinin receptors, previously designated CCK-A and CCK-B, are now designated CCK-1 and CCK-2. The CCK-1 or A receptor is primarily localized in the gastrointestinal system, whereas the CCK-2 or B receptor is located within the central nervous system [53].

The presence of food in the upper part of the small intestine promotes cholecystokinin secretion. Its secretion is especially stimulated by proteases and peptones, and long-chain fatty acids in the chyme and leads to reduced food intake by activating melanocortin pathway in the hypothalamus [54].

More than 30 years ago, Gibbs *et al.* [55] first demonstrated that exogenous administration of either purified or synthetic CCK-8 to the peritoneal cavity in experimental animals reduced the size of the meal. The response is dose-dependent, and it has been observed that cholecystokinin must be given just before the start of the meal to be effective. If administered more than 15 minutes before the animals start eating, the reduction in meal size is not observed [56]. Centrally administered cholecystokinin also leads to reduced food intake [57].

Experiments have shown that cholecystokinin is involved in the short-term regulation of food intake since repeated or prolonged administration of cholecystokinin to experimental animals has no effect on weight loss. When the size of each meal is reduced by this hormone, the animals compensate by increasing meals frequency. Although the effects of exogenous cholecystokinin are short, it also interacts with long-term energy balance signals such as leptin and insulin [58]. Thus, the anorexigenic effect of cholecystokinin can be enhanced by concomitant administration of low concentrations of leptin.

There has been a major interest in potential use of CCKA agonist in treatment of obesity. In experimental animals with ablated CCKA receptor, there is an increased requirement for larger meals leading to obesity, due to overexpression of NPY neurons in ARC [59] (Fig. **2**).

Peptide YY is a 36 amino acid long peptide secreted from the endocrine L cells of the distal intestines with the main role in supressing the appetite [60]. The active form of the hormone has the greatest affinity for Y2 receptors found in peripheral and central nervous systems, with high concentrations in the ARC of the hypothalamus [61].

The concentration of circulating PYY is the lowest in the fasting state, and increases after food intake in proportion to the calorific value of the meal. Plasma hormone levels rise within 30 minutes, after which a plateau is maintained for 1-2 hours, and circulating levels remain elevated for at least another 6 hours [62].

Circulating PYY levels were observed to be low in obese and higher in patients with anorexia nervosa compared to controls. Obese individuals have also been shown to have lower PYY values during fasting [63]. Obese people need to ingest a meal with higher caloric value, in order to excrete the same amount of PYY compared to controls [64]. Peripheral administration of PYY in healthy individuals results in reduced food intake and a longer sense of satiety and long-term weight loss [64].

Interestingly, contrary to peripheral administration, intracerebroventricular administration of PYY stimulates food intake possibly through the action of PYY on Y1 and Y5 receptors in PVN [65].

Glucagon-like peptide (GLP)-1 is an incretin hormone, released from the gut in response to food intake particularly carbohydrate rich food. It promotes insulin secretion and is widely used in the treatment of type 2 diabetes mellitus. The early peak of GLP-1 secretion occurs shortly after meal ingestion (approximately after 15 minutes) whereas the second and larger peak appears later and is thought to be derived from direct contact of nutrients with L cells [66]. This results in a reduction of food intake in humans either peripherally or centrally [67]. Exogenous GLP-1 reduces food intake and enhances satiety in humans, in both lean and obese individuals, but doses administered are usually much higher compared to amount of GLP-1 secreted after a meal. Infusions of synthetic human GLP-1 (7-36) during the consumption of breakfast enhanced fullness and satiety when compared to the placebo infusion [68]. During a later ad libitum lunch, food intake was also significantly reduced by the earlier GLP-1 infusion.

GLP-1 has been shown to cross the blood-brain barrier and binds to GLP-1 receptor (GLP-1R) in the hypothalamus [69]. It has been shown that peripheral injection of liraglutide directly stimulates POMC/CART neurons and inhibits NPY/AgRP neurons in the ARC resulting in a decrease of body weight [70] (Fig. 2). GLP-1 is also expressed in neurons of the nucleus of the solitary tract which project to the PVN and are activated by several factors that decrease food intake [71]. Furthermore, the GLP-1 receptor (GLP-1R) is expressed on vagal afferents and the peripheral satiety effect of GLP-1 is blocked by vagotomy [72]. These data point towards a mediation of GLP-1's food intake-reducing effect by the vagus nerve and hindbrain, as well as, by stimulation of anorexogenic and inhibition of orexigenic neurons in the arcuate nucleus.

PANCREATIC HORMONES

Insulin, a hormone secreted from beta cells of the Langerhans islets in the pancreas, has the role to regulate blood glucose levels. During and immediately after a meal (prandial level) or after glucose administration (stimulated level) insulin levels in the bloodstream are increased to allow glucose to be absorbed into peripheral tissue cells and organs. Increased insulin, after a meal, binds to insulin receptors expressed in the hypothalamus, especially in the arcuate nucleus and the dorsomedial hypothalamus where it activates anorexigenic POMC/CART neurons and at the same time inhibits orexigenic AgRP/NYP neurons [49] (Fig. 2).

Loch *et al.* [73] found that NPY-expressing neurons are critical in mediating the central actions of insulin in the regulation of appetite and energy homeostasis, since lack of insulin signaling in NPY neurons leads to increased body weight and adiposity attributable to significantly increased food intake and reduced energy expenditure.

The absence of insulin signaling in NPY neurons also leads to a significant up-regulation of hypothalamic NPY expression, which is consistent with the observed increase in appetite and reduced energy expenditure as well as reduced bone mass [74].

The action of insulin in AgRP neurons may play a more imporant role in controlling hepatic glucose production, whereas NPY neurons may play a significant role in the regulation of appetite and energy balance.

Pancreatic Polypeptide (PP) is released from PP cells in Langerhans pancreatic islets usually after a meal. It binds to Y receptors, with the highest affinity for Y4 receptors located in the hypothalamus and brainstem, exerting anorexigenic effects [75].

Plasma PP levels show variations; the lowest level is in the morning and the highest in the evening. The level of PP rises after a meal, in proportion to the caloric intake, and remains elevated for another 6 hours after a meal [65].

Interestingly, PP has both anorexigenic and orexigenic effects, depending on the route of administration Intracerebroventricular infusion of PP in experimental animals stimulates appetite and food intake while peripheral administration reduces food intake [65]. In subjects with normal weight, intravenous infusion of PP raised PP levels three times higher compared to postprandial PP levels in the same subjects after a meal and reduced food intake by 25% over 24 hours.

Amylin is also secreted by beta cells of the Langerhans islets. As insulin, its plasma levels rise significantly after a diet rich in nutrients, especially carbohydrates, and consequently fall during fasting period [76]. The amylin level is also proportional to the mass of adipose tissue [77]. It acts mainly as short-term satiation factor and decreases eating in rats after central and peripheral administration. Amylin regulates food intake by interacting with other endogenous regulators of eating, in particular with leptin, and has the ability to overcome leptin resistance in obesity [78]. Administration of amylin alone or in combination produces a clinically relevant weight loss in humans by slowing gastric emptying and reducing postprandial glucagon secretion [79].

ADIPOKINES

Leptin is a hormone synthesized in adipose tissue, with the main role to regulate food intake and energy consumption. The concentration of leptin in the blood is proportional to the amount of adipose tissue [80].

In the arcuate nucleus of the hypothalamus, leptin binds to its receptor (primarily ObRb isoform) [81], where it stimulates POMC/CART neurons to secrete α-MSH, resulting in decreased appetite, food intake, and increased energy expenditure. In addition, leptin inhibits AgRP / NYP neurons, further contributing to decreased appetite and food intake [82] (Fig. **3**).

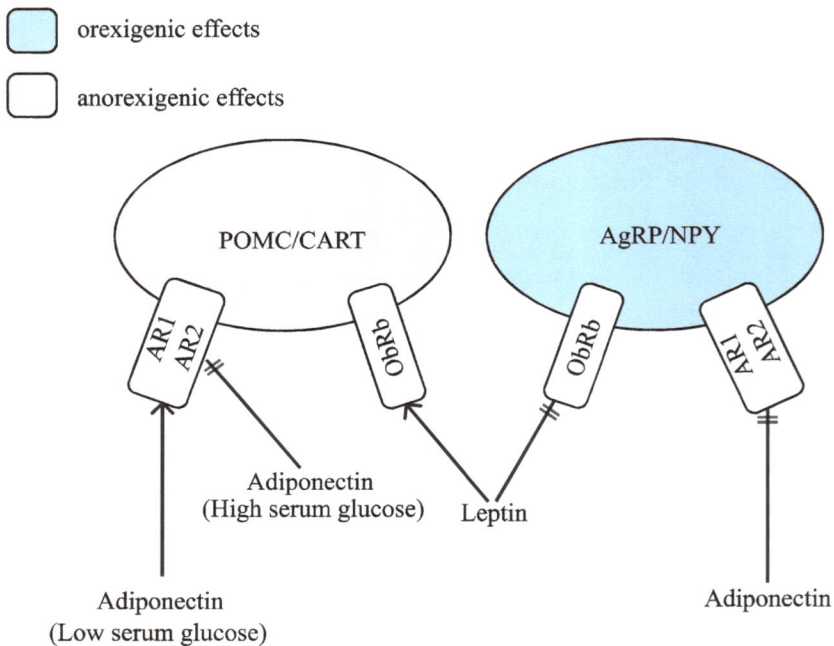

Fig. (3). Interaction between adipokines and arcuate neurons in regulation of food intake.
POMC/CART- proopiomelanocortin/cocaine- and amphetamine-regulated transcript neurons; AgRP/NPY-agouti related peptide/neuropeptide Y neurons; AR1-adiponectin receptor 1; AR2-adiponectin receptor 2; ObRb-long leptin receptor isoform.

Adiponectin is a protein that is primarily synthesized in adipose tissue, but it can be found in other tissues such as brown adipose tissue, skeletal muscle, liver, heart muscle and placenta. The adiponectin receptors, both adipoR1 and R2, are expressed in the brain including the arcuate nucleus of hypothalamus (both NPY and POMC neurons) suggesting its role in the regulation of food intake [83]. However, its effects on food intake are not quite understood. Two opposing mechanisms have been documented. Central administration of adiponectin promoted food in reefed rodents [84], while another report showed suppression of food intake in fasted rodents [85]. A recent study has shown that the direction of the action of adiponectin on anorexigenic proopiomelanocortin (POMC) neuron activity in ARC depends on the level of glucose. Adiponectin activates POMC neurons under low glucose, while it inactivates POMC neurons under elevated glucose conditions [86] (Fig. **3**). Blood glucose level changes mainly due to food intake and adiponectin may affect food-regulating neurons before and after meal differently. The effect of adiponectin on neuropeptide Y (NPY) / agouti related peptide (AgRP) neurons, which play a key role in promoting feeding, is essentially required for fully understanding its action on feeding. A recent study examined the effects of adiponectin on NPY neurons and found that adiponectin at physiological range promotes postsynaptic inhibition of NPY neurons, serving as a mild suppressor [87], while at pharmacologic concentrations, adiponectin has been shown to significantly inhibit NPY neuron activity, which could be used to treat hyperphagia and obesity [88].

CONCLUDING REMARKS

In conclusion, many hormones released from the pancreas and adipose tissue are involved in the regulation of food intake and inform the central nervous system of short- and long-term fluctuations in food intake. All of these signals are relayed to the central nervous system and integrate within the hypothalamus and brainstem that, through neuropeptides such as neuropeptide Y, AgRP, and melanocortin, modulate appetite, energy expenditure, and behavior.

CONSENT FOR PUBLICATION

Not applicable.

CONFLICT OF INTEREST

The authors confirm that this chapter content has no conflict of interest.

ACKNOWLEDGEMENTS

The authors would like to express their sincere thanks to the editor and anonymous reviewers for their time and valuable suggestions.

REFERENCES

[1]   Loiselle DS, Barclay CJ. The ineluctable constraints of thermodynamics in the aetiology of obesity. Clin Exp Pharmacol Physiol 2018; 45(3): 219-25.
[http://dx.doi.org/10.1111/1440-1681.12869] [PMID: 28994136]

[2]   Howell S, Kones R. "Calories in, calories out" and macronutrient intake: the hope, hype, and science

of calories. Am J Physiol Endocrinol Metab 2017; 313(5): E608-12.
[http://dx.doi.org/10.1152/ajpendo.00156.2017] [PMID: 28765272]

[3]   Bellisle F, Drewnowski A, Anderson GH, Westerterp-Plantenga M, Martin CK. Sweetness, satiation, and satiety. J Nutr 2012; 142(6): 1149S-54S.
[http://dx.doi.org/10.3945/jn.111.149583] [PMID: 22573779]

[4]   Strader AD, Woods SC. Gastrointestinal hormones and food intake. Gastroenterology 2005; 128(1): 175-91.
[http://dx.doi.org/10.1053/j.gastro.2004.10.043] [PMID: 15633135]

[5]   Henry BA, Clarke IJ. Adipose tissue hormones and the regulation of food intake. J Neuroendocrinol 2008; 20(6): 842-9.
[http://dx.doi.org/10.1111/j.1365-2826.2008.1730.x] [PMID: 18601708]

[6]   Tabe-Bordbar S, Anastasio TJ. Computational Analysis of the Hypothalamic Control of Food Intake. Front Comput Neurosci 2016; 10: 27.
[http://dx.doi.org/10.3389/fncom.2016.00027] [PMID: 27199725]

[7]   Chen Y, Lin YC, Kuo TW, Knight ZA. Sensory detection of food rapidly modulates arcuate feeding circuits. Cell 2015; 160(5): 829-41.
[http://dx.doi.org/10.1016/j.cell.2015.01.033] [PMID: 25703096]

[8]   Sohn JW. Network of hypothalamic neurons that control appetite. BMB Rep 2015; 48(4): 229-33.
[http://dx.doi.org/10.5483/BMBRep.2015.48.4.272] [PMID: 25560696]

[9]   Joly-Amado A, Cansell C, Denis RG, *et al.* The hypothalamic arcuate nucleus and the control of peripheral substrates. Best Pract Res Clin Endocrinol Metab 2014; 28(5): 725-37.
[http://dx.doi.org/10.1016/j.beem.2014.03.003] [PMID: 25256767]

[10]   Ferguson AV, Latchford KJ, Samson WK. The paraventricular nucleus of the hypothalamus - a potential target for integrative treatment of autonomic dysfunction. Expert Opin Ther Targets 2008; 12(6): 717-27.
[http://dx.doi.org/10.1517/14728222.12.6.717] [PMID: 18479218]

[11]   Hron BM, Ebbeling CB, Feldman HA, Ludwig DS. Hepatic, adipocyte, enteric and pancreatic hormones: response to dietary macronutrient composition and relationship with metabolism. Nutr Metab (Lond) 2017; 14: 44.
[http://dx.doi.org/10.1186/s12986-017-0198-y] [PMID: 28694840]

[12]   Rui L. Brain regulation of energy balance and body weight. Rev Endocr Metab Disord 2013; 14(4): 387-407.
[http://dx.doi.org/10.1007/s11154-013-9261-9] [PMID: 23990408]

[13]   Timper K, Brüning JC. Hypothalamic circuits regulating appetite and energy homeostasis: pathways to obesity. Dis Model Mech 2017; 10(6): 679-89.
[http://dx.doi.org/10.1242/dmm.026609] [PMID: 28592656]

[14]   Bertolini A, Tacchi R, Vergoni AV. Brain effects of melanocortins. Pharmacol Res 2009; 59(1): 13-47.
[http://dx.doi.org/10.1016/j.phrs.2008.10.005] [PMID: 18996199]

[15]   Huang HH, Chen CY. Alpha-melanocyte stimulating hormone in ghrelin-elicited feeding and gut motility. J Chin Med Assoc 2019; 82(2): 87-91.
[http://dx.doi.org/10.1097/JCMA.0000000000000007] [PMID: 30839496]

[16]   Balthasar N, Dalgaard LT, Lee CE, *et al.* Divergence of melanocortin pathways in the control of food intake and energy expenditure. Cell 2005; 123(3): 493-505.
[http://dx.doi.org/10.1016/j.cell.2005.08.035] [PMID: 16269339]

[17]   Huszar D, Lynch CA, Fairchild-Huntress V, *et al.* Targeted disruption of the melanocortin-4 receptor results in obesity in mice. Cell 1997; 88(1): 131-41.
[http://dx.doi.org/10.1016/S0092-8674(00)81865-6] [PMID: 9019399]

[18] Singh M, Mukhopadhyay K. Alpha-melanocyte stimulating hormone: an emerging anti-inflammatory antimicrobial peptide. BioMed Res Int 2014; 2014: 874610.
[http://dx.doi.org/10.1155/2014/874610] [PMID: 25140322]

[19] Holzer P, Reichmann F, Farzi A. Neuropeptide Y, peptide YY and pancreatic polypeptide in the gut-brain axis. Neuropeptides 2012; 46(6): 261-74.
[http://dx.doi.org/10.1016/j.npep.2012.08.005] [PMID: 22979996]

[20] Comeras LB, Herzog H, Tasan RO. Neuropeptides at the crossroad of fear and hunger: a special focus on neuropeptide Y. Ann N Y Acad Sci 2019; 1455(1): 59-80.
[http://dx.doi.org/10.1111/nyas.14179] [PMID: 31271235]

[21] Parker SL, Balasubramaniam A. Neuropeptide Y Y2 receptor in health and disease. Br J Pharmacol 2008; 153(3): 420-31.
[http://dx.doi.org/10.1038/sj.bjp.0707445] [PMID: 17828288]

[22] Hofmann S, Bellmann-Sickert K, Beck-Sickinger AG. Chemical modification of neuropeptide Y for human Y1 receptor targeting in health and disease. Biol Chem 2019; 400(3): 299-311.
[http://dx.doi.org/10.1515/hsz-2018-0364] [PMID: 30653463]

[23] Yi M, Li H, Wu Z, *et al.* A Promising Therapeutic Target for Metabolic Diseases: Neuropeptide Y Receptors in Humans. Cell Physiol Biochem 2018; 45(1): 88-107.
[http://dx.doi.org/10.1159/000486225] [PMID: 29310113]

[24] Yulyaningsih E, Zhang L, Herzog H, Sainsbury A. NPY receptors as potential targets for anti-obesity drug development. Br J Pharmacol 2011; 163(6): 1170-202.
[http://dx.doi.org/10.1111/j.1476-5381.2011.01363.x] [PMID: 21545413]

[25] Nguyen AD, Mitchell NF, Lin S, *et al.* Y1 and Y5 receptors are both required for the regulation of food intake and energy homeostasis in mice. PLoS One 2012; 7(6): e40191.
[http://dx.doi.org/10.1371/journal.pone.0040191] [PMID: 22768253]

[26] Batterham RL, Cowley MA, Small CJ, *et al.* Gut hormone PYY(3-36) physiologically inhibits food intake. Nature 2002; 418(6898): 650-4.
[http://dx.doi.org/10.1038/nature00887] [PMID: 12167864]

[27] Lin S, Shi YC, Yulyaningsih E, *et al.* Critical role of arcuate Y4 receptors and the melanocortin system in pancreatic polypeptide-induced reduction in food intake in mice. PLoS One 2009; 4(12): e8488.
[http://dx.doi.org/10.1371/journal.pone.0008488] [PMID: 20041129]

[28] Tiesjema B, Adan RA, Luijendijk MC, Kalsbeek A, la Fleur SE. Differential effects of recombinant adeno-associated virus-mediated neuropeptide Y overexpression in the hypothalamic paraventricular nucleus and lateral hypothalamus on feeding behavior. J Neurosci 2007; 27(51): 14139-46.
[http://dx.doi.org/10.1523/JNEUROSCI.3280-07.2007] [PMID: 18094253]

[29] de Backer MW, la Fleur SE, Adan RA. Both overexpression of agouti-related peptide or neuropeptide Y in the paraventricular nucleus or lateral hypothalamus induce obesity in a neuropeptide- and nucleus specific manner. Eur J Pharmacol 2011; 660(1): 148-55.
[http://dx.doi.org/10.1016/j.ejphar.2010.12.021] [PMID: 21211526]

[30] Farzi A, Reichmann F, Holzer P. The homeostatic role of neuropeptide Y in immune function and its impact on mood and behaviour. Acta Physiol (Oxf) 2015; 213(3): 603-27.
[http://dx.doi.org/10.1111/apha.12445] [PMID: 25545642]

[31] Li C, Wu X, Liu S, Zhao Y, Zhu J, Liu K. Roles of Neuropeptide Y in Neurodegenerative and Neuroimmune Diseases. Front Neurosci 2019; 13: 869.
[http://dx.doi.org/10.3389/fnins.2019.00869] [PMID: 31481869]

[32] Sternson SM. Hypothalamic survival circuits: blueprints for purposive behaviors. Neuron 2013; 77(5): 810-24.
[http://dx.doi.org/10.1016/j.neuron.2013.02.018] [PMID: 23473313]

[33]   Betley JN, Cao ZF, Ritola KD, Sternson SM. Parallel, redundant circuit organization for homeostatic control of feeding behavior. Cell 2013; 155(6): 1337-50.
[http://dx.doi.org/10.1016/j.cell.2013.11.002] [PMID: 24315102]

[34]   Essner RA, Smith AG, Jamnik AA, Ryba AR, Trutner ZD, Carter ME. AgRP Neurons Can Increase Food Intake during Conditions of Appetite Suppression and Inhibit Anorexigenic Parabrachial Neurons. J Neurosci 2017; 37(36): 8678-87.
[http://dx.doi.org/10.1523/JNEUROSCI.0798-17.2017] [PMID: 28821663]

[35]   Thomas MA, Xue B. Mechanisms for AgRP neuron-mediated regulation of appetitive behaviors in rodents. Physiol Behav 2018; 190: 34-42.
[http://dx.doi.org/10.1016/j.physbeh.2017.10.006] [PMID: 29031550]

[36]   Takase K, Kikuchi K, Tsuneoka Y, Oda S, Kuroda M, Funato H. Meta-analysis of melanin-concentrating hormone signaling-deficient mice on behavioral and metabolic phenotypes. PLoS One 2014; 9(6): e99961.
[http://dx.doi.org/10.1371/journal.pone.0099961] [PMID: 24924345]

[37]   Saito Y, Cheng M, Leslie FM, Civelli O. Expression of the melanin-concentrating hormone (MCH) receptor mRNA in the rat brain. J Comp Neurol 2001; 435(1): 26-40.
[http://dx.doi.org/10.1002/cne.1191] [PMID: 11370009]

[38]   Pissios P, Bradley RL, Maratos-Flier E. Expanding the scales: The multiple roles of MCH in regulating energy balance and other biological functions. Endocr Rev 2006; 27(6): 606-20.
[http://dx.doi.org/10.1210/er.2006-0021] [PMID: 16788162]

[39]   Saito Y, Nothacker HP, Wang Z, Lin SH, Leslie F, Civelli O. Molecular characterization of the melanin-concentrating-hormone receptor. Nature 1999; 400(6741): 265-9.
[http://dx.doi.org/10.1038/22321] [PMID: 10421368]

[40]   Sherwood A, Wosiski-Kuhn M, Nguyen T, *et al.* The role of melanin-concentrating hormone in conditioned reward learning. Eur J Neurosci 2012; 36(8): 3126-33.
[http://dx.doi.org/10.1111/j.1460-9568.2012.08207.x] [PMID: 22775118]

[41]   Kojima M, Hosoda H, Date Y, Nakazato M, Matsuo H, Kangawa K. Ghrelin is a growth-hormon--releasing acylated peptide from stomach. Nature 1999; 402(6762): 656-60.
[http://dx.doi.org/10.1038/45230] [PMID: 10604470]

[42]   Guo ZF, Ren AJ, Zheng X, *et al.* Different responses of circulating ghrelin, obestatin levels to fasting, re-feeding and different food compositions, and their local expressions in rats. Peptides 2008; 29(7): 1247-54.
[http://dx.doi.org/10.1016/j.peptides.2008.02.020] [PMID: 18400333]

[43]   Chen CY, Fujimiya M, Laviano A, Chang FY, Lin HC, Lee SD. Modulation of ingestive behavior and gastrointestinal motility by ghrelin in diabetic animals and humans. J Chin Med Assoc 2010; 73(5): 225-9.
[http://dx.doi.org/10.1016/S1726-4901(10)70048-4] [PMID: 20685586]

[44]   Rossi M, Kim MS, Morgan DG, *et al.* A C-terminal fragment of Agouti-related protein increases feeding and antagonizes the effect of alpha-melanocyte stimulating hormone *in vivo.* Endocrinology 1998; 139(10): 4428-31.
[http://dx.doi.org/10.1210/endo.139.10.6332] [PMID: 9751529]

[45]   Wren AM, Small CJ, Ward HL, *et al.* The novel hypothalamic peptide ghrelin stimulates food intake and growth hormone secretion. Endocrinology 2000; 141(11): 4325-8.
[http://dx.doi.org/10.1210/endo.141.11.7873] [PMID: 11089570]

[46]   Huang HH, Chen LY, Doong ML, Chang SC, Chen CY. α-melanocyte stimulating hormone modulates the central acyl ghrelin-induced stimulation of feeding, gastrointestinal motility, and colonic secretion. Drug Des Devel Ther 2017; 11: 2377-86.
[http://dx.doi.org/10.2147/DDDT.S143749] [PMID: 28860709]

[47] Somogyi V, Gyorffy A, Scalise TJ, *et al.* Endocrine factors in the hypothalamic regulation of food intake in females: a review of the physiological roles and interactions of ghrelin, leptin, thyroid hormones, oestrogen and insulin. Nutr Res Rev 2011; 24(1): 132-54.
[http://dx.doi.org/10.1017/S0954422411000035] [PMID: 21418732]

[48] Makris MC, Alexandrou A, Papatsoutsos EG, *et al.* Ghrelin and Obesity: Identifying Gaps and Dispelling Myths. A Reappraisal. In Vivo 2017; 31(6): 1047-50.
[PMID: 29102924]

[49] Shin AC, Filatova N, Lindtner C, *et al.* Insulin Receptor Signaling in POMC, but Not AgRP, Neurons Controls Adipose Tissue Insulin Action. Diabetes 2017; 66(6): 1560-71.
[http://dx.doi.org/10.2337/db16-1238] [PMID: 28385803]

[50] Howick K, Griffin BT, Cryan JF, Schellekens H. From Belly to Brain: Targeting the Ghrelin Receptor in Appetite and Food Intake Regulation. Int J Mol Sci 2017; 18(2): 273.
[http://dx.doi.org/10.3390/ijms18020273] [PMID: 28134808]

[51] Polak JM, Bloom SR, Rayford PL, Pearse AG, Buchan AM, Thompson JC. Identification of cholecystokinin-secreting cells. Lancet 1975; 2(7943): 1016-8.
[http://dx.doi.org/10.1016/S0140-6736(75)90297-4] [PMID: 53500]

[52] Beinfeld MC, Meyer DK, Brownstein MJ. Cholecystokinin in the central nervous system. Peptides 1981; 2 (Suppl. 2): 77-9.
[http://dx.doi.org/10.1016/0196-9781(81)90015-2] [PMID: 6283500]

[53] Herranz R. Cholecystokinin antagonists: pharmacological and therapeutic potential. Med Res Rev 2003; 23(5): 559-605.
[http://dx.doi.org/10.1002/med.10042] [PMID: 12789687]

[54] Woods SC. Gastrointestinal satiety signals I. An overview of gastrointestinal signals that influence food intake. Am J Physiol Gastrointest Liver Physiol 2004; 286(1): G7-G13.
[http://dx.doi.org/10.1152/ajpgi.00448.2003] [PMID: 14665437]

[55] Gibbs J, Young RC, Smith GP. Cholecystokinin decreases food intake in rats. J Comp Physiol Psychol 1973; 84(3): 488-95.
[http://dx.doi.org/10.1037/h0034870] [PMID: 4745816]

[56] Antin J, Gibbs J, Holt J, Young RC, Smith GP. Cholecystokinin elicits the complete behavioral sequence of satiety in rats. J Comp Physiol Psychol 1975; 89(7): 784-90.
[http://dx.doi.org/10.1037/h0077040] [PMID: 1176672]

[57] Zhang DM, Bula W, Stellar E. Brain cholecystokinin as a satiety peptide. Physiol Behav 1986; 36(6): 1183-6.
[http://dx.doi.org/10.1016/0031-9384(86)90498-1] [PMID: 3755245]

[58] Tsunoda Y, Yao H, Park J, Owyang C. Cholecystokinin synthesizes and secretes leptin in isolated canine gastric chief cells. Biochem Biophys Res Commun 2003; 310(3): 681-4.
[http://dx.doi.org/10.1016/j.bbrc.2003.08.154] [PMID: 14550255]

[59] Berna MJ, Tapia JA, Sancho V, Jensen RT. Progress in developing cholecystokinin (CCK)/gastrin receptor ligands that have therapeutic potential. Curr Opin Pharmacol 2007; 7(6): 583-92.
[http://dx.doi.org/10.1016/j.coph.2007.09.011] [PMID: 17997137]

[60] Suzuki K, Jayasena CN, Bloom SR. Obesity and appetite control. Exp Diabetes Res 2012; 2012: 824305.
[http://dx.doi.org/10.1155/2012/824305] [PMID: 22899902]

[61] Abbott CR, Small CJ, Kennedy AR, *et al.* Blockade of the neuropeptide Y Y2 receptor with the specific antagonist BIIE0246 attenuates the effect of endogenous and exogenous peptide YY(3-36) on food intake. Brain Res 2005; 1043(1-2): 139-44.
[http://dx.doi.org/10.1016/j.brainres.2005.02.065] [PMID: 15862527]

[62]   De Silva A, Bloom SR. Gut Hormones and Appetite Control: A Focus on PYY and GLP-1 as Therapeutic Targets in Obesity. Gut Liver 2012; 6(1): 10-20.
[http://dx.doi.org/10.5009/gnl.2012.6.1.10] [PMID: 22375166]

[63]   Sloth B, Holst JJ, Flint A, Gregersen NT, Astrup A. Effects of PYY1-36 and PYY3-36 on appetite, energy intake, energy expenditure, glucose and fat metabolism in obese and lean subjects. Am J Physiol Endocrinol Metab 2007; 292(4): E1062-8.
[http://dx.doi.org/10.1152/ajpendo.00450.2006] [PMID: 17148749]

[64]   Sloth B, Davidsen L, Holst JJ, Flint A, Astrup A. Effect of subcutaneous injections of PYY1-36 and PYY3-36 on appetite, ad libitum energy intake, and plasma free fatty acid concentration in obese males. Am J Physiol Endocrinol Metab 2007; 293(2): E604-9.
[http://dx.doi.org/10.1152/ajpendo.00153.2007] [PMID: 17566112]

[65]   Alhadeff AL, Golub D, Hayes MR, Grill HJ. Peptide YY signaling in the lateral parabrachial nucleus increases food intake through the Y1 receptor. Am J Physiol Endocrinol Metab 2015; 309(8): E759-66.
[http://dx.doi.org/10.1152/ajpendo.00346.2015] [PMID: 26330345]

[66]   Prinz P, Stengel A. Control of Food Intake by Gastrointestinal Peptides: Mechanisms of Action and Possible Modulation in the Treatment of Obesity. J Neurogastroenterol Motil 2017; 23(2): 180-96.
[http://dx.doi.org/10.5056/jnm16194] [PMID: 28096522]

[67]   Gutzwiller JP, Göke B, Drewe J, *et al.* Glucagon-like peptide-1: a potent regulator of food intake in humans. Gut 1999; 44(1): 81-6.
[http://dx.doi.org/10.1136/gut.44.1.81] [PMID: 9862830]

[68]   Flint A, Raben A, Astrup A, Holst J. Glucagon-Like Peptide 1 Promotes Satiety and Suppresses Energy Intake in Humans. Journal of Clinical Investigation 1998; 101(3): 515.

[69]   Merchenthaler I, Lane M, Shughrue P. Distribution of pre-pro-glucagon and glucagon-like peptide-1 receptor messenger RNAs in the rat central nervous system. J Comp Neurol 1999; 403(2): 261-80.
[http://dx.doi.org/10.1002/(SICI)1096-9861(19990111)403:2<261::AID-CNE8>3.0.CO;2-5] [PMID: 9886047]

[70]   Secher A, Jelsing J, Baquero AF, *et al.* The arcuate nucleus mediates GLP-1 receptor agonist liraglutide-dependent weight loss. J Clin Invest 2014; 124(10): 4473-88.
[http://dx.doi.org/10.1172/JCI75276] [PMID: 25202980]

[71]   Dailey MJ, Moran TH. Glucagon-like peptide 1 and appetite. Trends Endocrinol Metab 2013; 24(2): 85-91.
[http://dx.doi.org/10.1016/j.tem.2012.11.008] [PMID: 23332584]

[72]   Abbott CR, Monteiro M, Small CJ, *et al.* The inhibitory effects of peripheral administration of peptide YY(3-36) and glucagon-like peptide-1 on food intake are attenuated by ablation of the vagal-brainstem-hypothalamic pathway. Brain Res 2005; 1044(1): 127-31.
[http://dx.doi.org/10.1016/j.brainres.2005.03.011] [PMID: 15862798]

[73]   Loh K, Zhang L, Brandon A, *et al.* Insulin controls food intake and energy balance *via* NPY neurons. Mol Metab 2017; 6(6): 574-84.
[http://dx.doi.org/10.1016/j.molmet.2017.03.013] [PMID: 28580287]

[74]   Baldock PA, Sainsbury A, Couzens M, *et al.* Hypothalamic Y2 receptors regulate bone formation. J Clin Invest 2002; 109(7): 915-21.
[http://dx.doi.org/10.1172/JCI0214588] [PMID: 11927618]

[75]   Bewick GA. Bowels control brain: Gut hormones and obesity. Biochem Med (Zagreb) 2012; 22(3): 283-97.
[http://dx.doi.org/10.11613/BM.2012.032] [PMID: 23092061]

[76]   Hay DL, Chen S, Lutz TA, Parkes DG, Roth JD. Amylin: pharmacology, physiology, and clinical potential. Pharmacol Rev 2015; 67(3): 564-600.

[http://dx.doi.org/10.1124/pr.115.010629] [PMID: 26071095]

[77] Lutz TA. The role of amylin in the control of energy homeostasis. Am J Physiol Regul Integr Comp Physiol 2010; 298(6): R1475-84.
[http://dx.doi.org/10.1152/ajpregu.00703.2009] [PMID: 20357016]

[78] Lutz TA. Pancreatic amylin as a centrally acting satiating hormone. Curr Drug Targets 2005; 6(2): 181-9.
[http://dx.doi.org/10.2174/1389450053174596] [PMID: 15777188]

[79] Osto M, Wielinga PY, Alder B, Walser N, Lutz TA. Modulation of the satiating effect of amylin by central ghrelin, leptin and insulin. Physiol Behav 2007; 91(5): 566-72.
[http://dx.doi.org/10.1016/j.physbeh.2007.03.017] [PMID: 17481674]

[80] Hussain Z, Khan JA. Food intake regulation by leptin: Mechanisms mediating gluconeogenesis and energy expenditure. Asian Pac J Trop Med 2017; 10(10): 940-4.
[http://dx.doi.org/10.1016/j.apjtm.2017.09.003] [PMID: 29111188]

[81] Borba-Murad GR, Vardanega-Peicher M, Galende SB, *et al.* Central role of cAMP in the inhibition of glycogen breakdown and gluconeogenesis promoted by leptin and insulin in perfused rat liver. Pol J Pharmacol 2004; 56(2): 223-31.
[PMID: 15156073]

[82] Gavrila A, Chan JL, Miller LC, Heist K, Yiannakouris N, Mantzoros CS. Circulating melanin-concentrating hormone, agouti-related protein, and alpha-melanocyte-stimulating hormone levels in relation to body composition: alterations in response to food deprivation and recombinant human leptin administration. J Clin Endocrinol Metab 2005; 90(2): 1047-54.
[http://dx.doi.org/10.1210/jc.2004-1124] [PMID: 15546902]

[83] Guillod-Maximin E, Roy AF, Vacher CM, *et al.* Adiponectin receptors are expressed in hypothalamus and colocalized with proopiomelanocortin and neuropeptide Y in rodent arcuate neurons. J Endocrinol 2009; 200(1): 93-105.
[http://dx.doi.org/10.1677/JOE-08-0348] [PMID: 18971219]

[84] Kubota N, Yano W, Kubota T, *et al.* Adiponectin stimulates AMP-activated protein kinase in the hypothalamus and increases food intake. Cell Metab 2007; 6(1): 55-68.
[http://dx.doi.org/10.1016/j.cmet.2007.06.003] [PMID: 17618856]

[85] Coope A, Milanski M, Araújo EP, *et al.* AdipoR1 mediates the anorexigenic and insulin/leptin-like actions of adiponectin in the hypothalamus. FEBS Lett 2008; 582(10): 1471-6.
[http://dx.doi.org/10.1016/j.febslet.2008.03.037] [PMID: 18394428]

[86] Suyama S, Maekawa F, Maejima Y, Kubota N, Kadowaki T, Yada T. Glucose level determines excitatory or inhibitory effects of adiponectin on arcuate POMC neuron activity and feeding. Sci Rep 2016; 6: 30796.
[http://dx.doi.org/10.1038/srep30796]

[87] Suyama S, Lei W, Kubota N, Kadowaki T, Yada T. Adiponectin at physiological level glucose-independently enhances inhibitory postsynaptic current onto NPY neurons in the hypothalamic arcuate nucleus. Neuropeptides 2017; 65: 1-9.
[http://dx.doi.org/10.1016/j.npep.2017.03.003] [PMID: 28606559]

[88] Sun J, Gao Y, Yao T, *et al.* Adiponectin potentiates the acute effects of leptin in arcuate Pomc neurons. Mol Metab 2016; 5(10): 882-91.
[http://dx.doi.org/10.1016/j.molmet.2016.08.007] [PMID: 27689001]

CHAPTER 4

The Role of Meta-Inflammation in The Adipose Tissue Dysfunction and Obesity

Asija Začiragić[*]

Department of Human Physiology, Faculty of Medicine University of Sarajevo, Bosnia and Herzegovina

Abstract: The term "meta-inflammation" refers to chronic metabolic inflammation, which is thought to have an important role in the pathogenesis of numerous metabolic diseases. Majority of authors agree that inflammation, as a component of immune system, may serve as a link between obesity and numerous diseases. Hence, the role of meta-inflammation in the pathogenesis of obesity-related diseases is extensively investigated. Mitochondrial dysfunction in adipocytes is lately regarded as a primary cause of adipose tissue inflammation. This newly proposed hypothesis contradicts currently prevailing concept that "adipose tissue hypoxia" underlies adipose tissue dysfunction in obesity. Infiltration of adipose tissue by immune cells is one of the hallmarks of adipose tissue dysfunction. Based on the current knowledge, adipose tissue (AT) macrophages are considered to have a pivotal role in the development of adipose tissue inflammation and dysfunction. Macrophages that infiltrate the adipose tissue are divided into: pro-inflammatory (M1) and anti-inflammatory (M2) AT macrophages. Studies have shown that M1 AT macrophages contribute to insulin resistance by producing pro-inflammatory cytokines. Conversely, M2 AT macrophages are involved in the repair or remodeling of tissues. In obesity, adipose tissue becomes inflamed and goes through cellular remodeling. Adipocytes increase in number (hyperplasia) and size (hypertrophy), become infiltrated by macrophages and undergo fibrosis. Hypertrophic adipocytes secrete more pro-inflammatory molecules that lead to a shift of M2 to M1 AT macrophages. Adipose tissue dysfunction in obesity is characterized by changes on cellular and molecular level, which include immune cells such as T cells, B cells and dendritic cells. However, their role in meta-inflammation and adipose tissue dysfunction remains to be fully elucidated. Novel findings suggest that dysregulation of autophagy in adipose tissue has an important role in meta-inflammation. Studies have shown that there is a strong relationship between the prenatal and perinatal environment and obesity-related diseases. Childhood obesity is associated with meta-inflammation that affects not only adipose tissue but other organs as well. Since adipose tissue dysfunction in obesity plays a pivotal role in disturbing homeostatic processes in the human body, it is of essential importance that health care systems at the global level work on implementation of precautionary strategies in order to prevent the development and progression of meta-inflammation and obesity-related metabolic complications starting at early stages of life.

---

[*] **Corresponding author Asija Začiragić:** Department of Human Physiology, Faculty of Medicine University of Sarajevo, Bosnia and Herzegovina; Tel: +387 33 226 478, Ext: 525; E-mail: zarias@lol.ba

Keywords: Adipose tissue dysfunction, Adipose tissue dendritic cells, Anti-inflammatory cytokines, Autophagy, B cells, Macrophages, Macrophage polarization, Meta-inflammation, Obesity, Pro-inflammatory cytokines, T regulatory cells.

INTRODUCTION

In the past few decades, data from literature point to a significant association between increasingly prevalent metabolic diseases and chronic systemic low-grade inflammation. This notion has led to the formulation of the new term "meta-inflammation" that refers to chronic metabolic inflammation, which is thought to have an important role in the pathogenesis of numerous metabolic diseases. Adipose tissue, liver, pancreas and brain are considered to be metabolic organs affected by inflammatory changes with consequent disturbances of tissue homeostasis [1].

Obesity is characterized by abnormal and excessive accumulation of adipose tissue in the body. Novel findings suggest that obesity leads to local inflammation of adipose tissue, which, in turn, promotes chronic systemic low-grade inflammation with consequent metabolic diseases such as type 2 diabetes mellitus, cardiovascular and neurodegenerative diseases, various types of cancer, and nonalcoholic fatty liver disease, among others [2].

Currently, the research community seeks possible coalescing mechanism that underlays the pathogenesis of obesity-related diseases. The present notion points to a close association between nutrient overload and disturbances in mediators of inflammation and immunity on cellular and molecular level. The majority of authors agree that inflammation, as a component of immune system, may serve as a link between obesity and numerous diseases. Hence, the role of meta-inflammation in the pathogenesis of obesity-related diseases is extensively investigated.

Epidemiological studies have shown an association between insulin resistance and systemic, low-grade, chronic inflammation that is accompanied by elevated levels of serum C-reactive protein (CRP), an acute phase protein produced in the liver [3]. Nutritional excess can lead to increased synthesis of reactive oxygen species (ROS) leading to oxidative and endoplasmic reticulum stress as a result of increased circulating lipids (lipotoxicity) and glucose (glucotoxicity) [4, 5]. Lipotoxicity and glucotoxicity in time lead to β cell dysfunction and decreased insulin production. Eventually, exhaustion of β cells occurs, resulting in type 2 diabetes [6 - 8].

Woo *et al.* [9] recently proposed that mitochondrial dysfunction in adipocytes is a primary cause of adipose tissue inflammation. Although white adipocytes have a low abundance of mitochondria, latest evidence suggests that mitochondria are essential for maintaining metabolic homeostasis in white adipocytes since mitochondrial function is essential for adiponectin synthesis. This newly proposed hypothesis contradicts currently prevailing concept that "adipose tissue hypoxia" underlies adipose tissue dysfunction in obesity.

The main distinction between these two theories is that "adipose tissue hypoxia" theory argues that adipocytes are enlarged in obesity and since these enlarged adipocytes are distant from vasculature, hypoxia occurs in them resulting in decreased adiponectin production. Conversely, based on the theory suggested by Woo *et al.* [9] mitochondrial dysfunction leads to the accumulation of triglycerides resulting in hypertrophy of adipocytes, adipose tissue inflammation, and insulin resistance.

Adipose tissue dysfunction is characterized by the altered production of adipokines with predominance of those with pro-inflammatory properties. Further, increased adipogenesis and disturbed angiogenesis are also features of adipose tissue dysfunction alongside with excessive lipid storage, hypoxia and fibrosis with consequent necrosis [10 - 12] (Fig. **1**).

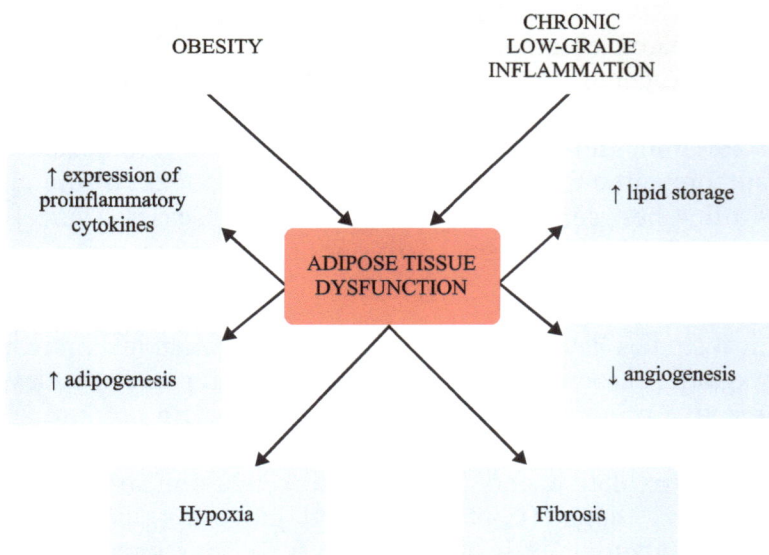

Fig. (1). Features of adipose tissue dysfunction associated with obesity and chronic low-grade inflammation.

PRO-INFLAMMATORY AND ANTI-INFLAMMATORY CYTOKINES IN OBESITY

Infiltration of adipose tissue by immune cells is one of the hallmarks of adipose tissue dysfunction. These immune cells include M1 and M2 macrophages, effector and memory T-cells, interleukin 10 producing FoxP3+ T regulatory cells, natural killer and natural killer T (NKT) cells, and granulocytes [13]. Based on the current knowledge, adipose tissue (AT) macrophages are considered to have pivotal role in the development of adipose tissue inflammation. Macrophages that infiltrate the adipose tissue are divided into: pro-inflammatory (M1) and anti-inflammatory (M2) AT macrophages. Studies have shown that M1 AT macrophages contribute to insulin resistance by producing pro-inflammatory cytokines, such as tumor necrosis factor (TNF)-α, interleukin (IL)-6, interleukin (IL)-15, interleukin (IL)-1, interleukin (IL)-18, and monocyte chemoattractant protein (MCP)-1. Conversely, M2 AT macrophages are involved in the repair or remodeling of tissues by the production of IL-10, IL-4, Il-13, arginase-1, and CD206. M2-like macrophages are predominantly present in the lean adipose tissue, and are considered to have important role in adipose tissue homeostasis. Conversely, M1-like macrophages are predominantly present in the obese adipose tissue and contribute to local and systemic insulin resistance. AT macrophages traits are mediated by adipokines and fatty acids secreted from adipocytes as well as by cytokines secreted from other immune cells in adipose tissue [14] (Fig. **2**).

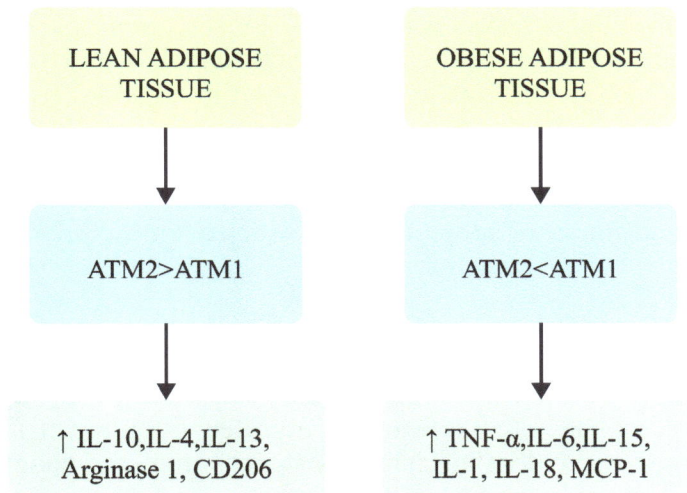

Fig. (2). Polarization of adipose tissue macrophages in lean and obese adipose tissue.
ATM2 - adipose tissue macrophage type 2; ATM1 - adipose tissue macrophage type 1, TNF α- tumor necrosis factor alpha; IL-interleukin; MCP- monocyte chemoattractant protein.

TNF-α is a cytokine that is thus far most extensively investigated in obesity, and metabolic diseases in general. The majority of studies have found an association between increased production of TNF-α and metabolic syndrome. However, there are few studies where this association was not proven. Based on current conception, increased expression of TNF- α is a consequence of obesity itself and not metabolic disturbances in human body. Another pro-inflammatory cytokine well studied in the context of obesity is IL-6. Although IL-6 by its actions on central nervous system (CNS), decreases food intake leading to a decrease in body weight, earlier studies have shown that IL-6 is one of the most potent stimulator of CRP liver production and consequent inflammation seen in obesity. Role of IL-15 as pro-inflammatory cytokines in obesity was also reported, and it has been shown that exercise and calorie restriction leads to decreased expression of IL-15. Furthermore, excess of fat can result in increased IL-1β production seen in insulin resistance and obesity. Adipocytes have been found to produce IL-18, and its increased production is seen in obesity and type 2 diabetes. IL-18 is considered to be a pro-inflammatory cytokine and studies have demonstrated that weight loss after bariatric surgery is followed by decrease in IL-18 production [3].

Whereas pro-inflammatory cytokines and their roles have been given much attention in the past few decades, the actions of anti-inflammatory cytokines in metabolic diseases and obesity are still understudied. Cytokines in adipose tissue with promising anti-inflammatory potential are predominantly produced by AT macrophages and have been reported to prevent and counterattack insulin resistance and metabolic disorders in general. Preservation of lean body mass and intake of unsaturated free fatty acids has been shown to activate M2 AT macrophages, which in turn by the production of interleukin (IL)-4, -10, and -13, and release of adiponectin protects against insulin resistance by direct suppression of inflammation. M2 AT macrophages also have the ability to promote positive homeostatic events, such as remodeling of adipose tissue leading to hypoxia prevention and clearance of apoptotic cells, which averts cellular necrosis [13, 15, 16].

Obesity is characterized by enlargement of AT macrophages that could be explained by several mechanisms. Firstly, recruitment-dependent mechanisms such as adipocyte death, chemokine release, and lipolysis of fatty acids might explain AT macrophages increase in obesity. Secondly, novel findings suggest that recruitment-independent mechanisms such as impaired apoptosis, increased proliferation and decreased withdrawal may explain an increase of AT macrophages in obesity [17]. In general, AT macrophages determine the "low-grade" chronic obesity-related inflammation by the production of specific inflammatory molecules.

The growing evidence point to the key role of adipose tissue as an active participant in the control of numerous pathological processes. As a potent endocrine organ, adipose tissue has been shown to have an impact on the pathogenesis of obesity-related metabolic and inflammatory conditions. The proven interplay between immune and metabolic system in obesity leads to the increased secretion of pro-inflammatory cytokines resulting in a chronic active inflammatory condition that leads to the development of obesity-related pathologies [18].

Findings from recent studies suggest that in individuals with normal BMI, the primary role of adipocytes is the regulation of metabolic homeostasis and storage of lipids. Under these conditions, there is a predominance of M2 AT macrophages, which secrete anti-inflammatory cytokines creating an anti-inflammatory milieu that protects from the development of inflammation and insulin resistance. This effect is thought to be the result of peroxisome proliferator-activated receptor-(PPAR)s and liver X receptor- (LXR) families activity, which counterattacks inflammation [19, 20]. Further, novel data point to the important anti-inflammatory role of a new adipokine, the lipocalin-2 (LCN2), which has been shown to increase secretion of adiponektin, upregulates PPARγ, increases the release of adiponectin and also antagonizes TNF-α actions on metabolic and inflammatory gene expression in AT macrophages [21].

In obesity, adipose tissue (AT) becomes inflamed and goes through cellular remodeling. Adipocytes increase in number (hyperplasia) and size (hypertrophy), become infiltrated by macrophages and undergo fibrosis. Hypertrophic adipocytes secrete more pro-inflammatory molecules that leads to shift of M2 to M1 AT macrophages. M1 macrophages tend to form crown-like structures constituted by necrotic-like adipocytes and adipocyte cellular fragments resulting in an increase of AT inflammation and its exacerbation [22]. Moreover, M1 AT macrophages release classical pro-inflammatory cytokines and inducible nitric oxide synthase (iNOS), an isoform of NOS enzyme that has inflammatory properties. However, the mechanisms responsible for the monocyte/macrophage attraction to AT is still largely unknown. It has been suggested that AT-endothelial cells contribute to this process. It seems that AT pro-inflammatory milieu in obesity activates endothelial cells, which in turn attract monocyte/macrophage cells to the AT. Furthermore, an association between adipogenesis and angiogenesis has been implied.

Another mechanism that remains unclear is what causes the shift of M2 AT macrophages to M1 AT macrophages in obesity. Different inflammatory phenotype of adipocytes from visceral and subcutaneous AT has been shown. Visceral AT has more pronounced pro-inflammatory capacity than subcutaneous AT. Also, based on the previously mentioned "adipose tissue hypoxia" theory, hyperplasia and hypertrophy of adipocytes in obesity cause hypoperfusion and lead to local hypoxia with the consequent secretion of pro-inflammatory cytokines.

Although AT macrophages are mainly divided into M1 and M2 classes, Russo *et al.* [23] recently proposed that this division is not that simple and that basically, there are more than two populations of AT macrophages, which have unique tissue distributions and functions, express specific markers and transcriptional profiles. The precise number of AT macrophages subsets is yet unknown and is constantly evolving. Furthermore, mechanisms of their activations are different, but data from literature point to different metabolic stimuli that have a role in this process, including high glucose and high insulin as well as free fatty acids. Although it is now evident that several AT macrophages subsets exist in obese AT, intracellular pathways, regulatory factors and transcriptional mechanisms that underlie functional differences remain to be fully clarified.

Heterogeneity and diversity of AT macrophages depends on their location, but is also different in the lean and obese setting. There are two major AT macrophages subtypes: monocyte derived/"recruited" macrophages and tissue resident macrophages. Based on the metabolic status, properties, number and localization of AT macrophages greatly differ [24, 25]. Animal studies have shown that AT macrophages population increases from 10% in lean AT to more than 50% in severe obese AT [26].

Resident AT macrophages are located between adipocytes and along AT vascular structures. They regulate adipocyte lipid metabolism by secreting catecholamines and IL-10, express anti-inflammatory cytokines and have a role in the clearance of apoptotic cells and in the resolution of inflammation. In the obese setting, recruitment of monocyte derived / "recruited" macrophages occurs and this recruited AT macrophages undergo a polarization shift toward pro-inflammatory phenotype [27]. Lumeng *et al.* [28] were the first to report macrophage polarization state in obesity when revealed a propensity for M1 inflammatory gene expression over that of M2 after high-fat intake.

Shifts in macrophage polarization are thought to contribute to obesity-induced insulin resistance. Anti-inflammatory, M2-like phenotypes, of the residing macrophages are present in lean AT [29]. In obesity, pro-inflammatory, M1-like macrophages are recruited into AT. Results of Shi *et al.* [30] have shown that during obesity, M1-like AT macrophages weakened insulin responses of adipocytes and boosted inflammatory responses through release of pro-inflammatory cytokines. Moreover, obesity stress not only enhanced infiltration of pro-inflammatory macrophages into AT, but also initiated the M2-like residing macrophages to undergo a phenotypic switch to M1 [28]. Studies have shown that T cells and adipocytes are also important mediators of macrophage polarization. Namely, T regulator cells have been reported to improve insulin response by promoting M2 polarization [31], whereas adipocytes in obesity mainly produce pro-inflammatory cytokines, which promotes M1-like polarization [32]. Additionally, epigenetic mechanisms play important role in regulation of macrophage polarization in obesity. Animal studies have reported that DNA methylation suppresses activation of M2 AT macrophages in obese mice, whereas inhibition of DNA methylation promoted M2 AT macrophages and decreased their inflammatory markers release [33].

Peripheral blood monocytes serve as a source for AT macrophages and are divided into three subsets: classical monocytes (CD14++ CD16-), intermediate monocytes (CD14++ CD16+), and non-classical monocytes (CD14+ CD16++). It has been proposed that CD14++ CD16- monocytes have pro-inflammatory properties, whereas CD14+ CD16++ monocytes have a patrolling roles and consequent anti-inflammatory features [34]. Studies have shown that pro-inflammatory AT macrophages correlate with high BMI as well as with the production of reactive oxygen species [35]. Anti-inflammatory cytokines released by resident AT macrophages within lean AT preserve insulin sensitivity by neutralizing inflammatory responses [36]. Conversely, in obese AT production of pro-inflammatory cytokines by recruited macrophages occurs alongside with diminished adipocyte function [37].

According to novel findings, macrophage infiltration, activation and polarization are the key initiators of meta-inflammation. Altered macrophage polarization not only contributes to local tissue pathology in obesity, but also has a widespread influence in promoting insulin resistance and its consequent symptoms. Earlier study by Fujisaka *et al.* [14] has shown that insulin resistance is associated with both the number of M1 macrophages and the M1-to-M2 ratio. However, underlying mechanisms and actions of macrophage polarization on physiological functions and pathological alterations in obesity remain to be fully elucidated.

The role of meta-inflammation in adipose tissue dysfunction and obesity has been supported by recent findings which suggest that pro-inflammatory AT macrophages rely on glycolysis for their metabolic demands, whereas anti-inflammatory AT macrophages rely on oxidative phosphorylation pathways [38 - 40]. In lean AT, cytokines release occurs as the consequence of glycolysis, fatty acid oxidation, and glutaminolysis. In obese AT, although both oxidative phosphorylation and glycolysis pathways are activated, glycolysis is regarded responsible mostly for the higher cytokine production by AT macrophages [41].

These findings support important association between metabolism and inflammation in obesity setting.

Adipose tissue macrophages participate in apoptosis of adipocytes by indorsing the clearance of fragmented cellular contents *via* lysosomal activation and phagocytosis [42]. In lean AT, this AT macrophages role is regarded important for overall tissue health and maintenance of AT homeostasis. Contrary, in obese AT most recruited AT macrophages tend to accumulate especially around dying adipocytes. It has been speculated that in obese setting metabolic capacity of AT macrophages in debris clearance could be diminished resulting in a maladaptive inflammatory response [43].

Another important feature of AT macrophages is their role in adipogenesis (new adipose tissue cell formation) and angiogenesis [44, 45]. Studies have shown that recruited macrophages have the ability to promote endothelial cell and consequent new vessel formation. This action of recruited macrophages occurs *via* TNF-α and platelet-derived growth factor (PDGF) that are regarded as angiogenic factors and have been reported to be mediators of endothelial cell tube formation and capillary maturation [45 - 47].

THE ROLE OF IMMUNE CELLS IN ADIPOSE TISSUE DYSFUNCTION

Inflammatory responses in obesity tend to be low-grade and chronic unlike acute inflammation, which represents defense mechanism triggered by injury, pathogen infection, or cancer that aims to restore tissue function and homeostasis. This low-grade/chronic inflammation is not followed by clinical signs of acute inflammation and is often referred as subclinical inflammation. It occurs in AT and has been shown to lead to decrease in systemic insulin sensitivity. Although chronic inflammation is low-grade in its nature it still affects numerous metabolic pathways and has a key role in the development of insulin resistance [48]. Since inflammation is regarded as a part of immune system, observed interconnections between inflammatory responses, immune system and metabolism have in recent years led to conception of a new biomedical field called immunometabolism.

Adipose tissue dysfunction in obesity is followed by activation and increase of the number of adipose tissue T cells (ATTs) as well as increase of CD8+-to-CD4+ T-cell ratio, while the number of the T regulatory cells (Tregs) decreases [49]. These ATTs changes in obesity are linked with the development of insulin resistance. The down-regulation of Treg cells together with an increased infiltration of T cells and NK cells in AT has been linked with inflammation in obesity in both animal and human studies [50, 51].

The importance of B lymphocytes in the regulation of AT inflammation and glucose homeostasis is less understood. However, animal studies have shown that B lymphocytes are recruited to AT shortly after the initiation of a high-fat diet. This recruitment occurs prior to the infiltration of AT with T cell [52]. Also, studies involving patients with type 2 diabetes have shown that there is increased B-cell activation in these patients followed by their dysregulated function with increase in pro-inflammatory IL-8 expression and down-regulation of anti-inflammatory IL-10 cytokines [53].

Other types of cells that are regarded important in adipose tissue remodeling in obesity are adipose tissue dendritic cells (ATDCs). Earlier studies often confused AT macrophages and ATDCs since they share expression of markers such as CD11b, F4/80, and CD11c [54, 55]. However, transcriptional profiling of AT macrophages and ATDCs has shown their distinct expression profiles and functions. The importance of ADDCs in meta-inflammation and insulin resistance remains largely unknown, although both AT macrophages and ATDCs quantitative surge in obesity have been reported [56, 57]. A positive correlation between high BMI and ATDCs increase has been found in humans [58]. In obesity setting, the majority of authors regard ATDCs as pro-inflammatory and link them with the development of insulin resistance [23]. However, the exact role of ATDCs in obesity-related inflammation remains to be fully elucidated (Fig. **3**).

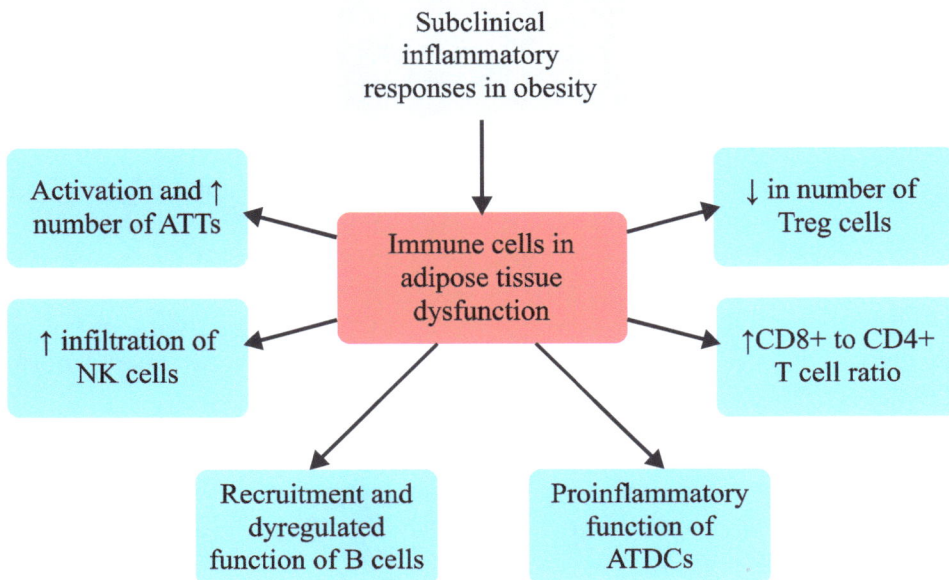

Fig. (3). Immune cells in adipose tissue dysfunction.
ATTs- adipose tissue T cells; Treg - T regulatory cells; NK- natural killer cells; ATDCs- adipose tissue dendritic cells.

THE ROLE OF AUTOPHAGY IN OBESITY AND META-INFLAMMATION

Novel findings suggest that dysregulation of autophagy in adipose tissue has an important role in the development of obesity and insulin resistance. Autophagy represents a cluster of lysosomal degradation processes with the pivotal role in the regulation of tissue differentiation, nutrient availability and organelle recycling. In human body, autophagy has numerous physiological but also pathophysiological functions. Recent studies have shown the important role of autophagy not only in energy homeostasis and organism as a whole but also on the cellular level. Moreover, dysregulation of autophagy has been reported to be related to diseases such as obesity, insulin resistance, diabetes mellitus and osteoporosis [59].

In the adipose tissue, autophagy has been found to regulate its physiological functions, adipose tissue mass, as well as adipose tissue differentiation. Moreover, it has been demonstrated that autophagy plays an important role in mediating biological responses by adipokines such as adiponectin and leptin. Adiponectin induces autophagy in the liver, heart, vascular system, muscle and chondrocytes. Recent studies have found that activation of autophagy by adiponectin may be one of the possible explanations for its cytoprotective effects. Furthermore, novel findings suggest that activation of autophagy plays a significant role in the anti-inflammatory responses exerted by adiponectin [60].

Leptin has been found to induce autophagy in lung, brain, heart and chondrocytes. Gan *et al.* [61] have reported that leptin inhibits endoplasmic reticulum stress-mediated autophagy in adipose tissue. The same authors also reported that endoplasmic reticulum stress-mediated autophagy is required for inflammation suggesting that leptin inhibits inflammatory responses by suppressing autophagy induction. In obesity, leptin levels increase and adiponectin levels decrease. Numerous studies have shown that obesity is associated with increased risk for various types of cancer and leptin has been shown to promote tumor growth. These effects may be explained by the ability of leptin to activate autophagy in cancer cells. This leptin-induced autophagy in cancer cells has been reported to suppress apoptosis [60].

It has also been shown that different cell types in AT regulate autophagy in dissimilar ways. An animal study on adipocyte-specific autophagy-deficient mouse model has reported decreased susceptibility to high fat diet-induced obesity and altered adipogenesis [62] Dysregulated autophagy associated with nutrient-induced endoplasmic reticulum stress has been shown as an early event in the activation of inflammatory processes seen in obesity. Liu *et al.* [63] reported that pro-inflammatory macrophage polarization is enhanced by impaired macrophage autophagy, while Grijavla *et al.* [64] argue that autophagy is unessential for macrophage-mediated lipid homeostasis in adipose tissue. Studies in humans have shown increased autophagy gene expression in AT of obese subjects [65]. Conversely, a recent investigation found that autophagy ablation in adipocytes induces insulin resistance [66]. Furthermore, enhanced autophagy was reported in non-healthy individuals and diabetic obese subjects compared to healthy controls [67], while Soussi *et al.* [68] found decreased autophagy in healthy obese subjects. The observed discrepancy might be explained by different regulation of autophagy in diverse adipose tissue cells, as well as by different distribution of AT in overweight and obese subjects.

Although recent studies point to diverse roles of autophagic pathways in the regulation of AT function, the exact impact of autophagy in AT biology, and especially in the induction of meta-inflammation in obesity remains unclear. Further studies are needed that will explain the complex nature of autophagy in AT biology in normal weight and obese individuals.

CONCLUDING REMARKS

Experimental studies have demonstrated that an increase in body weight and overall adiposity can occur early in animals fed high content of fat. Moreover, inflammatory changes in AT can be found in these animals within first three days of this kind of diet [69, 70]. However, the causes of these early manifestations of obesity remain to be resolved. In those animals that are continuously fed a high content of fat, adiposity and weight gain progress followed by hyperlipidemia and insulin resistance observed in AT, liver and muscle. Resulting obesity is accompanied with apoptosis, endoplasmic reticulum stress, reduction in adiponectin release, and AT macrophages polarization. All of these changes favor the development of low-grade/chronic inflammation in AT [48].

Moreover, animal and epidemiological studies have shown that there is a strong relationship between the and perinatal environment and obesity-related diseases [71]. Challis *et al.* [72] have reported that inflammatory mechanisms may impact the in utero programming of nutrient metabolism, since pregnancy is regarded as a physiologic inflammatory state. Maternal obesity is linked with endotoxemia and AT macrophages accumulation. These two conditions have been shown to affect the developing fetus predisposing it to obesity development in later stages of life [73]. However, it remains to be elucidated how precisely maternal and paternal factors influence the epigenetic programming of metabolism genes that may result in adult obesity.

Human studies have shown that meta-inflammation can occur in early phases of life. Childhood obesity is associated with meta-inflammation that affects not only

AT but other organs as well [74]. Unraveling mechanisms that trigger childhood meta-inflammation are of utmost importance since this can lead to successful preventive strategies in combating increasing prevalence of childhood and adult obesity. Since AT dysfunction in obesity plays a pivotal role in disturbing homeostatic processes in the human body, it is of vital importance that health care systems at the global level work on the implementation of precautionary strategies in order to prevent the development and progression of obesity-related metabolic complications starting at early stages of life.

CONSENT FOR PUBLICATION

Not applicable.

CONFLICT OF INTEREST

The authors confirm that this chapter content has no conflict of interest.

ACKNOWLEDGEMENTS

The authors would like to express their sincere thanks to the editor and anonymous reviewers for their time and valuable suggestions.

REFERENCES

[1]　Hotamisligil GS. Inflammation, metaflammation and immunometabolic disorders. Nature 2017; 542(7640): 177-85.
[http://dx.doi.org/10.1038/nature21363] [PMID: 28179656]

[2]　Karczewski J, Śledzińska E, Baturo A, *et al.* Obesity and inflammation. Eur Cytokine Netw 2018; 29(3): 83-94.
[http://dx.doi.org/10.1684/ecn.2018.0415] [PMID: 30547890]

[3]　Rakotoarivelo V, Variya B, Ilangumaran S, Langlois MF, Ramanathan S. Inflammation in human adipose tissues-Shades of gray, rather than white and brown. Cytokine Growth Factor Rev 2018; 44: 28-37.
[http://dx.doi.org/10.1016/j.cytogfr.2018.10.001] [PMID: 30301598]

[4]　Ouchi N, Parker JL, Lugus JJ, Walsh K. Adipokines in inflammation and metabolic disease. Nat Rev Immunol 2011; 11(2): 85-97.
[http://dx.doi.org/10.1038/nri2921] [PMID: 21252989]

[5]　Kahn BB. Type 2 diabetes: when insulin secretion fails to compensate for insulin resistance. Cell 1998; 92(5): 593-6.
[http://dx.doi.org/10.1016/S0092-8674(00)81125-3] [PMID: 9506512]

[6]　Harding HP, Ron D. Endoplasmic reticulum stress and the development of diabetes: a review. Diabetes 2002; 51 (Suppl. 3): S455-61.
[http://dx.doi.org/10.2337/diabetes.51.2007.S455] [PMID: 12475790]

[7]　Prentki M, Nolan CJ. Islet beta cell failure in type 2 diabetes. J Clin Invest 2006; 116(7): 1802-12.
[http://dx.doi.org/10.1172/JCI29103] [PMID: 16823478]

[8]　Weir GC, Bonner-Weir S. Five stages of evolving beta-cell dysfunction during progression to diabetes. Diabetes 2004; 53 (Suppl. 3): S16-21.

[http://dx.doi.org/10.2337/diabetes.53.suppl_3.S16] [PMID: 15561905]

[9]   Woo CY, Jang JE, Lee SE, Koh EH, Lee KU. Mitochondrial Dysfunction in Adipocytes as a Primary Cause of Adipose Tissue Inflammation. Diabetes Metab J 2019; 43(3): 247-56.
[http://dx.doi.org/10.4093/dmj.2018.0221] [PMID: 30968618]

[10]   Unamuno X, Gómez-Ambrosi J, Rodríguez A, Becerril S, Frühbeck G, Catalán V. Adipokine dysregulation and adipose tissue inflammation in human obesity. Eur J Clin Invest 2018; 48(9): e12997.
[http://dx.doi.org/10.1111/eci.12997] [PMID: 29995306]

[11]   Pellegrinelli V, Carobbio S, Vidal-Puig A. Adipose tissue plasticity: how fat depots respond differently to pathophysiological cues. Diabetologia 2016; 59(6): 1075-88.
[http://dx.doi.org/10.1007/s00125-016-3933-4] [PMID: 27039901]

[12]   Virtue S, Vidal-Puig A. Adipose tissue expandability, lipotoxicity and the Metabolic Syndrome--an allostatic perspective. Biochim Biophys Acta 2010; 1801(3): 338-49.
[http://dx.doi.org/10.1016/j.bbalip.2009.12.006] [PMID: 20056169]

[13]   Guzik TJ, Skiba DS, Touyz RM, Harrison DG. The role of infiltrating immune cells in dysfunctional adipose tissue. Cardiovasc Res 2017; 113(9): 1009-23.
[http://dx.doi.org/10.1093/cvr/cvx108] [PMID: 28838042]

[14]   Fujisaka S, Usui I, Bukhari A, *et al.* Regulatory mechanisms for adipose tissue M1 and M2 macrophages in diet-induced obese mice. Diabetes 2009; 58(11): 2574-82.
[http://dx.doi.org/10.2337/db08-1475] [PMID: 19690061]

[15]   Lumeng CN, Saltiel AR. Inflammatory links between obesity and metabolic disease. J Clin Invest 2011; 121(6): 2111-7.
[http://dx.doi.org/10.1172/JCI57132] [PMID: 21633179]

[16]   Esser N, Legrand-Poels S, Piette J, Scheen AJ, Paquot N. Inflammation as a link between obesity, metabolic syndrome and type 2 diabetes. Diabetes Res Clin Pract 2014; 105(2): 141-50.
[http://dx.doi.org/10.1016/j.diabres.2014.04.006] [PMID: 24798950]

[17]   Hill AA, Reid Bolus W, Hasty AH. A decade of progress in adipose tissue macrophage biology. Immunol Rev 2014; 262(1): 134-52.
[http://dx.doi.org/10.1111/imr.12216] [PMID: 25319332]

[18]   Balistreri CR, Caruso C, Candore G. The role of adipose tissue and adipokines in obesity-related inflammatory diseases. Mediators Inflamm 2010; 2010: 802078.
[http://dx.doi.org/10.1155/2010/802078] [PMID: 20671929]

[19]   Moller DE, Berger JP. Role of PPARs in the regulation of obesity-related insulin sensitivity and inflammation. Int J Obes Relat Metab Disord 2003; 27 (Suppl. 3): S17-21.
[http://dx.doi.org/10.1038/sj.ijo.0802494] [PMID: 14704738]

[20]   Joseph SB, Castrillo A, Laffitte BA, Mangelsdorf DJ, Tontonoz P. Reciprocal regulation of inflammation and lipid metabolism by liver X receptors. Nat Med 2003; 9(2): 213-9.
[http://dx.doi.org/10.1038/nm820] [PMID: 12524534]

[21]   Zhang J, Wu Y, Zhang Y, Leroith D, Bernlohr DA, Chen X. The role of lipocalin 2 in the regulation of inflammation in adipocytes and macrophages. Mol Endocrinol 2008; 22(6): 1416-26.
[http://dx.doi.org/10.1210/me.2007-0420] [PMID: 18292240]

[22]   Bourlier V, Zakaroff-Girard A, Miranville A, *et al.* Remodeling phenotype of human subcutaneous adipose tissue macrophages. Circulation 2008; 117(6): 806-15.
[http://dx.doi.org/10.1161/CIRCULATIONAHA.107.724096] [PMID: 18227385]

[23]   Russo L, Lumeng CN. Properties and functions of adipose tissue macrophages in obesity. Immunology 2018; 155(4): 407-17.
[http://dx.doi.org/10.1111/imm.13002] [PMID: 30229891]

[24] Weisberg SP, McCann D, Desai M, Rosenbaum M, Leibel RL, Ferrante AW Jr. Obesity is associated with macrophage accumulation in adipose tissue. J Clin Invest 2003; 112(12): 1796-808.
[http://dx.doi.org/10.1172/JCI200319246] [PMID: 14679176]

[25] Xu H, Barnes GT, Yang Q, *et al.* Chronic inflammation in fat plays a crucial role in the development of obesity-related insulin resistance. J Clin Invest 2003; 112(12): 1821-30.
[http://dx.doi.org/10.1172/JCI200319451] [PMID: 14679177]

[26] Li P, Lu M, Nguyen MT, *et al.* Functional heterogeneity of CD11c-positive adipose tissue macrophages in diet-induced obese mice. J Biol Chem 2010; 285(20): 15333-45.
[http://dx.doi.org/10.1074/jbc.M110.100263] [PMID: 20308074]

[27] Lumeng CN, DelProposto JB, Westcott DJ, Saltiel AR. Phenotypic switching of adipose tissue macrophages with obesity is generated by spatiotemporal differences in macrophage subtypes. Diabetes 2008; 57(12): 3239-46.
[http://dx.doi.org/10.2337/db08-0872] [PMID: 18829989]

[28] Lumeng CN, Bodzin JL, Saltiel AR. Obesity induces a phenotypic switch in adipose tissue macrophage polarization. J Clin Invest 2007; 117(1): 175-84.
[http://dx.doi.org/10.1172/JCI29881] [PMID: 17200717]

[29] Nguyen MT, Favelyukis S, Nguyen AK, *et al.* A subpopulation of macrophages infiltrates hypertrophic adipose tissue and is activated by free fatty acids *via* Toll-like receptors 2 and 4 and JNK-dependent pathways. J Biol Chem 2007; 282(48): 35279-92.
[http://dx.doi.org/10.1074/jbc.M706762200] [PMID: 17916553]

[30] Shi H, Kokoeva MV, Inouye K, Tzameli I, Yin H, Flier JS. TLR4 links innate immunity and fatty acid-induced insulin resistance. J Clin Invest 2006; 116(11): 3015-25.
[http://dx.doi.org/10.1172/JCI28898] [PMID: 17053832]

[31] Vieira-Potter VJ. Inflammation and macrophage modulation in adipose tissues. Cell Microbiol 2014; 16(10): 1484-92.
[http://dx.doi.org/10.1111/cmi.12336] [PMID: 25073615]

[32] Maachi M, Piéroni L, Bruckert E, *et al.* Systemic low-grade inflammation is related to both circulating and adipose tissue TNFalpha, leptin and IL-6 levels in obese women. Int J Obes Relat Metab Disord 2004; 28(8): 993-7.
[http://dx.doi.org/10.1038/sj.ijo.0802718] [PMID: 15211360]

[33] Li C, Xu MM, Wang K, Adler AJ, Vella AT, Zhou B. Macrophage polarization and meta-inflammation. Transl Res 2018; 191: 29-44.
[http://dx.doi.org/10.1016/j.trsl.2017.10.004] [PMID: 29154757]

[34] Yang J, Zhang L, Yu C, Yang XF, Wang H. Monocyte and macrophage differentiation: circulation inflammatory monocyte as biomarker for inflammatory diseases. Biomark Res 2014; 2(1): 1.
[http://dx.doi.org/10.1186/2050-7771-2-1] [PMID: 24398220]

[35] Nakajima S, Koh V, Kua LF, *et al.* Accumulation of CD11c+CD163+ Adipose Tissue Macrophages through Upregulation of Intracellular 11β-HSD1 in Human Obesity. J Immunol 2016; 197(9): 3735-45.
[http://dx.doi.org/10.4049/jimmunol.1600895] [PMID: 27698011]

[36] Chawla A, Nguyen KD, Goh YP. Macrophage-mediated inflammation in metabolic disease. Nat Rev Immunol 2011; 11(11): 738-49.
[http://dx.doi.org/10.1038/nri3071] [PMID: 21984069]

[37] Jaitin DA, Adlung L, Thaiss CA, *et al.* Lipid-associated macrophages control metabolic homeostasis in trem2-dependent manner. Cell 2019; 178(3): 686-698. e14.
[http://dx.doi.org/10.1016/j.cell.2019.05.054] [PMID: 31257031]

[38] Boscá L, González-Ramos S, Prieto P, *et al.* Metabolic signatures linked to macrophage polarization: from glucose metabolism to oxidative phosphorylation. Biochem Soc Trans 2015; 43(4): 740-4.

[http://dx.doi.org/10.1042/BST20150107] [PMID: 26551722]

[39] Jha AK, Huang SC, Sergushichev A, *et al.* Network integration of parallel metabolic and transcriptional data reveals metabolic modules that regulate macrophage polarization. Immunity 2015; 42(3): 419-30.
[http://dx.doi.org/10.1016/j.immuni.2015.02.005] [PMID: 25786174]

[40] O'Neill LA, Pearce EJ. Immunometabolism governs dendritic cell and macrophage function. J Exp Med 2016; 213(1): 15-23.
[http://dx.doi.org/10.1084/jem.20151570] [PMID: 26694970]

[41] Boutens L, Hooiveld GJ, Dhingra S, Cramer RA, Netea MG, Stienstra R. Unique metabolic activation of adipose tissue macrophages in obesity promotes inflammatory responses. Diabetologia 2018; 61(4): 942-53.
[http://dx.doi.org/10.1007/s00125-017-4526-6] [PMID: 29333574]

[42] Neels JG, Olefsky JM. Inflamed fat: what starts the fire? J Clin Invest 2006; 116(1): 33-5.
[http://dx.doi.org/10.1172/JCI27280] [PMID: 16395402]

[43] Lumeng CN, Deyoung SM, Bodzin JL, Saltiel AR. Increased inflammatory properties of adipose tissue macrophages recruited during diet-induced obesity. Diabetes 2007; 56(1): 16-23.
[http://dx.doi.org/10.2337/db06-1076] [PMID: 17192460]

[44] Odegaard JI, Chawla A. Alternative macrophage activation and metabolism. Annu Rev Pathol 2011; 6: 275-97.
[http://dx.doi.org/10.1146/annurev-pathol-011110-130138] [PMID: 21034223]

[45] Pang C, Gao Z, Yin J, Zhang J, Jia W, Ye J. Macrophage infiltration into adipose tissue may promote angiogenesis for adipose tissue remodeling in obesity. Am J Physiol Endocrinol Metab 2008; 295(2): E313-22.
[http://dx.doi.org/10.1152/ajpendo.90296.2008] [PMID: 18492768]

[46] Cho CH, Koh YJ, Han J, *et al.* Angiogenic role of LYVE-1-positive macrophages in adipose tissue. Circ Res 2007; 100(4): e47-57.
[http://dx.doi.org/10.1161/01.RES.0000259564.92792.93] [PMID: 17272806]

[47] Ligresti G, Aplin AC, Zorzi P, Morishita A, Nicosia RF. Macrophage-derived tumor necrosis factor-alpha is an early component of the molecular cascade leading to angiogenesis in response to aortic injury. Arterioscler Thromb Vasc Biol 2011; 31(5): 1151-9.
[http://dx.doi.org/10.1161/ATVBAHA.111.223917] [PMID: 21372301]

[48] Sun S, Ji Y, Kersten S, Qi L. Mechanisms of inflammatory responses in obese adipose tissue. Annu Rev Nutr 2012; 32: 261-86.
[http://dx.doi.org/10.1146/annurev-nutr-071811-150623] [PMID: 22404118]

[49] Winer S, Chan Y, Paltser G, *et al.* Normalization of obesity-associated insulin resistance through immunotherapy. Nat Med 2009; 15(8): 921-9.
[http://dx.doi.org/10.1038/nm.2001] [PMID: 19633657]

[50] Deiuliis J, Shah Z, Shah N, *et al.* Visceral adipose inflammation in obesity is associated with critical alterations in tregulatory cell numbers. PLoS One 2011; 6(1): e16376.
[http://dx.doi.org/10.1371/journal.pone.0016376] [PMID: 21298111]

[51] O'Rourke RW, Metcalf MD, White AE, *et al.* Depot-specific differences in inflammatory mediators and a role for NK cells and IFN-gamma in inflammation in human adipose tissue. Int J Obes 2009; 33(9): 978-90.
[http://dx.doi.org/10.1038/ijo.2009.133] [PMID: 19564875]

[52] Duffaut C, Galitzky J, Lafontan M, Bouloumié A. Unexpected trafficking of immune cells within the adipose tissue during the onset of obesity. Biochem Biophys Res Commun 2009; 384(4): 482-5.
[http://dx.doi.org/10.1016/j.bbrc.2009.05.002] [PMID: 19422792]

[53] Jagannathan M, McDonnell M, Liang Y, *et al.* Toll-like receptors regulate B cell cytokine production

in patients with diabetes. Diabetologia 2010; 53(7): 1461-71.
[http://dx.doi.org/10.1007/s00125-010-1730-z] [PMID: 20383694]

[54]   Gautier EL, Shay T, Miller J, *et al.* Gene-expression profiles and transcriptional regulatory pathways that underlie the identity and diversity of mouse tissue macrophages. Nat Immunol 2012; 13(11): 1118-28.
[http://dx.doi.org/10.1038/ni.2419] [PMID: 23023392]

[55]   Ginhoux F, Liu K, Helft J, *et al.* The origin and development of nonlymphoid tissue CD103+ DCs. J Exp Med 2009; 206(13): 3115-30.
[http://dx.doi.org/10.1084/jem.20091756] [PMID: 20008528]

[56]   Wu H, Perrard XD, Wang Q, *et al.* CD11c expression in adipose tissue and blood and its role in diet-induced obesity. Arterioscler Thromb Vasc Biol 2010; 30(2): 186-92.
[http://dx.doi.org/10.1161/ATVBAHA.109.198044] [PMID: 19910635]

[57]   Yekollu SK, Thomas R, O'Sullivan B. Targeting curcusomes to inflammatory dendritic cells inhibits NF-κB and improves insulin resistance in obese mice. Diabetes 2011; 60(11): 2928-38.
[http://dx.doi.org/10.2337/db11-0275] [PMID: 21885868]

[58]   Bertola A, Ciucci T, Rousseau D, *et al.* Identification of adipose tissue dendritic cells correlated with obesity-associated insulin-resistance and inducing Th17 responses in mice and patients. Diabetes 2012; 61(9): 2238-47.
[http://dx.doi.org/10.2337/db11-1274] [PMID: 22596049]

[59]   Kim KH, Lee MS. Autophagy--a key player in cellular and body metabolism. Nat Rev Endocrinol 2014; 10(6): 322-37.
[http://dx.doi.org/10.1038/nrendo.2014.35] [PMID: 24663220]

[60]   Park PH. Autophagy induction: a critical event for the modulation of cell death/survival and inflammatory responses by adipokines. Arch Pharm Res 2018; 41(11): 1062-73.
[http://dx.doi.org/10.1007/s12272-018-1082-7] [PMID: 30264324]

[61]   Gan L, Liu Z, Luo D, *et al.* Reduced endoplasmic reticulum stress-mediated autophagy is required for leptin alleviating inflammation in adipose tissue. Front Immunol 2017; 8: 1507.
[http://dx.doi.org/10.3389/fimmu.2017.01507] [PMID: 29250056]

[62]   Zhang Y, Goldman S, Baerga R, Zhao Y, Komatsu M, Jin S. Adipose-specific deletion of autophagy-related gene 7 (atg7) in mice reveals a role in adipogenesis. Proc Natl Acad Sci USA 2009; 106(47): 19860-5.
[http://dx.doi.org/10.1073/pnas.0906048106] [PMID: 19910529]

[63]   Liu K, Zhao E, Ilyas G, *et al.* Impaired macrophage autophagy increases the immune response in obese mice by promoting proinflammatory macrophage polarization. Autophagy 2015; 11(2): 271-84.
[http://dx.doi.org/10.1080/15548627.2015.1009787] [PMID: 25650776]

[64]   Grijalva A, Xu X, Ferrante AW Jr. Autophagy is dispensable for macrophage-mediated lipid homeostasis in adipose tissue. Diabetes 2016; 65(4): 967-80.
[http://dx.doi.org/10.2337/db15-1219] [PMID: 26868294]

[65]   Haim Y, Blüher M, Slutsky N, *et al.* Elevated autophagy gene expression in adipose tissue of obese humans: A potential non-cell-cycle-dependent function of E2F1. Autophagy 2015; 11(11): 2074-88.
[http://dx.doi.org/10.1080/15548627.2015.1094597] [PMID: 26391754]

[66]   Cai J, Pires KM, Ferhat M, *et al.* Autophagy ablation in adipocytes induces insulin resistance and reveals roles for lipid peroxide and Nrf2 signaling in adipose-liver crosstalk. Cell Rep 2018; 25(7): 1708-17. e5.
[http://dx.doi.org/10.1016/j.celrep.2018.10.040]

[67]   Romero M, Zorzano A. Role of autophagy in the regulation of adipose tissue biology. Cell Cycle 2019; 18(13): 1435-45.
[http://dx.doi.org/10.1080/15384101.2019.1624110] [PMID: 31135269]

[68] Soussi H, Reggio S, Alili R, *et al.* DAPK2 Downregulation Associates With Attenuated Adipocyte Autophagic Clearance in Human Obesity. Diabetes 2015; 64(10): 3452-63.
[http://dx.doi.org/10.2337/db14-1933] [PMID: 26038578]

[69] Kleemann R, van Erk M, Verschuren L, *et al.* Time-resolved and tissue-specific systems analysis of the pathogenesis of insulin resistance. PLoS One 2010; 5(1): e8817.
[http://dx.doi.org/10.1371/journal.pone.0008817] [PMID: 20098690]

[70] Radonjic M, de Haan JR, van Erk MJ, *et al.* Genome-wide mRNA expression analysis of hepatic adaptation to high-fat diets reveals switch from an inflammatory to steatotic transcriptional program. PLoS One 2009; 4(8): e6646.
[http://dx.doi.org/10.1371/journal.pone.0006646] [PMID: 19680557]

[71] Monasta L, Batty GD, Cattaneo A, *et al.* Early-life determinants of overweight and obesity: a review of systematic reviews. Obes Rev 2010; 11(10): 695-708.
[http://dx.doi.org/10.1111/j.1467-789X.2010.00735.x] [PMID: 20331509]

[72] Challis JR, Lockwood CJ, Myatt L, Norman JE, Strauss JF III, Petraglia F. Inflammation and pregnancy. Reprod Sci 2009; 16(2): 206-15.
[http://dx.doi.org/10.1177/1933719108329095] [PMID: 19208789]

[73] Basu S, Haghiac M, Surace P, *et al.* Pregravid obesity associates with increased maternal endotoxemia and metabolic inflammation. Obesity (Silver Spring) 2011; 19(3): 476-82.
[http://dx.doi.org/10.1038/oby.2010.215] [PMID: 20930711]

[74] Singer K, Lumeng CN. The initiation of metabolic inflammation in childhood obesity. J Clin Invest 2017; 127(1): 65-73.
[http://dx.doi.org/10.1172/JCI88882] [PMID: 28045405]

CHAPTER 5

Meta-inflammation, Obesity and Cardiometabolic Syndrome

Amela Derviševic[*]

Department of Human Physiology, Faculty of Medicine, University of Sarajevo . Sarajevo, Bosnia and Herzegovina

Abstract: The pathophysiological consequences of obesity are largely based on morphofunctional changes in visceral adipose tissue. By disrupting all phases of adipogenesis, visceral obesity causes adipocyte dysfunction with changes in the adipokine secretion pattern and the onset of local low-grade chronic inflammation or meta-inflammation. Anatomical position of visceral adipose tissue allows direct drainage of proinflammatory and prothrombotic adipocytokines into the portal bloodstream and liver, which play a key role in the pathogenesis of insulin resistance, metabolic and cardiovascular disorders, forming a complex cardiometabolic syndrome. The emergence of insulin resistance followed by atherogenic dyslipidemia results in an increase in extracellular concentrations of free fatty acids and the expansion of ectopic fat depots primarily in the liver, pancreas, heart, kidneys, skeletal muscles and bones. Large insulin-resistant fat cells of ectopic fat depots contribute to the development of insulin resistance and low-grade systemic inflammation by endocrine, paracrine, and autocrine secretion of proinflammatory molecules such as: interleukin- (IL) - 6, tumor necrosis factor-alpha (TNF-α), IL-8, IL-1, and others, causing a complex clinical disorder which yields a number of interrelated risk factors and long-term cardiometabolic disease risk increase.

Keywords: Adipose tissue, Cardiometabolic syndrome, Ectopic fat depots, Insulin resistance, Meta-inflammation, Obesity.

INTRODUCTION

According to the World Health Organization (WHO), obesity is an abnormal and excessive fat accumulation that may impair health [1]. An intensive study on the problem of obesity finds validation in the high prevalence of this disorder as well as its numerous comorbidities that may result from the increase in adipose tissue mass or the endocrine and paracrine effect of adipose tissue cell products [2].

[*] **Corresponding author Amela Derviševic:** Department of Human Physiology, Faculty of Medicine, University of Sarajevo . Sarajevo, Bosnia and Herzegovina; Tel: +387 33 226 478, Ext. 528; E-mail: amela.dervisevic@mf.unsa.ba

The etiology of obesity is complex and multifactorial. It is reflected in the interaction of genetic, epigenetic, behavioral, social and environmental factors, which, while acting on energy homeostasis, lead to a distortion of the balance between energy intake and consumption over a long period of time [3].

Today, the most commonly used form for diagnosis of obesity is the assessment of nutrition estimated from the Body Mass Index (BMI), which is calculated as the ratio of body mass expressed in kilograms (kg) and squared body height expressed in meters (m). According to the applicable criteria, adults with a BMI of 25 to 29 kg/m² are considered to be overweight, while those with a BMI equal to or greater than 30 kg/m² are considered obese [4].

Although increasing BMI is highly associated with progressive increase in cardiometabolic risk [5], it may not always be a precise parameter [6]. The specific distribution of adipose tissue is the enlargement of adipose tissue in different body compartments, and it is much more important for risk assessment. Recent findings have shown that every section of adipose tissue could be considered as a separate department of endocrine tissue with a unique proteomic profile [7].

Waist circumference (WC) is the simple, efficient and inexpensive anthropometric method showing a good correlation with abdominal fat mass and cardiometabolic disease risk [8]. The main disadvantage of WC is that it cannot separate assessment of visceral from subcutaneous adipose tissue [9], and that the accuracy of outcomes depends on the exact measurement protocol [10].

Relating to their function and morphology, adipose tissue is classified into brown adipose tissue (BAT), beige adipose tissue and white adipose tissue (WAT) [11].

BAT in its classic form, is present in newborns, where it provides thermal protection after birth [12]. In adults, BAT is present in a small percentage in the cervical, supraclavicular, and paravertebral regions [13]. Recent research has proven that the level of BAT activity is inversely associated with BMI, body fat percentage and age. BAT participates in 3-5% of basal metabolic rate [14], and it is very important in maintaining whole-body glucose and energy homeostasis [15].

Beige/brite adipose tissue cells are phenotypically between white and brown adipocytes, but despite that fact, it is more likely that beige fat is thermogenic and functionally more similar to brown fat [16].

White adipose tissue is by location broadly classified as follows: subcutaneous adipose tissue (SAT) and visceral adipose tissue (VAT) [17]. Subcutaneous WAT adipose tissue (located under the skin) forms around 65-70% of total adipose tissue [18].

The primary role of SAT is the regulation of storage and mobilization of energy in the form of fat. In this adipose tissue, excess energy is stored in the form of triglycerides (TGs), which, when cells and tissues are in need of energy, can be mobilized in the form of non-steroidal fatty acids (NEFA) [19].

Visceral adipose tissue is deposited in or around internal organs (liver, pancreas, kidneys) [20], skeletal muscles and blood vessels, in order to provide physical and mechanical protection [21]. Intraabdominal VAT fat deposits in normally nourished individuals make up 10-20% of total fat in men and 5-10% of total fat in women [22], while the intramuscular (12%) and thoracic VAT (2%) components are significantly lower [18].

According to adipose tissue disposition, obesity can be classified as subcutaneous (peripheral) and visceral (central) type. Peripheral obesity is also known as women obesity (gynoid) or obesity of lower body parts, while central obesity is labeled as men obesity (android) or obesity of upper body parts [23].

Obesity leads to disorders in the level of lipid storage capacity for subcutaneous adipose tissue (hypertrophy and adipocyte dysfunction), which results in so-called "*spillover*" FFAs and their secondary deposition in VAT and ectopic depots around visceral organs [24].

An increase in VAT mass leads to a central type of obesity in both sexes and also to an increase in the risk of developing diseases related to obesity, such as type 2 diabetes mellitus (T2DM), metabolic syndrome (MetS) and heart disease [23].

Proliferative capacity of VAT adipocytes is lower comparing to SAT adipocytes [25], which makes them more hypertrophic, more dysfunctional, and also they are necrotizing faster, triggering a more intense inflammatory response [26]. In adult women, visceral fat is known to increase up to four times, from 25 to 65 years of age, which increases the overall cardiometabolic risk [27].

Even in non-obese individuals, an increase in visceral adipose tissue is associated with the development of coronary artery disease and an increased risk of a heart attack [28]. A 10-year study of the effects of visceral obesity on the development of T2DM has shown that this type of obesity precedes the T2DM, even independently of insulin levels, glycaemia, BMI, and family medical history [29]. Visceral adipose tissue is associated with reduced utilization of FFA by skeletal muscle [30]. Unlike subcutaneous, visceral obesity is associated with serum total cholesterol and TG concentrations [31], and contributes to the formation of a lipid profile that promotes fat accumulation in blood vessels [32].

A crucial reason for this role of visceral adipose tissue, in addition to its great metabolic and endocrine activity, is the anatomical localization that allows the direct secretion of the synthesized molecules and metabolites into the portal bloodstream and then into the liver [33].

OBESITY-INDUCED INFLAMMATION

For many years, it has been known that fat is not only a passive depot, but also a complex and active metabolic organ consisting of adipocytes as basic cells, connective tissue matrix, nerve fibers, blood vessels, inflammatory and immune cells [33].

The environment surrounding adipocytes is very precise in its capillary network density, macrophage concentration, and factors with high tissue growth potential, which makes adipose tissue the only organ of the human body capable of expansion at any time in life [34]. Adipocytes, as the basic functional units of adipose tissue, synthesize series of hormones, cytokines, growth factors, and other humoral factors labeled as adipokines, which are different from each other, not only by molecular mass or structure, but also within physiological functions. Adipokines mechanism of action is local, with autocrine and paracrine secretion, but they can also manifest their activity in circulation by endocrine controlled secretion using neuroendocrine mechanisms [19]. Secretory activity, including membrane, cytoplasmic and nuclear adipocyte receptors, provides a significant role of adipose tissue in the regulation of energetic, neuroendocrine, immunological and cardiovascular homeostasis [35]. Besides adipocytes, in adipose tissue, stroma cells and vascular bed cells are also metabolically active [36]. The process of adipocyte self-renewal (adipogenesis) is a continuous process, and it lasts a lifetime, which is shown by the existence of preadipocytes in adipose tissue and the death of adipocytes by apoptosis [37].

It is considered that 50% of subcutaneous adipocytes regenerate every 8 (9.5) years, whereas, in visceral adipose tissue, approximately 10% of adipocytes are replaced by the new one each and every year [38].

Obesity induced by energetic misbalance, genetic factors, and environmental factors in adipose tissue causes its dysfunction, adiposopathy, or sick fat [37]. Morphological and functional changes in adipose tissue cells are presented as possible indicators for inflammatory response whose initiation and amplification has systemic effect classified as chronic, and it is called metabolic (meta) inflammation [39]. Metabolic inflammation can be defined as a long term, low-grade inflammatory process induced by impaired nutrients and energy balance [40]. Molecular mechanisms, which represent the basis of inflammatory response activation in dysfunctional depots of adipose tissue, are very complex.

A positive energy balance leads to the deposition of excess energy in the form of fat. The capacity of adipose tissue for fat deposition can be increased by adipocyte hyperplasia (the formation of new adipocytes from stromal preadipocyte differentiation) or hypertrophy (the massive enlargement of existing adipocytes) [19]. The contribution of hyperplasia in fat depots mass increase is limited, genetically controlled and insufficient, which is why hypertrophy of adipose cells is taking over the need for fat depots [41].

Adipocyte hypertrophy causes decreased perfusion with consequent hypoxia in enlarged fat depots, which in adipocytes, extracellular matrix and macrophage cells induces the expression of pro-inflammatory mediators, cytokines and numerous proangiogenetic genes and contributes to the development of microcirculatory disorders and local apoptosis [42] (Fig. **1**).

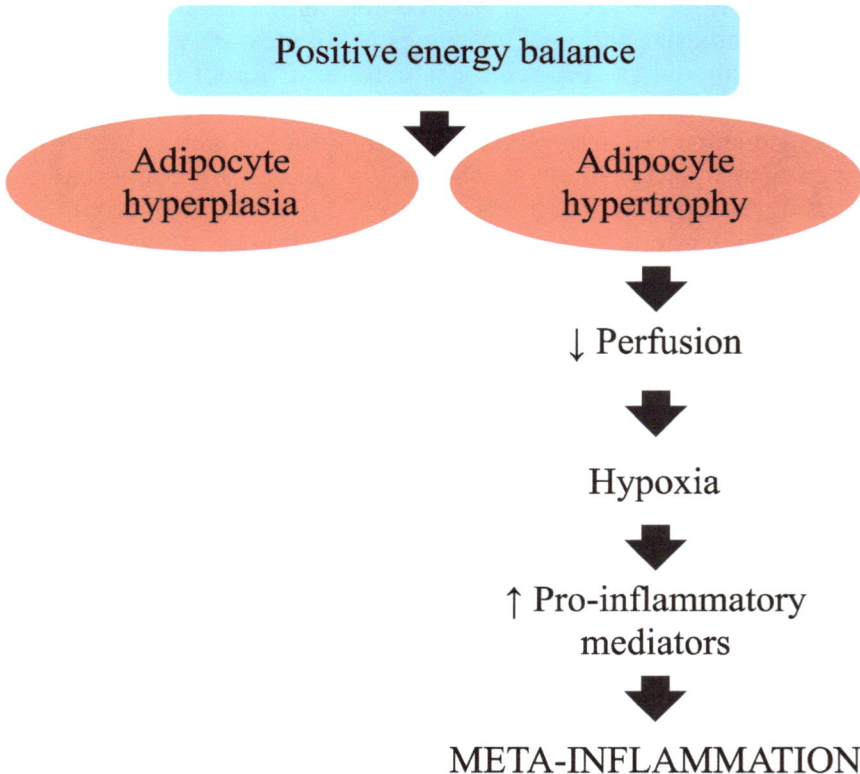

Fig. (1). Cascade of events in adipose tissue from positive energy balance to meta-inflammation.

VAT is thought to be responsible for the onset of meta-inflammation in obesity, because it secretes more pro-inflammatory cytokines per gram than SAT [43]. Surgical removal of SAT alone does not lead to a decrease in the level of pro-inflammatory cytokines [44], which is a consequence of a decrease in VAT mass [45].

Hypertrophic adipocytes are exposed to increased cytotoxic stress, most commonly in the endoplasmic reticulum and mitochondria, which is associated with increased free radical production and oxidative stress [46]. Early symptoms of adipose tissue dysfunction, low perfusion and hypoxia, leads to many changes in adipocytes, stromal cells and vascular bed cells whose effects are subsequently reflected on the whole-body level, thereby affecting metabolic health [47]. Activation and migration of macrophages in adipose tissue are initial events when it comes to obesity-induced inflammation. Signal mechanism from dysfunctional adipocytes activates and changes the status of local macrophages. In adipose tissue, local macrophages form aggregates around necrotic adipocytes, lipid crown-like structures (LCLS) and they produce chemokines, which preserve the inflammatory process [48].

DYSFUNCTION OF ADIPOSE TISSUE AND LINKED CARDIOMETABOLIC CONSEQUENCES

Besides well-known statements emphasizing the significance of obesity level and specific distribution of adipose tissue, the importance of cardiometabolic consequences of dysfunctional adipose tissue in the emergence of obesity-linked diseases is increasing. Mechanism of action of various metabolic stressors in adiposopathy results in the release of pro-inflammatory cytokines, TNF-α, IL-1ß, IL-6, CRP, leptin, resistin, retinol-binding protein 4 (RbP4), lipocalin 2, IL-18, angiopoietin-like protein 2 (ANGPTL2), CC-chemokine ligand 2 (CCL2), CXC-chemokine ligand 5 (CXCL5) and nicotinamide phospho ribosyltransferase (NAmPT), while the synthesis of anti-inflammatory factors, adiponectin and secreted frizzled-related protein 5 (sFRP5) are reduced [49].

Disruption of the endocrine function of adipocytes, primarily visceral adipose tissue, leads to the development of numerous cardiometabolic abnormalities, such as: insulin resistance (IR), T2DM [50], hypertension, hyperlipoproteinemia, atherosclerotic cardiovascular disease (CVD) and contributeS to the development of cardiometabolic syndrome (CMS) [51] (Fig. **2**).

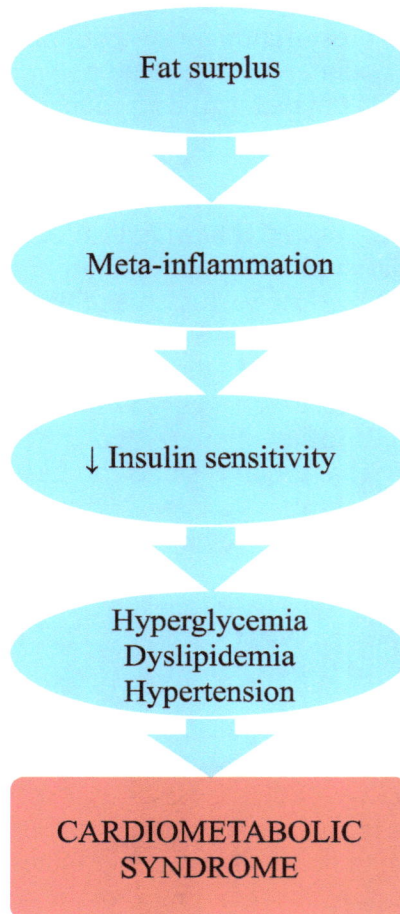

Fig. (2). The association between fat surplus and cardiometabolic syndrome.

Cardiometabolic syndrome, previously and more commonly known as metabolic syndrome (MS) or insulin resistance syndrome [52], is a set of different, partially or fully expressed metabolic abnormalities that increase an individual's risk of developing cardiovascular disease and/or T2DM. The main components of MS are: impaired glucose metabolism, visceral obesity, dyslipidemia and hypertension [53].

Based on the 2005 International Diabetes Federation (IDF) guidelines, the criteria for diagnosing MS are the presence of visceral obesity (WC for the European population ≥ 94 cm in men and ≥ 80 cm in women) and the existence of two of the following criteria: serum TG levels ≥ 1.70 mmol/l; HDL-cholesterol < 1.00

mmol/l in men and < 1.30 mmol/l in women; blood pressure ≥ 130/85 mmHg and fasting glycemia ≥ 5.6 mmol/ and/or previously diagnosed T2DM [54].

Insulin resistance is defined as a weaker response to insulin than normal, and it often leads to hyperinsulinemia in order to maintain homeostasis of glycemia [55]. Reduced insulin sensitivity is considered to be the most significant characteristic of CMS, and presents both a cause and a consequence of the development of most metabolic and hemodynamic disorders associated with CMS [56].

Adipocyte-mediated inflammatory pathways in adipose tissue are crossing with insulin signaling pathways. Pro-inflammatory cytokines secreted by adipocytes of obese individuals and the inflammation induced by these cytokines contribute greatly to insulin resistance [57].

The main link between chronic adipose inflammation and insulin resistance is the increased concentration of FFA in the bloodstream which are the product of lipolytic processes induced by pro-inflammatory cytokines and chemokines that take place in VAT. Lipolysis and the onset of FFA can also be induced by IR in adipocytes, which overall increases the release of FFA into the circulation and lead to the development of insulin resistance [58]. Increased circulating FFA themselves promote the development of IR in the three major insulin-sensitive tissues (skeletal muscle, liver and adipose tissue) by disrupting insulin signaling in target tissue cells directly, blocking insulin receptors [59].

The decreased ability of insulin to achieve adequate glucose utilization in tissues at physiological concentrations leads to a compensatory increase in pancreatic islet mass, an increase in the secretory capacity of pancreatic β-cells, and hyperinsulinemia [60]. Persistent hyperinsulinemia is associated with a decreased ability of insulin to suppress the gluconeogenesis process in the liver, while the FFA can enhance this process. In addition, a decreased insulin receptor count in the liver slows insulin clearance by the liver (and possibly kidney and other sites) and contributes to hyperinsulinemia, which, with increased FFA from visceral adipose tissue, causes fatty liver infiltration, increased very-low-density lipoprotein (VLDL) synthesis, and formation of dyslipidemia [61].

The prominent dyslipidemia is a central metabolic consequence of adipose tissue dysfunction, which, in addition to an increase in systemic levels of FFA and VLDL, is characterized by an increase in the concentration of triglycerides, and low-density lipoprotein (LDL) cholesterol (LDL-C) level, with a low high-density lipoprotein (HDL) cholesterol (HDL-C) and apolipoprotein A-I (apoA-I) concentration [62]. Obesity, primarily visceral, results in overall fat accumulation,

accumulation of triglycerides in the liver, and the development of non-alcoholic fatty liver disease (NAFLD) [63].

Increased activity of hormone-sensitive lipase (HSL) in adipocytes increases the concentration of FFA in the blood and their influx into the liver. In the liver, increased β-oxidation of FFA and lipid deposition in hepatocytes (steatosis) cause damage to mitochondria and endoplasmic reticulum over time due to the production of reactive oxygen species (ROS) from the FFA metabolism *via* oxidation, lipotoxicity, and hepatocyte necrosis and apoptosis [64].

Hepatic steatosis leads to increased nuclear factor kappa-light-chain-enhancer of activated B cells (NK-κβ) signaling in the liver, which then induces the production of local and systemic inflammatory cytokines, primarily TNF-α, leading to chronic liver damage accompanied by progressive fibrosis [65]. According to both human and murine studies, in the liver, TNF-α induces total TGs production, as demonstrated by the increase of TG-containing VLDL particles after TNF-α administration [66].

Possible contributing factors to the development of hepatic inflammation and NAFLD are intestinal-producing lipopolysaccharide endotoxins. These compounds are responsible for the induction of oxidative stress and the production of cytokines, especially TNF-α [67]. According to experimental data, elevated leptin levels and reduced adiponectin levels observed in obesity also contribute to the development and progression of NAFLD [68].

Skeletal muscle tissue is the "intersection" of the pathways of FFA and glucose metabolism, which, in addition to the liver, is the most important organ in the development of IR. The accumulation of lipotoxic FFA in skeletal muscle causes incomplete β-oxidation and the accumulation of toxic lipolysis products, which activate the NK-κβ signal transduction pathway, alter the activity of insulin receptor substrates 1 (IRS-1) of dependent phosphatidylinositol (PI)-3 kinases, and cause IR formation [69]. Insulin resistance decreases the metabolic capacity of muscle in the use of glucose and lipids for energy production, which increases fat deposition in muscle and further reduces insulin sensitivity [70]. Lipotoxic products and IR lead to mitochondrial damage, oxidative stress and myocyte apoptosis.

Skeletal muscle mitochondria have a large respiratory reserve and are resistant to stress at a moderate FFA influx. Physical activity increases the metabolic capacity of skeletal muscle, decreases cellular stress and slows the development of IR [71, 72], which is why paradoxically, despite high muscle fat, trained athletes remain insulin sensitive (athlete's paradox) [73].

In addition to its association with other risk factors, excessive accumulation and dysfunction of visceral adipose tissue also affect myocardial function and morphology. Epicardial adipose tissue (EAT) is a deposit of adipose tissue between the myocardium and the visceral pericardium, without a structure or fascia separating it from the myocardium and the epicardial vessels [74]. It is characterized by its high capacity for metabolism and storage of fat, which is why it is an important local source of FFAs for the myocardium during periods of energy deficiency [75].

In addition, adipocytes in the EAT are rapidly subjected to the browning process and they are able to provide thermal protection [76]. In obesity, hypertrophy of EAT, hypoxia, inflammation, IR, myocardial remodeling ("cardiac steatosis") and transmural damage of blood vessels endothelium ("inside out") occurs [77]. Obesity increases the stroke and minute volume of the heart, leading to increased cardiac output and subsequent hypertrophy and dilation of the left ventricle (LV) and enlargement of the left atrium (LA) with common diastolic ventricular dysfunction [78].

Although obesity is associated with a higher incidence of CVD, the fact is that mildly obese and overweight patients with CVD have a better prognosis than their leaner counterparts with the same CVD and this has been termed the obesity paradox [78]. The phenomenon of the obesity paradox is seen in many forms of CVD [79], in addition to other diseases, such as end-stage renal disease, human immunodeficiency and various pulmonary diseases [80, 81].

Arterial hypertension associated with obesity and IR is present in most people with CMS. Diminished tissue sensitivity to insulin can be viewed as the most important factor in the genesis of hypertension *via* several mechanisms: increased sodium reabsorption in the kidney tubules, activation of the sympathetic nervous system, and alteration in vascular resistance through increased calcium concentration in smooth muscle cells [82].

The insulin resistance state causes endothelial cell dysfunction by decreasing nitric oxide (NO) synthesis and increasing the release of pro-coagulant factors leading to thrombocyte activation [83]. Compensatory hyperinsulinemia in obesity contributes to the enhancement of vasoconstriction, inflammation, increased sodium, and water retention, resulting in the elevation of blood pressure [84].

In obese subjects with insulin resistance, the vasodilatory effect of insulin achieved by the stimulation of increased production of NO from vascular endothelial cells is absent [85], while the effect on renal sodium reabsorption is still retained, and that is contributing to the development of hypertension [86].

Increased insulin levels cause an increase in angiotensinogen secretion in adipocytes of obese individuals, which subsequently results in the activation of the renin-angiotensin-aldosterone system (RAAS) in addition to sodium retention and extracellular fluid volume growth [87]. In addition, it decreases uric acid clearance in the kidneys and increases the retention of salt and water [88].

Leptin contributes to the development of hypertension in obesity, acting on the hypothalamus and increasing CV sympathetic activity. Hyperinsulinemia may also be caused activation of the sympathetic nervous system in different tissues, including the kidneys. The increased circulating levels of FFA from visceral fat depots in obese subjects play a role in the overactivity of the sympathetic nervous system and, ultimately, the rise in blood pressure [89]. Accumulating evidence indicate that in obese patients, ghrelin and adiponectin increase sympathetic activity and cause obesity-induced hypertension [90, 91].

Chronic inflammation in obese individuals presents a significant risk factor for the incidence of prothrombotic conditions, multivariable pathogenesis considering the direct relationship between the features causing the insulin resistance, abdominal obesity, atherogenic dyslipidemia, as well as hypertension, and early onset of endothelial dysfunction [92].

The lack of the physiological inhibitory effect of insulin on the aggregation of thrombocytes has been shown in obese individuals [93].

The dysfunction of thrombocytes in obesity results in the increased activation and thus aggregation, furthering the prothrombotic state [94].

In central obesity, thrombocytes show impaired response to the physiological antiaggregation effects of NO, prostacyclin, and their effectors [95].

The dysfunction of endothelial cells in obese patients increases the syntheses of several thrombocyte activations and aggregation markers: thrombocyte microparticles; thromboxane (TX) B2 metabolites, soluble P-selectin; and platelet-derived CD40L, and decreases the synthesis of aggregation inhibitors [91].

Changes in the coagulation process in obese individuals are associated with increased activity of certain coagulation factors, as following: fibrinogen, von Willebrand factor (vWF), tissue factor (TF), factor VII and factor VIII [96].

A disorder in the process of hemostasis present in obese individuals is a prolonged clot lysis time (CLT), which partly occurs due to an increase in the synthesis of plasminogen activator -1 (PAI-1) inhibitors. Higher plasma concentration of PAI-

1 in obese individuals is mostly the result of over-synthesis in adipocytes caused by proinflammatory cytokines, and endothelial dysfunction, which increased PAI-1 synthesis in endothelial cells [97].

Obesity affects bone homeostasis *via* activities of several adipose tissue-derived molecules, which modulate bone metabolism acting on either bone formation or resorption [98]. The effects of hyperleptinemia on bone metabolism are complex, both negative and positive, and might depend on its site and mode of action. Peripheral administration of leptin could increase bone mass by inhibiting bone resorption and increasing bone formation. On the other hand, leptin inhibits bone formation through the effects on the central nervous system [98]. Eleveted leptin levels in human obesity are associated with a reduction of bone formation biomarkers, especially osteocalcin [99].

Furthermore, low levels of adiponectin in obesity decrease bone mass by suppressing osteoblastogenesis and activating osteoclastogenesis which indicates that a rise in adiponectin levels, caused by fat reduction, may have a positive effect on bone formation stimulating the proliferation, differentiation, and mineralization of osteoblastic cells [100].

The hormone resistin increases osteoblast proliferation, cytokine release, and osteoclast differentiation [101]. According to a recent study, in obesity-associated inflammation, leptin acts by immunomodulatory stimulation of lymphocytopoiesis and mobilization of monocytes and neutrophil granulocytes from the bone marrow and promotes the proliferation of myeloid precursors [102]. Alongside the leptin, adiponectin promotes proliferation and suppresses the differentiation of hematopoietic cells, maintaining their undifferentiated state [103].

In the obese state, subclinical low-grade inflammation, together with systemic and local oxidative stress, play a pivotal role in the initiation or progression of obesity-related glomerulopathy [104].

The glomerular hyperfiltration found in obesity is closely related to increasing renal hemodynamic parameters, including glomerular pressure, filtration fraction, RAAS activity, and sodium and glucose absorption in the proximal renal tubules [105]. Glomerular hyperfiltration, over time, leads to a compensatory structural abnormality in glomeruli, such as glomerulomegaly, which is a histological hallmark of obesity-related glomerulopathy [106]. Obesity-induced glomerulo-megaly may cause glomerular podocytes function changes, mesangial cell proliferation, matrix accumulation and progressive renal fibrosis leading to focal segmental glomerulosclerosis (FSGS) [107].

THE PHENOMENON OF OBESITY WITHOUT CARDIOMETABOLIC COMPLICATIONS

Studies have shown that between 10% and 30% of obese individuals are actually metabolically (or cardiometabolic) healthy [108]. In this context, the term "metabolically healthy obese" (MHO) applies to individuals who are obese (BMI $\geq 30 \text{ kg/m}^2$) with no or little cardiometabolic risk complications [109].

However, despite the high prevalence of metabolically healthy obese (MHO) individuals, there is still no exact accepted definition nor the criteria used to determine whether an obese person is metabolically healthy [110].

Based on the criteria used, the incidence of metabolically healthy individuals in the obese population varies up to 47% when classified based on the absence of the MS as defined by the National Cholesterol Education Program Adult Treatment Panel III [111].

The most commonly used criteria for defining MHO are having two or less of the following five MS components: hypertension, high plasma TG concentration, low HDL-C concentration, high fasting blood glucose, and large waist circumference; or having none or just one abnormal component excluding waist circumference [111].

In some studies, markers of homeostasis model assessment of insulin resistance (HOMA-IR) and systemic inflammation markers such as C reactive protein (CRP) are also included as criteria to define MHO [112].

A large number of clinical and metabolic characteristics have been identified in MHO individuals, which differentiate them from obese individuals with metabolic manifestations.

The differences in metabolic response between MHO individuals and obese individuals at metabolic risk have not been fully discovered, and the involvement of numerous factors such as ethnic, genetic, biochemical, hormonal or neurohumoral is assumed [113].

Despite elevated fat mass, MHO phenotype can be characterized by normal or high levels of insulin sensitivity, normotension, normal lipid, hormonal, liver enzymes, immune and inflammation markers profile [113].

Moreover, recent data from the literature point that MHO individuals have a lower fasting respiratory quotient, that is, greater cardiorespiratory fitness and physical activity, compared with metabolically unhealthy obese (MUO) subjects [114] (Fig. **3**).

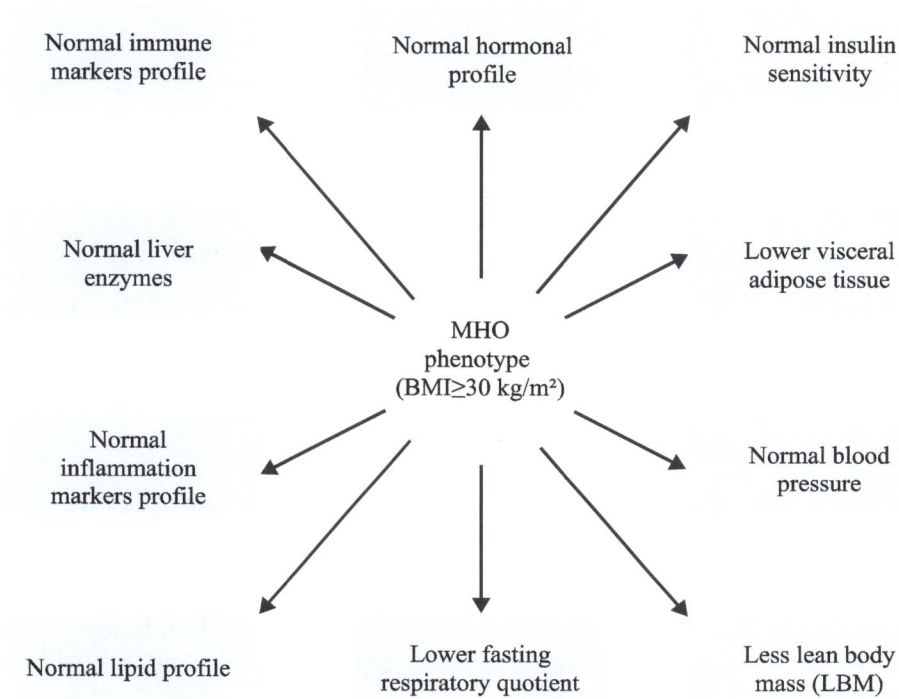

Fig. (3). The characteristics of the MHO phenotype.

It has not yet been determined whether MHO are protected from the increased risk of developing cardiometabolic complications associated with obesity compared with normal-weight subjects, or if there is a delay in the progression of complications in this subpopulation of obese individuals [115].

Some studies show that MHO individuals exhibit certain phenotypic differences relative to obese individuals with metabolic risk - most commonly, they are having a lower visceral adipose tissue and a less lean body mass (LBM) compared with at-risk obese individuals [113].

MHO - METABOLICALLY HEALTHY OBESE; BMI - BODY MASS INDEX

Metabolically healthy obese individuals have up to 54% less visceral fat stores than other obese and lower muscle fat infiltration compared with MUO subjects [116, 117]. On the other hand, in MHO individuals, insulin-sensitive subcutaneous adipose tissue increases and expand, ectopic fat depots are reduced, macrophage infiltration is reduced and the person is in low risk of MS development [118].

Furthermore, obese that belong to this group have a lower fatty liver index and lower concentrations of hepatic enzymes compared with MUO individuals [117].

This is in line with the main role of ectopic liver adipose tissue, which is important in maintaining an insulin-resistant state in obese individuals independently of visceral fat and intramuscular lipid depots [119].

Results from various studies indicate significantly lower levels of high-sensitivity C-reactive protein and alpha-1 antitrypsin in metabolically healthy obese individuals compared to other obese individuals [120]. Moreover, in metabolically healthy subjects, the concentration of IL-6, the main inducer of hepatic CRP synthesis, has also been lower [121].

The fundamental mechanisms underlying the different metabolic profiles of MHO and MUO individuals remain poorly understood [122].

Evidence from meta-analyses and prospective studies has clearly established that MHO individuals have half of the risk for developing T2DM and cardiovascular diseases compared with MUO subjects [123], but their risk is still higher than in metabolically healthy lean people [124].

In view of the foregoing, it is clear that MHO should not be treated as a benign condition and that individual obesity treatment should be considered in MHO subjects to reduce the risk of cardiometabolic consequences [124].

CONCLUDING REMARKS

Besides well-known statements emphasizing the significance of obesity level and specific distribution of adipose tissue, the importance of metabolic consequences of dysfunctional adipose tissue in the emergence of cardiometabolic risk is increasing.

The mechanism of action of various metabolic stressors in dysfunctional adipose tissue results in the release of various pro-inflammatory cytokines, including IL-6 and TNF-α, and contributes to the development of obesity-associated inflammation, also called meta-inflammation.

Meta-inflammation is associated with numerous metabolic abnormalities such as: insulin resistance, type 2 diabetes mellitus, hypertension, hyperlipoproteinemia, and vascular disease, contributing to the development of the cardiometabolic syndrome.

CONSENT FOR PUBLICATION

Not applicable.

CONFLICT OF INTEREST

The authors confirm that this chapter content has no conflict of interest.

ACKNOWLEDGEMENTS

The authors would like to express their sincere thanks to the editor and anonymous reviewers for their time and valuable suggestions.

REFERENCES

[1]   Müller MJ, Geisler C. Defining obesity as a disease. Eur J Clin Nutr 2017; 71(11): 1256-8.
[http://dx.doi.org/10.1038/ejcn.2017.155] [PMID: 28952604]

[2]   Longo M, Zatterale F, Naderi J, *et al.* Adipose tissue dysfunction as determinant of obesity-associated metabolic complications. Int J Mol Sci 2019; 20(9): 2358.
[http://dx.doi.org/10.3390/ijms20092358] [PMID: 31085992]

[3]   Tsigos C, Hainer V, Basdevant A, *et al.* Management of obesity in adults: European clinical practice guidelines. Obes Facts 2008; 1(2): 106-16.
[http://dx.doi.org/10.1159/000126822] [PMID: 20054170]

[4]   World Health Organization. Obesity: Preventing and Managing the Global Epidemic. Report of a WHO Consultation. WHO Technical Report Series, No 894. Geneva: World Health Organization 2000.

[5]   Berrington de Gonzalez A, Hartge P, Cerhan JR, *et al.* Body-mass index and mortality among 1.46 million white adults. N Engl J Med 2010; 363(23): 2211-9.
[http://dx.doi.org/10.1056/NEJMoa1000367] [PMID: 21121834]

[6]   Blundell JE, Dulloo AG, Salvador J, Frühbeck G. Beyond BMI--phenotyping the obesities. Obes Facts 2014; 7(5): 322-8.
[http://dx.doi.org/10.1159/000368783] [PMID: 25485991]

[7]   Yang X, Smith U. Adipose tissue distribution and risk of metabolic disease: does thiazolidinedione-induced adipose tissue redistribution provide a clue to the answer? Diabetologia 2007; 50(6): 1127-39.
[http://dx.doi.org/10.1007/s00125-007-0640-1] [PMID: 17393135]

[8]   Klein S, Allison DB, Heymsfield SB, *et al.* Waist circumference and cardiometabolic risk: a consensus statement from SHAPING America's health: association for weight management and obesity prevention; NAASO, The obesity society; the American Society for Nutrition; and the American Diabetes Association. Am J Clin Nutr 2007; 85(5): 1197-202.
[http://dx.doi.org/10.1093/ajcn/85.5.1197] [PMID: 17490953]

[9]   Onat A, Avci GS, Barlan MM, Uyarel H, Uzunlar B, Sansoy V. Measures of abdominal obesity assessed for visceral adiposity and relation to coronary risk. Int J Obes Relat Metab Disord 2004; 28(8): 1018-25.
[http://dx.doi.org/10.1038/sj.ijo.0802695] [PMID: 15197408]

[10]   Millar SR, Perry IJ, Van den Broeck J, Phillips CM. Optimal central obesity measurement site for

assessing cardiometabolic and type 2 diabetes risk in middle-aged adults. PLoS One 2015; 10(6): e0129088.
[http://dx.doi.org/10.1371/journal.pone.0129088] [PMID: 26042771]

[11]   Lizcano F. The Beige Adipocyte as a Therapy for Metabolic Diseases. Int J Mol Sci 2019; 20(20): 5058.
[http://dx.doi.org/10.3390/ijms20205058] [PMID: 31614705]

[12]   Luo L, Liu M. Adipose tissue in control of metabolism. J Endocrinol 2016; 231(3): R77-99.
[http://dx.doi.org/10.1530/JOE-16-0211] [PMID: 27935822]

[13]   Gesta S, Tseng YH, Kahn CR. Developmental origin of fat: tracking obesity to its source. Cell 2007; 131(2): 242-56.
[http://dx.doi.org/10.1016/j.cell.2007.10.004] [PMID: 17956727]

[14]   van Marken Lichtenbelt W. Brown adipose tissue and the regulation of nonshivering thermogenesis. Curr Opin Clin Nutr Metab Care 2012; 15(6): 547-52.
[http://dx.doi.org/10.1097/MCO.0b013e3283599184] [PMID: 23037904]

[15]   Chondronikola M, Volpi E, Børsheim E, et al. Brown adipose tissue improves whole-body glucose homeostasis and insulin sensitivity in humans. Diabetes 2014; 63(12): 4089-99.
[http://dx.doi.org/10.2337/db14-0746] [PMID: 25056438]

[16]   Wu J, Cohen P, Spiegelman BM. Adaptive thermogenesis in adipocytes: is beige the new brown? Genes Dev 2013; 27(3): 234-50.
[http://dx.doi.org/10.1101/gad.211649.112] [PMID: 23388824]

[17]   Gulyaeva O, Dempersmier J, Sul HS. Genetic and epigenetic control of adipose development. Biochim Biophys Acta Mol Cell Biol Lipids 2019; 1864(1): 3-12.
[http://dx.doi.org/10.1016/j.bbalip.2018.04.016] [PMID: 29704660]

[18]   Misra A, Vikram NK. Clinical and pathophysiological consequences of abdominal adiposity and abdominal adipose tissue depots. Nutrition 2003; 19(5): 457-66.
[http://dx.doi.org/10.1016/S0899-9007(02)01003-1] [PMID: 12714101]

[19]   Freedland ES. Role of a critical visceral adipose tissue threshold (CVATT) in metabolic syndrome: implications for controlling dietary carbohydrates: a review. Nutr Metab (Lond) 2004; 1(1): 12.
[http://dx.doi.org/10.1186/1743-7075-1-12] [PMID: 15530168]

[20]   Yuan JC, Yogarajah T, Lim SK, Yvonne Tee GB, Khoo BY. Pilot study and bioinformatics analysis of differentially expressed genes in adipose tissues of rats with excess dietary intake. Mol Med Rep 2020; 21(5): 2063-72.
[http://dx.doi.org/10.3892/mmr.2020.11012] [PMID: 32323762]

[21]   Bays H. Central obesity as a clinical marker of adiposopathy; increased visceral adiposity as a surrogate marker for global fat dysfunction. Curr Opin Endocrinol Diabetes Obes 2014; 21(5): 345-51.
[http://dx.doi.org/10.1097/MED.0000000000000093] [PMID: 25106000]

[22]   Lee MJ, Wu Y, Fried SK. Adipose tissue heterogeneity: implication of depot differences in adipose tissue for obesity complications. Mol Aspects Med 2013; 34(1): 1-11.
[http://dx.doi.org/10.1016/j.mam.2012.10.001] [PMID: 23068073]

[23]   Aras Ş, Üstünsoy S, Armutçu F. Indices of Central and Peripheral Obesity; Anthropometric Measurements and Laboratory Parameters of Metabolic Syndrome and Thyroid Function. Balkan Med J 2015; 32(4): 414-20.
[http://dx.doi.org/10.5152/balkanmedj.2015.151218] [PMID: 26740903]

[24]   Castro AV, Kolka CM, Kim SP, Bergman RN. Obesity, insulin resistance and comorbidities? Mechanisms of association. Arq Bras Endocrinol Metabol 2014; 58(6): 600-9.
[http://dx.doi.org/10.1590/0004-2730000003223] [PMID: 25211442]

[25]   Baglioni S, Cantini G, Poli G, et al. Functional differences in visceral and subcutaneous fat pads originate from differences in the adipose stem cell. PLoS One 2012; 7(5): e36569.

[http://dx.doi.org/10.1371/journal.pone.0036569] [PMID: 22574183]

[26]   Joe AW, Yi L, Even Y, Vogl AW, Rossi FM. Depot-specific differences in adipogenic progenitor abundance and proliferative response to high-fat diet. Stem Cells 2009; 27(10): 2563-70.
[http://dx.doi.org/10.1002/stem.190] [PMID: 19658193]

[27]   Hunter GR, Lara-Castro C, Byrne NM, Zakharkin SO, St Onge M-P, Allison Db. Weight loss needed to maintain visceral adipose tissue during aging. Int J Body Compos Res 2005; 3(2): 55-61.

[28]   Nakamura T, Tokunaga K, Shimomura I, *et al.* Contribution of visceral fat accumulation to the development of coronary artery disease in non-obese men. Atherosclerosis 1994; 107(2): 239-46.
[http://dx.doi.org/10.1016/0021-9150(94)90025-6] [PMID: 7980698]

[29]   Boyko EJ, Fujimoto WY, Leonetti DL, Newell-Morris L. Visceral adiposity and risk of type 2 diabetes: a prospective study among Japanese Americans. Diabetes Care 2000; 23(4): 465-71.
[http://dx.doi.org/10.2337/diacare.23.4.465] [PMID: 10857936]

[30]   Colberg SR, Simoneau JA, Thaete FL, Kelley DE. Skeletal muscle utilization of free fatty acids in women with visceral obesity. J Clin Invest 1995; 95(4): 1846-53.
[http://dx.doi.org/10.1172/JCI117864] [PMID: 7706491]

[31]   Fujioka S, Matsuzawa Y, Tokunaga K, Tarui S. Contribution of intra-abdominal fat accumulation to the impairment of glucose and lipid metabolism in human obesity. Metabolism 1987; 36(1): 54-9.
[http://dx.doi.org/10.1016/0026-0495(87)90063-1] [PMID: 3796297]

[32]   Nieves DJ, Cnop M, Retzlaff B, *et al.* The atherogenic lipoprotein profile associated with obesity and insulin resistance is largely attributable to intra-abdominal fat. Diabetes 2003; 52(1): 172-9.
[http://dx.doi.org/10.2337/diabetes.52.1.172] [PMID: 12502509]

[33]   Ibrahim MM. Subcutaneous and visceral adipose tissue: structural and functional differences. Obes Rev 2010; 11(1): 11-8.
[http://dx.doi.org/10.1111/j.1467-789X.2009.00623.x] [PMID: 19656312]

[34]   Ahima RS. Adipose tissue as an endocrine organ. Obesity (Silver Spring) 2006; 14(5) (Suppl. 5): 242S-9S.
[http://dx.doi.org/10.1038/oby.2006.317] [PMID: 17021375]

[35]   Harwood HJ Jr. The adipocyte as an endocrine organ in the regulation of metabolic homeostasis. Neuropharmacology 2012; 63(1): 57-75.
[http://dx.doi.org/10.1016/j.neuropharm.2011.12.010] [PMID: 22200617]

[36]   Asterholm Wernstedt, C Tao, TS Morley, *et al.* Adipocyte inflammation is essential for healthy adipose tissue expansion and remodeling. Cell Metab 2014; 20(1): 103-18.

[37]   Bays HE. Adiposopathy is "sick fat" a cardiovascular disease? J Am Coll Cardiol 2011; 57(25): 2461-73.
[http://dx.doi.org/10.1016/j.jacc.2011.02.038] [PMID: 21679848]

[38]   Spalding KL, Arner E, Westermark PO, *et al.* Dynamics of fat cell turnover in humans. Nature 2008; 453(7196): 783-7.
[http://dx.doi.org/10.1038/nature06902] [PMID: 18454136]

[39]   Monteiro R, Azevedo I. Chronic inflammation in obesity and the metabolic syndrome. Mediators Inflamm 2010; 2010: 289645.
[http://dx.doi.org/10.1155/2010/289645] [PMID: 20706689]

[40]   Gregor MF, Hotamisligil GS. Inflammatory mechanisms in obesity. Annu Rev Immunol 2011; 29: 415-45.
[http://dx.doi.org/10.1146/annurev-immunol-031210-101322] [PMID: 21219177]

[41]   Jo J, Gavrilova O, Pack S, *et al.* Hypertrophy and/or Hyperplasia: Dynamics of Adipose Tissue Growth. PLOS Comput Biol 2009; 5(3): e1000324.
[http://dx.doi.org/10.1371/journal.pcbi.1000324] [PMID: 19325873]

[42] Meiliana A, Dewi NM, Wijaya A. Adipose tissue, inflammation (meta☐inflammation) and obesity management. Indonesian Biomed J 2015; 7(3): 129-46.
[http://dx.doi.org/10.18585/inabj.v7i3.185]

[43] Fain JN. Release of interleukins and other inflammatory cytokines by human adipose tissue is enhanced in obesity and primarily due to the nonfat cells. Vitam Horm 2006; 74: 443-77.
[http://dx.doi.org/10.1016/S0083-6729(06)74018-3] [PMID: 17027526]

[44] Klein S, Fontana L, Young VL, *et al.* Absence of an effect of liposuction on insulin action and risk factors for coronary heart disease. N Engl J Med 2004; 350(25): 2549-57.
[http://dx.doi.org/10.1056/NEJMoa033179] [PMID: 15201411]

[45] Ziccardi P, Nappo F, Giugliano G, *et al.* Reduction of inflammatory cytokine concentrations and improvement of endothelial functions in obese women after weight loss over one year. Circulation 2002; 105(7): 804-9.
[http://dx.doi.org/10.1161/hc0702.104279] [PMID: 11854119]

[46] Alicka M, Marycz K. The effect of chronic inflammation and oxidative and endoplasmic reticulum stress in the course of metabolic syndrome and its therapy. Stem Cells Int 2018; 2018(9): 4274361.
[http://dx.doi.org/10.1155/2018/4274361] [PMID: 30425746]

[47] Goossens GH, Blaak EE. Adipose tissue dysfunction and impaired metabolic health in human obesity: a matter of oxygen? Front Endocrinol (Lausanne) 2015; 6: 55.
[http://dx.doi.org/10.3389/fendo.2015.00055] [PMID: 25964776]

[48] Johnson AR, Milner JJ, Makowski L. The inflammation highway: metabolism accelerates inflammatory traffic in obesity. Immunol Rev 2012; 249(1): 218-38.
[http://dx.doi.org/10.1111/j.1600-065X.2012.01151.x] [PMID: 22889225]

[49] Ouchi N, Parker JL, Lugus JJ, Walsh K. Adipokines in inflammation and metabolic disease. Nat Rev Immunol 2011; 11(2): 85-97.
[http://dx.doi.org/10.1038/nri2921] [PMID: 21252989]

[50] Chen Y, He D, Yang T, *et al.* Relationship between body composition indicators and risk of type 2 diabetes mellitus in Chinese adults. BMC Public Health 2020; 20(1): 452.
[http://dx.doi.org/10.1186/s12889-020-08552-5] [PMID: 32252701]

[51] Lee L, Sanders RA. Metabolic syndrome. Pediatr Rev 2012; 33(10): 459-66.
[http://dx.doi.org/10.1542/pir.33-10-459] [PMID: 23027600]

[52] Schulman IH, Zhou MS. Vascular insulin resistance: a potential link between cardiovascular and metabolic diseases. Curr Hypertens Rep 2009; 11(1): 48-55.
[http://dx.doi.org/10.1007/s11906-009-0010-0] [PMID: 19146801]

[53] Dragsbæk K, Neergaard JS, Laursen JM, *et al.* Metabolic syndrome and subsequent risk of type 2 diabetes and cardiovascular disease in elderly women: Challenging the current definition. Medicine (Baltimore) 2016; 95(36): e4806.
[http://dx.doi.org/10.1097/MD.0000000000004806] [PMID: 27603394]

[54] The IDF consensus worldwide definition of the metabolic syndrome. [Last accessed on 2018 Avg 01].
http://www.idf.org/webdata/docs/IDF_Meta_def_final.pdf

[55] Eckel RH, Grundy SM, Zimmet PZ. The metabolic syndrome. Lancet 2005; 365(9468): 1415-28.
[http://dx.doi.org/10.1016/S0140-6736(05)66378-7] [PMID: 15836891]

[56] Tran LT, Yuen VG, McNeill JH. The fructose-fed rat: a review on the mechanisms of fructose-induced insulin resistance and hypertension. Mol Cell Biochem 2009; 332(1-2): 145-59.
[http://dx.doi.org/10.1007/s11010-009-0184-4] [PMID: 19536638]

[57] Stafeev IS, Vorotnikov AV, Ratner EI, Menshikov MY, Parfyonova YV. Latent Inflammation and Insulin Resistance in Adipose Tissue. Int J Endocrinol 2017; 2017: 5076732.
[http://dx.doi.org/10.1155/2017/5076732] [PMID: 28912810]

[58]   Karpe F, Dickmann JR, Frayn KN. Fatty acids, obesity, and insulin resistance: time for a reevaluation. Diabetes 2011; 60(10): 2441-9.
[http://dx.doi.org/10.2337/db11-0425] [PMID: 21948998]

[59]   Zatterale F, Longo M, Naderi J, *et al.* Chronic Adipose Tissue Inflammation Linking Obesity to Insulin Resistance and Type 2 Diabetes. Front Physiol 2020; 10: 1607.
[http://dx.doi.org/10.3389/fphys.2019.01607] [PMID: 32063863]

[60]   Rachdaoui N. Insulin: The friend and the foe in the development of type 2 diabetes mellitus. Int J Mol Sci 2020; 21(5): 1770.
[http://dx.doi.org/10.3390/ijms21051770] [PMID: 32150819]

[61]   Stears A, O'Rahilly S, Semple RK, Savage DB. Metabolic insights from extreme human insulin resistance phenotypes. Best Pract Res Clin Endocrinol Metab 2012; 26(2): 145-57.
[http://dx.doi.org/10.1016/j.beem.2011.09.003] [PMID: 22498245]

[62]   Zhang T, Chen J, Tang X, Luo Q, Xu D, Yu B. Interaction between adipocytes and high-density lipoprotein:new insights into the mechanism of obesity-induced dyslipidemia and atherosclerosis. Lipids Health Dis 2019; 18(1): 223.
[http://dx.doi.org/10.1186/s12944-019-1170-9] [PMID: 31842884]

[63]   Fabbrini E, Sullivan S, Klein S. Obesity and nonalcoholic fatty liver disease: biochemical, metabolic, and clinical implications. Hepatology 2010; 51(2): 679-89.
[http://dx.doi.org/10.1002/hep.23280] [PMID: 20041406]

[64]   Trauner M, Arrese M, Wagner M. Fatty liver and lipotoxicity. Biochim Biophys Acta 2010; 1801(3): 299-310.
[http://dx.doi.org/10.1016/j.bbalip.2009.10.007] [PMID: 19857603]

[65]   Cai D, Yuan M, Frantz DF, *et al.* Local and systemic insulin resistance resulting from hepatic activation of IKK-beta and NF-kappaB. Nat Med 2005; 11(2): 183-90.
[http://dx.doi.org/10.1038/nm1166] [PMID: 15685173]

[66]   Popa C, Netea MG, van Riel PL, van der Meer JW, Stalenhoef AF. The role of TNF-alpha in chronic inflammatory conditions, intermediary metabolism, and cardiovascular risk. J Lipid Res 2007; 48(4): 751-62.
[http://dx.doi.org/10.1194/jlr.R600021-JLR200] [PMID: 17202130]

[67]   Harte AL, da Silva NF, Creely SJ, *et al.* Elevated endotoxin levels in non-alcoholic fatty liver disease. J Inflamm (Lond) 2010; 7: 15.
[http://dx.doi.org/10.1186/1476-9255-7-15] [PMID: 20353583]

[68]   Tsochatzis E, Papatheodoridis GV, Archimandritis AJ. The evolving role of leptin and adiponectin in chronic liver diseases. Am J Gastroenterol 2006; 101(11): 2629-40.
[http://dx.doi.org/10.1111/j.1572-0241.2006.00848.x] [PMID: 16952281]

[69]   Koves TR, Ussher JR, Noland RC, *et al.* Mitochondrial overload and incomplete fatty acid oxidation contribute to skeletal muscle insulin resistance. Cell Metab 2008; 7(1): 45-56.
[http://dx.doi.org/10.1016/j.cmet.2007.10.013] [PMID: 18177724]

[70]   Abdul-Ghani MA, DeFronzo RA. Pathogenesis of insulin resistance in skeletal muscle. J Biomed Biotechnol 2010; 2010: 476279.
[http://dx.doi.org/10.1155/2010/476279] [PMID: 20445742]

[71]   Friedrichsen M, Mortensen B, Pehmøller C, Birk JB, Wojtaszewski JF. Exercise-induced AMPK activity in skeletal muscle: role in glucose uptake and insulin sensitivity. Mol Cell Endocrinol 2013; 366(2): 204-14.
[http://dx.doi.org/10.1016/j.mce.2012.06.013] [PMID: 22796442]

[72]   Al-Khalili L, Bouzakri K, Glund S, Lönnqvist F, Koistinen HA, Krook A. Signaling specificity of interleukin-6 action on glucose and lipid metabolism in skeletal muscle. Mol Endocrinol 2006; 20(12): 3364-75.

[http://dx.doi.org/10.1210/me.2005-0490] [PMID: 16945991]

[73]   Li X, Li Z, Zhao M, *et al.* Skeletal muscle lipid droplets and the athlete's paradox. Cells 2019; 8(3): 249.
[http://dx.doi.org/10.3390/cells8030249] [PMID: 30875966]

[74]   Bertaso AG, Bertol D, Duncan BB, Foppa M. Epicardial fat: definition, measurements and systematic review of main outcomes. Arq Bras Cardiol 2013; 101(1): e18-28.
[http://dx.doi.org/10.5935/abc.20130138] [PMID: 23917514]

[75]   Sacks HS, Fain JN, Cheema P, *et al.* Inflammatory genes in epicardial fat contiguous with coronary atherosclerosis in the metabolic syndrome and type 2 diabetes: changes associated with pioglitazone. Diabetes Care 2011; 34(3): 730-3.
[http://dx.doi.org/10.2337/dc10-2083] [PMID: 21289232]

[76]   Yao X, Shan S, Zhang Y, Ying H. Recent progress in the study of brown adipose tissue. Cell Biosci 2011; 1: 35.
[http://dx.doi.org/10.1186/2045-3701-1-35] [PMID: 22035495]

[77]   Albakri A. Obesity cardiomyopathy: a review of literature on clinical status and meta-analysis of diagnostic and clinical management. Med Clin Arch 2018; 2(3): 6-13.
[http://dx.doi.org/10.15761/MCA.1000134]

[78]   Lavie CJ, De Schutter A, Parto P, *et al.* Obesity and prevalence of cardiovascular diseases and prognosis-the obesity paradox updated. Prog Cardiovasc Dis 2016; 58(5): 537-47.
[http://dx.doi.org/10.1016/j.pcad.2016.01.008] [PMID: 26826295]

[79]   Lavie CJ. Obesity and prognosis-just one of many cardiovascular paradoxes? Prog Cardiovasc Dis 2014; 56(4): 367-8.
[http://dx.doi.org/10.1016/j.pcad.2013.10.017] [PMID: 24438727]

[80]   Park J, Ahmadi S-F, Streja E, *et al.* Obesity paradox in end-stage kidney disease patients. Prog Cardiovasc Dis 2014; 56(4): 415-25.
[http://dx.doi.org/10.1016/j.pcad.2013.10.005] [PMID: 24438733]

[81]   Lavie CJ, De Schutter A, Milani RV. Healthy obese *versus* unhealthy lean: the obesity paradox. Nat Rev Endocrinol 2015; 11(1): 55-62.
[http://dx.doi.org/10.1038/nrendo.2014.165] [PMID: 25265977]

[82]   Soleimani M. Insulin resistance and hypertension: new insights. Kidney Int 2015; 87(3): 497-9.
[http://dx.doi.org/10.1038/ki.2014.392] [PMID: 25723632]

[83]   Ormazabal V, Nair S, Elfeky O, Aguayo C, Salomon C, Zuñiga FA. Association between insulin resistance and the development of cardiovascular disease. Cardiovasc Diabetol 2018; 17(1): 122.
[http://dx.doi.org/10.1186/s12933-018-0762-4] [PMID: 30170598]

[84]   Zhou MS, Schulman IH, Raij L. Vascular inflammation, insulin resistance, and endothelial dysfunction in salt-sensitive hypertension: role of nuclear factor kappa B activation. J Hypertens 2010; 28(3): 527-35.
[http://dx.doi.org/10.1097/HJH.0b013e3283340da8] [PMID: 19898250]

[85]   Zhou MS, Wang A, Yu H. Link between insulin resistance and hypertension: What is the evidence from evolutionary biology? Diabetol Metab Syndr 2014; 6(1): 12.
[http://dx.doi.org/10.1186/1758-5996-6-12] [PMID: 24485020]

[86]   Rocchini AP, Katch V, Kveselis D, *et al.* Insulin and renal sodium retention in obese adolescents. Hypertension 1989; 14(4): 367-74.
[http://dx.doi.org/10.1161/01.HYP.14.4.367] [PMID: 2676858]

[87]   Straub RH. Evolutionary medicine and chronic inflammatory state--known and new concepts in pathophysiology. J Mol Med (Berl) 2012; 90(5): 523-34.
[http://dx.doi.org/10.1007/s00109-012-0861-8] [PMID: 22271169]

[88] Muscelli E, Natali A, Bianchi S, *et al.* Effect of insulin on renal sodium and uric acid handling in essential hypertension. Am J Hypertens 1996; 9(8): 746-52.
[http://dx.doi.org/10.1016/0895-7061(96)00098-2] [PMID: 8862220]

[89] Lobato NS, Filgueira FP, Akamine EH, Tostes RC, Carvalho MH, Fortes ZB. Mechanisms of endothelial dysfunction in obesity-associated hypertension. Braz J Med Biol Res 2012; 45(5): 392-400.
[http://dx.doi.org/10.1590/S0100-879X2012007500058] [PMID: 22488221]

[90] Pöykkö SM, Kellokoski E, Hörkkö S, Kauma H, Kesäniemi YA, Ukkola O. Low plasma ghrelin is associated with insulin resistance, hypertension, and the prevalence of type 2 diabetes. Diabetes 2003; 52(10): 2546-53.
[http://dx.doi.org/10.2337/diabetes.52.10.2546] [PMID: 14514639]

[91] Iwashima Y, Katsuya T, Ishikawa K, *et al.* Hypoadiponectinemia is an independent risk factor for hypertension. Hypertension 2004; 43(6): 1318-23.
[http://dx.doi.org/10.1161/01.HYP.0000129281.03801.4b] [PMID: 15123570]

[92] Samad F, Ruf W. Inflammation, obesity, and thrombosis. Blood 2013; 122(20): 3415-22.
[http://dx.doi.org/10.1182/blood-2013-05-427708] [PMID: 24092932]

[93] Gerrits AJ, Koekman CA, van Haeften TW, Akkerman JW. Platelet tissue factor synthesis in type 2 diabetic patients is resistant to inhibition by insulin. Diabetes 2010; 59(6): 1487-95.
[http://dx.doi.org/10.2337/db09-1008] [PMID: 20200314]

[94] Santilli F, Vazzana N, Liani R, Guagnano MT, Davì G. Platelet activation in obesity and metabolic syndrome. Obes Rev 2012; 13(1): 27-42.
[http://dx.doi.org/10.1111/j.1467-789X.2011.00930.x] [PMID: 21917110]

[95] Russo I, Traversa M, Bonomo K, *et al.* In central obesity, weight loss restores platelet sensitivity to nitric oxide and prostacyclin. Obesity (Silver Spring) 2010; 18(4): 788-97.
[http://dx.doi.org/10.1038/oby.2009.302] [PMID: 19834474]

[96] Tichelaar YI, Kluin-Nelemans HJ, Meijer K. Infections and inflammatory diseases as risk factors for venous thrombosis. A systematic review. Thromb Haemost 2012; 107(5): 827-37.
[http://dx.doi.org/10.1160/TH11-09-0611] [PMID: 22437808]

[97] Morange PE, Alessi MC. Thrombosis in central obesity and metabolic syndrome: mechanisms and epidemiology. Thromb Haemost 2013; 110(4): 669-80.
[http://dx.doi.org/10.1160/TH13-01-0075] [PMID: 23765199]

[98] Greco EA, Lenzi A, Migliaccio S. The obesity of bone. Ther Adv Endocrinol Metab 2015; 6(6): 273-86.
[http://dx.doi.org/10.1177/2042018815611004] [PMID: 26623005]

[99] Suh HS, Hwang IC, Lee KS, Kim KK. Relationships between serum osteocalcin, leptin and the effect of weight loss by pharmacological treatment in healthy, nonsmoking Korean obese adults. Clin Chim Acta 2013; 418: 17-21.
[http://dx.doi.org/10.1016/j.cca.2012.11.029] [PMID: 23247052]

[100] Jürimäe J, Rembel K, Jürimäe T, Rehand M. Adiponectin is associated with bone mineral density in perimenopausal women. Horm Metab Res 2005; 37(5): 297-302.
[http://dx.doi.org/10.1055/s-2005-861483] [PMID: 15971153]

[101] Thommesen L, Stunes AK, Monjo M, *et al.* Expression and regulation of resistin in osteoblasts and osteoclasts indicate a role in bone metabolism. J Cell Biochem 2006; 99(3): 824-34.
[http://dx.doi.org/10.1002/jcb.20915] [PMID: 16721825]

[102] Francisco V, Pino J, Campos-Cabaleiro V, *et al.* Obesity, fat mass and Immune system: Role for Leptin. Front Physiol 2018; 9: 640.
[http://dx.doi.org/10.3389/fphys.2018.00640] [PMID: 29910742]

[103]   Wang H, Leng Y, Gong Y. Bone marrow fat and hematopoiesis. Front Endocrinol (Lausanne) 2018; 9: 694.
[http://dx.doi.org/10.3389/fendo.2018.00694] [PMID: 30546345]

[104]   Tang J, Yan H, Zhuang S. Inflammation and oxidative stress in obesity-related glomerulopathy. Int J Nephrol 2012; 2012: 608397.
[http://dx.doi.org/10.1155/2012/608397] [PMID: 22567283]

[105]   Naderpoor N, Lyons JG, Mousa A, *et al.* Higher glomerular filtration rate is related to insulin resistance but not to obesity in a predominantly obese non-diabetic cohort. Sci Rep 2017; 7: 45522. [published correctionappears in Sci Rep. 2018 Mar 19;8:46962].
[http://dx.doi.org/10.1038/srep45522] [PMID: 28368024]

[106]   Lee J, Kim HJ, Cho B, *et al.* Abdominal adipose tissue was associated with glomerular hyperfiltration among non-diabetic and normotensive adults with a normal Body Mass Index. PLoS One 2015; 10(10): e0141364.
[http://dx.doi.org/10.1371/journal.pone.0141364] [PMID: 26495973]

[107]   Chen HM, Liu ZH, Zeng CH, Li SJ, Wang QW, Li LS. Podocyte lesions in patients with obesity-related glomerulopathy. Am J Kidney Dis 2006; 48(5): 772-9.
[http://dx.doi.org/10.1053/j.ajkd.2006.07.025] [PMID: 17059996]

[108]   van Vliet-Ostaptchouk JV, Nuotio ML, Slagter SN, *et al.* The prevalence of metabolic syndrome and metabolically healthy obesity in Europe: a collaborative analysis of ten large cohort studies. BMC Endocr Disord 2014; 14: 9.
[http://dx.doi.org/10.1186/1472-6823-14-9] [PMID: 24484869]

[109]   Tsatsoulis A, Paschou SA. Metabolically obesity: criteria, epidemiology, contraversis, snd consequences. Curr Obes Rep 2020; 9(2): 109-20.
[http://dx.doi.org/10.1007/s13679-020-00375-0] [PMID: 32301039]

[110]   Bala C, Craciun AE, Hancu N. Updating the concept of metabolically healthy obesity. Acta Endocrinol (Bucur) 2016; 12(2): 197-205.
[http://dx.doi.org/10.4183/aeb.2016.197] [PMID: 31149087]

[111]   National Cholesterol Education Program (NCEP) Expert Panel on Detection, Evaluation, and Treatment of High Blood Cholesterol in Adults (Adult Treatment Panel III). Third report of the national cholesterol education program (NCEP) expert panel on detection, evaluation, and treatment of high blood cholesterol in adults (adult treatment panel III) final report. Circulation 2002; 106(25): 3143-421.
[http://dx.doi.org/10.1161/circ.106.25.3143] [PMID: 12485966]

[112]   Cătoi AF, Pârvu AE, Andreicuț AD, *et al.* Metabolically healthy *versus* unhealthy morbidly obese: chronic inflammation, nitro-oxidative stress, and insulin resistance. Nutrients 2018; 10(9): 1199.
[http://dx.doi.org/10.3390/nu10091199] [PMID: 30200422]

[113]   Primeau V, Coderre L, Karelis AD, *et al.* Characterizing the profile of obese patients who are metabolically healthy. Int J Obes 2011; 35(7): 971-81.
[http://dx.doi.org/10.1038/ijo.2010.216] [PMID: 20975726]

[114]   Pujia A, Gazzaruso C, Ferro Y, *et al.* Individuals with metabolically healthy overweight/obesity have higher fat utilization than metabolically unhealthy individuals. Nutrients 2016; 8(1): 1.
[http://dx.doi.org/10.3390/nu8010002] [PMID: 26742056]

[115]   Kissebah AH, Vydelingum N, Murray R, *et al.* Relation of body fat distribution to metabolic complications of obesity. J Clin Endocrinol Metab 1982; 54(2): 254-60.
[http://dx.doi.org/10.1210/jcem-54-2-254] [PMID: 7033275]

[116]   Stefan N, Kantartzis K, Machann J, *et al.* Identification and characterization of metabolically benign obesity in humans. Arch Intern Med 2008; 168(15): 1609-16.
[http://dx.doi.org/10.1001/archinte.168.15.1609] [PMID: 18695074]

[117] Messier V, Karelis AD, Robillard ME, *et al.* Metabolically healthy but obese individuals: relationship with hepatic enzymes. Metabolism 2010; 59(1): 20-4.
[http://dx.doi.org/10.1016/j.metabol.2009.06.020] [PMID: 19709695]

[118] Phillips CM. Metabolically healthy obesity across the life course: epidemiology, determinants, and implications. Ann N Y Acad Sci 2017; 1391(1): 85-100.
[http://dx.doi.org/10.1111/nyas.13230] [PMID: 27723940]

[119] Snel M, Jonker JT, Schoones J, *et al.* Ectopic fat and insulin resistance: pathophysiology and effect of diet and lifestyle interventions. Int J Endocrinol 2012; 2012: 983814.
[http://dx.doi.org/10.1155/2012/983814] [PMID: 22675355]

[120] Karelis AD, Faraj M, Bastard JP, *et al.* The metabolically healthy but obese individual presents a favorable inflammation profile. J Clin Endocrinol Metab 2005; 90(7): 4145-50.
[http://dx.doi.org/10.1210/jc.2005-0482] [PMID: 15855252]

[121] Shin MJ, Hyun YJ, Kim OY, Kim JY, Jang Y, Lee JH. Weight loss effect on inflammation and LDL oxidation in metabolically healthy but obese (MHO) individuals: low inflammation and LDL oxidation in MHO women. Int J Obes 2006; 30(10): 1529-34.
[http://dx.doi.org/10.1038/sj.ijo.0803304] [PMID: 16552406]

[122] Loos RJ. Integrating publicly available genome-wide association data to study the genetic basis of metabolically healthy obese and metabolically obese but normal-weight individuals. Diabetes 2014; 63(12): 4004-7.
[http://dx.doi.org/10.2337/db14-1358] [PMID: 25414016]

[123] Magkos F. Metabolically healthy obesity: what's in a name? Am J Clin Nutr 2019; 110(3): 533-9.
[http://dx.doi.org/10.1093/ajcn/nqz133] [PMID: 31240297]

[124] Blüher M. Metabolically healthy obesity. Endocr Rev 2020; 41(3): 405-20.

CHAPTER 6

Gender Differences in Obesity - Related Type 2 Diabetes: Possible Role of Meta-inflammation

Nermina Babić[*]

Department of Human Physiology, Faculty of Medicine, University of Sarajevo, Sarajevo, Bosnia and Herzegovina

Abstract: Biological and psychosocial differences between men and women affect the epidemiology and pathophysiology of many diseases, including type 2 diabetes mellitus (T2DM). Obesity is a major risk factor for T2DM. Sex hormones, estrogens, and androgens contribute to gender differences in obesity-related T2DM since they regulate not only biological characteristics but also adipose tissue function and metabolism. Obesity, in particular visceral obesity, is characterized by systemic low-grade inflammation or meta-inflammation. Meta-inflammation that occurs locally in adipose tissue becomes systemic *via* the release of various active inflammatory cytokines and acute-phase proteins, including TNF- α, interleukins 1β, 6, 17, and C-reactive protein (CRP) into the bloodstream and consequently leads to insulin resistance. Understanding the differences between sex and gender is equally important in the prevention of obesity-related T2DM, its diagnosis and therapy. The initial stages of meta-inflammation involve adipocyte hypertrophy, hypoxia and cellular stress. Studies on the role of gender differences in obesity-induced inflammatory response have shown that males have a greater inflammatory response in adipose tissue, increased adipocyte apoptosis and macrophage infiltration, greater accumulation of pro-inflammatory adipose tissue macrophages and increased expression of inflammatory cytokines. These data suggest that adipose tissue in males is more susceptible to inflammation when compared to females and that this might lead to a higher incidence of insulin resistance. It is still debated whether oxidative stress is more pronounced in women than in men with T2DM. However, in female patients with T2DM, serum levels of IL-6, TNF-α and CRP were significantly higher compared to males with T2DM. Gender differences have a major impact on the development and the progression of obesity-related T2DM and its complications. Future studies should contribute to a better understanding of gender differences in obesity-related T2DM and differences in the inflammatory response between men and women to establish prevention and treatment of diabetes by gender-related guidelines.

Keywords: Adipose tissue, Gender differences, Obesity, Sex hormones, Type 2 diabetes mellitus.

[*] **Corresponding author Nermina Babić**: Department of Human Physiology, Faculty of Medicine, University of Sarajevo, Sarajevo, Bosnia and Herzegovina; Tel: +387 33 226 478, Ext. 523; E-mail: nermina.babic@mf.unsa.ba

Asija Začiragić (Ed.)

INTRODUCTION

Obesity is a chronic inflammatory disease characterized by the accumulation of excess fat in an amount that has negative effects on health. Excessive energy intake and reduced physical activity are the most important causes of obesity [1]. Although food intake is precisely controlled by physiological mechanisms, numerous environmental, psychological, and social factors can cause eating disorders. Obesity is a major risk factor for type 2 diabetes mellitus (T2DM) [2]. The current data point to a significant impact of gender on the prevalence of obesity and T2DM [3]. At a younger age, the prevalence of diabetes is higher in men than in women, but the prevalence of diabetes increases significantly in postmenopausal women due to estrogen deficiency [4]. Women have greater difficulty in achieving target haemoglobin A1c (HbA1c) levels and their glycemic control is worse than in men [5]. Because the development of T2DM complications is directly associated with glycemic control, it follows that women have more common and more severe diabetes-related complications than men [6]. Obesity-related T2DM accompanied by complications represents a significant clinical as well as an economic problem due to high treatment costs [5, 7].

Sex and gender differences affect the epidemiology and pathophysiology of many diseases, including T2DM [8]. It is clear that gender differences should also be considered in the treatment of diabetes mellitus, as well as the influence of many other factors such as psychological factors, treatment response, differences in the glucose and energy homeostasis between men and women.

Distinguishing sex from gender can be difficult, so the term sex-gender is sometimes interchangeably used in the literature [9]. The term sex differences describe biological differences between males and females, including variations in sex hormones and their effects. The word gender refers to the psychosocial differences between the sexes such as societal norms, roles, lifestyles, relationships, cultural and behavioural expectations associated with being a man or woman [3, 10].

The problem with recognizing sex-gender differences is related to the fact that in most clinical and epidemiological studies, women are underrepresented. For years, in both human and animal studies, only males were included due to the unwanted effects of sex hormones. The results of those studies conducted on male sex/gender were simply applied to women. Many of the physiological values in the human body are based on research involving only healthy young men [9]. Also, most guidelines for the treatment of diabetes mellitus and various other diseases are based on the studies conducted mainly in adult men.

Understanding the differences between sex and gender is equally important in the prevention of obesity-related T2DM, its diagnosis and therapy.

DIABETES MELLITUS TYPE 2

Diabetes mellitus is a condition of chronic hyperglycemia, characterized by impaired metabolism of carbohydrates, proteins and fats resulting from a defect in insulin secretion and/or insulin action [11]. The most common form of diabetes is type 2 diabetes mellitus (T2DM), affecting mainly adults. It represents between 85 and 90% of all cases of diabetes [11, 12]. An increasing number of children are overweight and inactive, so T2DM is increasingly being diagnosed in young adults and children [13].

Type 2 diabetes mellitus is a fast-growing disease and a significant global health problem because it affects a large population worldwide [14, 15]. The etiology of T2DM is multifactorial. The development of the disease is associated with a family history of diabetes [16]. The incidence of disease increases with age, obesity, lack of exercise, unhealthy diet and stress [2, 17]. Genetic background and physical inactivity are two primary etiological components [18]. Most patients with this form of diabetes are obese or have an increased percentage of abdominal body fat [19].

Chronic hyperglycemia mainly affects eyes, nerves, kidneys and heart, causing damage to them and if untreated, leads to severe complications, such as ketoacidosis as acute and retinopathy, neuropathy, nephropathy, and cardiovascular diseases as chronic complications [2, 20, 21]. It has been found that patients with diabetes mellitus have a two- to threefold greater risk of cardiovascular disease as complications of the underlying disease [22]. Additionally, diabetes mellitus associated with cardiovascular complications is a major clinical problem as more than 75% of patients with diabetes die from cardiovascular diseases [23].

Persistent hyperglycemia is confirmed as the primary cause of diabetic complications, so the risk of complications depends on glycemic control and the duration of disease. The disorders that commonly occur with diabetes, especially high blood pressure and lipid abnormalities, exacerbate many diabetic complications [24].

PATHOGENESIS OF OBESITY-RELATED TYPE 2 DIABETES MELLITUS AND INSULIN RESISTANCE

The main pathophysiological characteristics of T2DM are impaired insulin secretion, decreased glucose uptake, insulin resistance in peripheral tissues (liver, muscle and fat) and increased hepatic glucose production [25].

This form of diabetes often remains undiagnosed for many years because many patients exhibit normal glucose tolerance at the beginning of their disease. There is increased production and secretion of insulin from pancreatic β-cells. So, hyperinsulinemia is present in a so-called "compensated" phase. As long as β-cells are able to increase insulin secretion and while there is a major reserve of these cells in the pancreas, normal glucose tolerance will be maintained. Over time, β-cell exhaustion develops, and they become unable to produce adequate amounts of insulin to maintain normal insulin secretion. This is followed by a relative, rather than absolute, insulin deficiency in peripheral tissues [26, 27]. At first, impaired glucose tolerance (IGT) occurs, characterized by elevated postprandial glucose, and later, due to increased liver glucose production, persistent hyperglycemia ensues [28].

Impaired insulin secretion and peripheral insulin resistance precedes the development of T2DM, and occur even 5 to 10 years before diabetes. The term insulin resistance refers to an impairment in insulin action in tissues that are the principal targets of glucose and lipid metabolism [29]. Those insulin-sensitive tissues are skeletal muscle, adipocytes, and liver. In these tissues, insulin resistance has major effects [30]. It reduces glucose uptake, impairs glycogen synthesis, and protein catabolism in skeletal muscles. In adipocytes, it inhibits lipoprotein lipase activity due to increased release of free fatty acids (FFA) and inflammatory cytokines as tumour necrosis factor- alpha (TNF-α), interleukin 6 (IL-6), and leptin from adipose tissue [29].

In normal physiological conditions, the liver acts as a buffer in maintaining glucose homeostasis by keeping blood glucose concentration within its normal range. After a meal, when blood glucose concentration is high, glucose enters hepatocytes and is converted into glycogen. Between meals, when blood glucose concentration falls below normal, stored glycogen is cleaved into glucose and released [31]. However, impaired insulin action in the liver leads to insulin resistance that is followed by reduced glycogen synthesis, gluconeogenesis, and hyperglycemia. At the same time, increases FFA derived from adipose tissue stimulates hepatic lipogenesis and very-low-density lipoprotein (VLDL) and triglyceride (TG) overproduction [32].

Numerous factors such as obesity, especially visceral adiposity, and a sedentary lifestyle affect the development of insulin resistance and T2DM [33]. Obesity, however, is a major cause of insulin resistance. Insulin resistance is triggered by cellular disturbances, such as inflammation, lipotoxicity, glucotoxicity, and oxidative stress that lead to impaired insulin and insulin-like growth factor 1 (IGF-1) receptor action by multiple mechanisms [34]. An important mechanism that induces insulin resistance in obesity is the inflammatory reaction in adipose tissue [35].

OBESITY

Obesity and overweight are defined as conditions of excessive fat accumulation in the body that presents a health risk [36]. The prevalence of overweight and obesity is rapidly rising worldwide, both in developing and developed countries, making it a major public health problem [37]. The epidemic of overweight and obesity has led to an increase in obesity-related diseases such as T2DM, metabolic syndrome, hypertension, dyslipidemia, cardiovascular disease, non-alcoholic fatty liver disease, some types of cancers *etc* [38]. All of these diseases represent important clinical problems but also constitute an enormous economic problem due to their high health costs. Studies have shown that the dysfunction of adipose tissue has an important role in these diseases [39, 40].

In recent years, it has been debated whether obesity is a disease. Our current knowledge about adipose tissue supports the fact that obesity is a chronic inflammatory disease, closely related to T2DM, heart disease, and cancer [41, 42]. Many studies have been conducted to identify factors that influence the development of obesity and obesity-induced diseases. Since the discovery that the ob gene encodes for the synthesis of leptin, an interest in the effects of genetics on obesity development has grown [43]. Although genetics play a significant role in body weight regulation, positive energy balance is a crucial factor in the development of obesity [44]. Excess energy intake and reduced energy expenditure because of sedentary lifestyle are the most important etiologic factors for obesity. In obese individuals, appetite and caloric ingestion may be impaired. Obese individuals have elevated plasma leptin levels and leptin resistance, which can be caused by impairment in leptin synthesis by adipocytes, impairment in leptin binding protein, and impairment of the brain leptin receptor [43, 45].

Obesity is characterized by a body mass index (BMI) greater than 30 kg/m^2. However, BMI does not directly provide information about the amount of body fat, nor does it take into account the individual's body structure, the proportion of muscle and bone mass, so its use is limited [46, 47]. Waist circumference (WC) and waist-to-hip ratio are better indices of abdominal fat distribution [48]. Abdominal obesity is defined as waist circumference >88 cm for women, and >102 cm for men. Those values also indicate a very high risk for the development of cardiovascular disease [46, 49].

ADIPOSE TISSUE

For many years, adipose tissue was only considered as energy storage, a thermal insulator, and mechanical support, but is now recognized as an endocrine and secretory organ. It secretes numerous bioactive substances and hormones, adipokines, through which it is involved in the control of food intake, the regulation of energy homeostasis, thermogenesis, immune and neuroendocrine processes in the organism [35].

It has been suggested that more than 600 secretory proteins are secreted from adipose tissue and several of them play an important role in glucose homeostasis [50]. There are two structurally and functionally differentiated types of adipose tissue in humans: white and brown. Brown adipose tissue (BAT), specialized in heat production, is found at birth but is almost absent in adult humans. Recent studies using PET-CT scans have shown that BAT can be found in adults in the fascial plane, in the ventral trunk, and sternocleidomastoid muscles. They also reported sex differences in the BAT mass, women having more BAT than men [51, 52].

Adult adipose tissue is predominantly white and is divided into two major depots: subcutaneous, located under the skin, and visceral which is concentrated in the abdominal cavity around internal organs [53]. Subcutaneous adipose tissue compromises approximately 80% of total body fat and can be divided into peripheral and central subcutaneous fat and, superficial and deep subcutaneous fat. Visceral adipose tissue compromises approximately 20% of total body fat and is generally considered as "bad" fat [35, 54]. This tissue is characterized by higher secretion of pro-inflammatory cytokines and lower secretion of adiponectin than subcutaneous fat. It secretes adipokines into the portal blood stream where they enter the liver, which is why its metabolic effect is greater than subcutaneous adipose tissue, which secretes adipokines into the central blood stream [46]. Visceral adipose tissue is associated with insulin resistance [55], high triglyceride levels, high blood pressure, and increased risk of diabetes and cardiovascular diseases [56].

There are additional fat depots that are usually called ectopic fat. They include pericardial, perivascular, epicardial, intramuscular, and intrahepatic fat depots. They play a major role in cardiovascular disease, the local inflammatory response, as well as in insulin resistance [57]. In individuals with central (abdominal) obesity who have a large amount of visceral fat, ectopic depots are more abundant.

Adipose tissue is composed of adipocytes, cells specialized in the storage of triglyceride fat, but also contains many different cell types called the stromal vascular fraction of cells, such as adipocytes precursors, fibroblasts, vascular cells, neuronal cells, and a variety of immune cells such as adipose tissue macrophages [58]. Excessive accumulation of adipose tissue in obese individuals is caused mainly by an enlargement of pre-existing, fully differentiated adipocytes storing an excess of fat [59, 60]. Excessive fat accumulation leads to adipocyte hypertrophy and hyperplasia, which significantly affects their metabolic properties. The change in the number and activity of adipocytes activates firstly the local inflammatory response and later on systemic inflammatory response [61].

META-INFLAMMATION IN OBESITY

Overweight and obesity, mostly visceral obesity is characterized by systemic low-grade inflammation. This metabolic-triggered inflammation is referred to as "meta-inflammation" or "metaflammation" [59, 60].

Research over the past few decades has shown that the main source of obesity-related inflammation is white adipose tissue. The initial signal for the inflammatory response of adipose tissue is believed to be chronic over-nutrition and excessive caloric intake [38, 62]. As a result of the difference between energy intake and output, adipocytes accumulate large amounts of fatty acids and expand. Excessive accumulation of adipose tissue is associated with metabolic stress responses in adipocytes followed by activation of the innate immune system [59, 60]. An inflammatory response is likely to be limited or absent if excessive fat accumulates mainly in superficial subcutaneous adipose tissue. However, if fat accumulates in abdominal and ectopic depots, a low-grade inflammatory response will develop [54].

Chronic low-grade inflammation that occurs locally in the adipose tissue becomes systemic by releasing various pro-inflammatory mediators into the bloodstream and consequently leads to insulin resistance [63].

It is thought that insulin resistance is a major cause of developing obesity-related T2DM and other endocrine and metabolic disorders associated with obesity. In obesity, adipose tissue is the primary site of inflammation but is not the only source of cytokine production. The liver, pancreas, brain, and probably muscles also participate in the inflammatory response.

Obesity-induced inflammation has significant differences compared to classic inflammation [59, 64]. Obesity-induced inflammation does not occur as a consequence of infection or injury. The inflammatory trigger is metabolic and is caused by excessive nutrient intake. The inflammatory state in obesity-induced inflammation is accompanied by a reduced metabolic rate, while classic inflammation is always associated with an increased local or systemic metabolic rate. Its duration is longer than in classic inflammation. When compared to classic inflammation, which is frequently transient and resolves quickly, obesity-induced inflammation is progressive and persistent over time. While classic inflammation is characterized by a local reaction, obesity-induced inflammation is characterized by systemic inflammation of insulin-sensitive tissues followed by elevated levels of active circulating inflammatory cytokines and acute-phase proteins, including TNF- α, interleukins 1β, 6, and 17, and C-reactive protein (CRP) [59, 64] (Fig. 1).

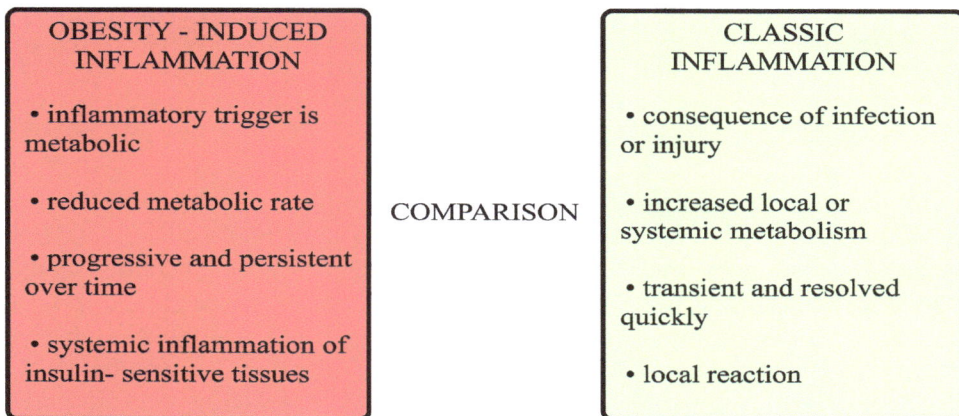

OBESITY - INDUCED INFLAMMATION		CLASSIC INFLAMMATION
• inflammatory trigger is metabolic • reduced metabolic rate • progressive and persistent over time • systemic inflammation of insulin- sensitive tissues	COMPARISON	• consequence of infection or injury • increased local or systemic metabolism • transient and resolved quickly • local reaction

Fig. (1). Comparison between obesity-induced and classic inflammation.

MECHANISMS OF META-INFLAMMATION IN OBESITY

The exact mechanisms underlying the initial stages of obesity-induced, low-grade inflammatory processes is unclear, but it is believed that it can involve: adipocyte hypertrophy, hypoxia, and cellular stress [41].

Hypertrophic and hyperplastic adipocytes secrete various cytokines and chemokines that attract monocytes from the circulation into adipose tissue where they differentiate into macrophages [65]. Cytokines such as TNF-α, monocyte chemotactic protein 1 (MCP-1), and macrophage inhibitory factor 1 (MIF-1) are able to attract macrophages and lymphocytes. They also play a central role in the activation of immune cells [66]. These pro-inflammatory mediators are initially secreted by adipocytes, but as adipose tissue expands, they are also secreted by infiltrated macrophages. So, the infiltration of adipose tissue is mainly composed of macrophages and secondarily cytotoxic T lymphocytes. There are few mast cells and neutrophils, while eosinophils and several subsets of T lymphocytes are reduced [67].

Among the immune cells, polarized macrophage activation appears to play a pivotal role in local and systemic chronic inflammation [68]. Macrophages in adipose tissue are mostly derived from the bone marrow. Their number is increased in obesity. In comparing lean to obese adipose tissue, the number of macrophages increases from 10% to up to 40% [66, 69].

In adipose tissue, there are two types of macrophages: pro-inflammatory a "classically-activated" phenotype of macrophages (M1), and anti-inflammatory, an "alternatively-activated" phenotype (M2). In adipose tissue of obese individuals, the number of M1 macrophages is increased, while the number of M2 macrophages is decreased. By increasing M1 macrophages, the amount of pro-inflammatory cytokines also increases. In addition to classical M1 and M2 macrophages, adipose tissue also consists of a mixed macrophages population with a pro-inflammatory phenotype that promotes adipose tissue fibrosis and insulin resistance [66, 70, 71]. Activated M1 macrophages are potent effectors cells that secrete pro-inflammatory factors such as TNF-α, IL-1β, IL-6, IL-12, IL-18, IL-23, and MCP-1. These cytokines, particularly TNF-α, IL-1β, and IL-6 are important inflammatory mediators and can directly induce and enhance insulin resistance in adipocytes, muscle, and liver cells [2]. M1 macrophages also induce production of nitric oxide (NO) and reactive oxygen species (ROS) which play important regulatory roles in obesity-associated chronic inflammation [71]. M2 macrophages have an anti-inflammatory phenotype. They secrete a high amount of anti-inflammatory cytokines such as IL-10 and TGF-β, as well as low amount of pro-inflammatory cytokines. They help regenerate, heal damaged tissues, and maintain tissue homeostasis [35, 72].

In addition to cytokines, metabolic signals, such as FFAs activate the innate immune system through the activation of pattern recognition receptors leading to stimulation of inflammatory signalling cascades [60].

The renin-angiotensin system (RAS) that is activated locally and systemically in obese individuals may also contribute to immune cell activation and inflammation [73].

Expansion of adipose tissue and adipocyte hypertrophy may be associated with local hypoxia because of poor vascularisation. Consequently, hypoxia occurs in adipocytes that are located away from blood vessels. Hypoxic conditions result in necrosis and cell death. Macrophages in adipose tissue are overrepresented around dead adipocytes arranged in cell aggregates referred to as "crown-like structures" [64, 74]. They remove dying cells and contribute to tissue angiogenesis. Fatty acids stored in hypertrophic adipocytes may cause lipid peroxidation that induces oxidative stress and consequently rises reactive oxygen species [75]. These molecules attract many immunological cells which are followed by a rise in TNF-α and leptin levels, and a decrease in adiponectin and IL-10 levels.

Eventually, by releasing various pro-inflammatory mediators into the bloodstream, the inflammation that occurs locally in adipose tissue becomes systemic, affecting other insulin-dependent tissue. The progressive insulin resistance develops as a central pathophysiological consequence. Furthermore, as long-term consequences of low-grade inflammation, inflammatory processes in other tissues and organs occur. The inflammation of pancreatic islets plays an important role in obesity-related T2DM. A lot of mechanisms may induce inflammation and β-cell dysfunction, such as chronic hyperglycemia, chronic hyperlipidemia, oxidative stress and, inflammatory cytokines [18].

GENDER DIFFERENCES IN GLYCEMIC CONTROL AND FOOD INTAKE

Gender differences arise from the socio-cultural backgrounds, such as behavioural differences, exposure to specific environmental factors, various forms of nutrition, lifestyles or prevention, and treatment attitudes [3].

Under normal conditions, there are gender differences in both fasting plasma glucose levels and plasma glucose levels during the oral glucose tolerance test (OGTT). Healthy men have higher levels of fasting plasma glucose and healthy women have higher levels of 2h plasma glucose during OGTT. These differences might be explained in part by the fact that men have greater muscle mass and faster gut glucose absorption compared to women [76]. It is possible that insulin sensitivity and pancreatic β-cell function are also different between men and women [77].

Gender differences are responsible for differences in the neural control of energy homeostasis. Food intake and body weight are controlled by various brain areas like the ventromedial hypothalamus, lateral hypothalamus, and arcuate nucleus [78]. Animal studies have shown that the influence of the ventromedial hypothalamus on control of food intake and body weight gain differs between male and female rats. Lesions to the ventromedial hypothalamus resulted in increased food intake and body weight gain in both male and female rats. Food intake was, however, more prominent in females, while body weight gain was more prominent in male rats. Therefore, it was suggested that the ventromedial hypothalamus in male rats exerts less influence on food intake but rather favours adipose tissue accumulation. It is also assumed that changes in energy homeostasis in ventromedial hypothalamus lesion are primarily due to neural control driven by increased parasympathetic and decreased sympathetic activity and not hyperphagia [79].

In the normal physiological state, leptin is involved in the regulation of energy balance and food intake. It inhibits appetite by acting on neurons in the hypothalamus. Also, in peripheral tissues, leptin promotes lipid oxidation and mitochondrial biogenesis and accelerates energy expenditure by signals and regulating factors derived from the brain. Leptin production is elevated in obesity, but its actions are impaired due to hypothalamic leptin resistance [80, 81].

Adiponectin is a cytokine that improves insulin sensitivity by increasing the oxidation of fatty acids and reducing the production of glucose in the liver. In contrast to leptin, its plasma level is decreased in obese individuals [81, 82].

Glycemic control in diabetes has been shown to reduce the risk of long-term complications. Compared with diabetic men, women usually have poorer glycemic control and are less likely to achieve target HbA1c levels. Alterations in energy and glucose homeostasis, treatment response, and psychological factors could be possible reasons for these gender differences [5, 83].

GENDER DIFFERENCES IN THE ETIOLOGY AND EPIDEMIOLOGY OF OBESITY-RELATED T2DM

Biological and psychosocial differences between men and women have a major impact on the development, progression of obesity-related T2DM and their complications.

The incidence of diabetes increases with age in both sexes and more than half of diabetes patients are middle-aged [2]. The overall number of women with T2DM is 10% higher than in men, although global diabetes prevalence is higher in men. This is primarily due to the fact that females are more likely to be diagnosed with diabetes after the age of menopause and the number of elderly women is higher than elderly men [12].

The number of women with impaired glucose tolerance (IGT) is higher than in men, accounting up to about 20% of cases [9]. Conversely, impaired fasting glucose (IFG) is more prevalent in men. These differences might be influenced by gonadal hormones [84].

A previous prospective study found that the occurrence of T2DM in both sexes was accompanied by an increased in the liver enzymes alanine aminotransferase (ALT), aspartate aminotransferase (AST), and/or glutamyl transferase (GGT). Comparing to other enzymes, GGT is most strongly association with T2DM, since GGT is more closely associated with fatty liver, oxidative stress, and insulin resistance [3, 85].

Risk factors more prevalent in women are elevated triglycerides and physical inactivity, whereas smoking, alcohol consumption and systolic hypertension are more common in men [86, 87].

Differences in genetic polymorphisms between genders might also play a role in the etiology and development of diabetes [88]. Physiological conditions specific to women, such as pregnancy and menopause, have an impact on appetite and weight regulation, which lead to an elevated obesity risk. A recent study conducted in China reported that women in the early menopausal period, those less than 45 years old, have a higher risk of diabetes compared to women during menopause, which usually starts at the age of 50 [89].

Obesity is a major and independent diabetes risk factor. In general, the prevalence of obesity is higher in women than in men [89]. It should be noted that obese women have a higher risk for T2DM compared to obese men, but the explanation for these differences remains unclear. It may be related to amount and distribution of fat [90, 91].

GENDER DIFFERENCES IN IMMUNOLOGICAL RESPONSE

Studies about gender differences in immunological response are limited because most of the studies were performed on male subjects. In general, women tolerate the immune response to infection better compared to men [92].

The results of some previous studies have shown that males have a greater inflammatory responses in adipose tissue. A study on the animal models showed increased adipocyte apoptosis and macrophage infiltration in males, whereas female animals had increased ability to expand adiposity [39] (Fig. **2**).

Another animal study, which included male mice on a fatty diet, has shown greater accumulation of pro-inflammatory adipose tissue macrophages (M1) and increased expression of inflammatory cytokines [93]. These data suggest that adipose tissue in males is more susceptible to inflammation compared to females, which could lead to a higher incidence of insulin resistance [93, 94].

Medrikova *et al*. [95] have shown similar results in their study. Long-term high-fat diets in female mice induced increased capacity for adipocyte enlargement and reduced adipose tissue macrophage infiltration, possibly indicating higher adipocyte insulin sensitivity in females. This result is unexpected because it is generally believed that adipocyte hypertrophy is associated with macrophage infiltration and adipose tissue inflammation. Despite sexual dimorphism in macrophage infiltration and inflammatory marker gene expression in adipose tissue, plasma levels of TNF-α, interleukin-6, interleukin-1β, and MCP-1 in male and female mice were similar [95, 96].

Clinical studies also indicate that men and women with polycystic ovary syndrome have more adipose tissue macrophages compared to premenopausal women [39].

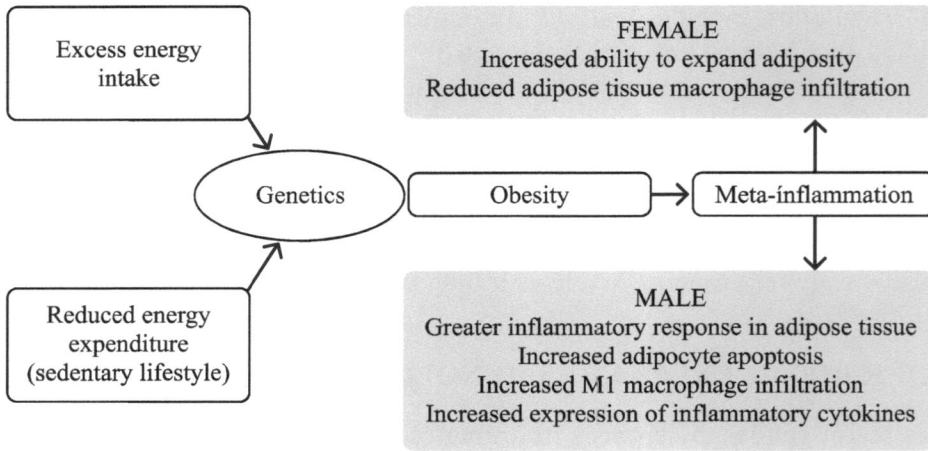

Fig. (2). Gender differences in immunological response in adipose tissue.

Oxidative stress plays an important role in the progression of diabetes and in the development of T2DM-related complications. Some studies indicate that oxidative stress is higher in women than in men with T2DM [9], but there is evidence that in both subcutaneous and gonadal fat tissue, oxidative stress markers are increased in males [39].

Inflammatory biomarkers, such as TNF, IL-6, and CRP, are elevated in insulin resistance and could predict the development of T2DM [97]. Plasma levels of TNF-α increase with age. It was reported that TNF-α and IL-6 induce insulin resistance by inhibiting lipoprotein lipase [98]. Accumulation of body fat leads to increased production of these cytokines that stimulate the production of CRP in the liver [99].

Some previous studies have explored sex differences in inflammatory cytokines in T2DM. Akash *et al.* [100] showed that serum levels of IL-6, TNF-α, and CRP in female diabetic patients were significantly higher compared to male diabetic patients and concluded that female diabetic patients were more prone to the increased levels of inflammatory biomarkers than male diabetic patients. They also found a significant association between inflammatory biomarkers and the development of insulin resistance. Serum level of TNF-α in females and serum levels of TNF-α and CRP in males had higher predictive values in the development of insulin resistance.

C-reactive protein is a sensitive marker of systemic inflammation. Elevated CRP levels are often observed in the elderly, overweight, and obese patients, and people who are less physically active [101]. Most studies have confirmed a significant role of CRP in cardiovascular risk assessment [102]. A recent study found that CRP was significantly higher in T2DM patients than in non-diabetic subjects, but there was no significant difference in CRP levels between diabetic males and females [101]. In another study, CRP and IL-6 levels in T2DM patients were significantly elevated compared to healthy subjects, but there was no association with T2DM duration, age, or gender [103].

In our previous study, we observed that serum CRP concentration was significantly higher in female compared to male patients with T2DM. The observed difference was explained as a result of obesity which is generally more frequently seen in women [99].

A study that involved newly diagnosed patients with T2DM found that 40% of patients had elevated levels of CRP that were independently associated with central obesity mainly in women. Interestingly, the administration of statins reduced the risk of elevated CRP, but only in women. These findings point to the importance of gender-specific treatment of patients with T2DM [104].

ADIPOSE TISSUE AS A MODULATOR OF META-INFLAMMATORY RESPONSES IN MEN AND WOMEN

By secreting many cytokines, adipose tissue plays an important role in sex-gender differences in meta-inflammatory responses. Additionally, the differing locations of fat stores in men and women may contribute to gender differences in meta-inflammation.

Intra-abdominal visceral adipose tissue is more likely to enhance the development of metabolic disorders, such as metabolic syndrome, insulin resistance, and T2DM compared to subcutaneous adipose tissue. Men accumulate more visceral fat, which is stored in the abdominal depot giving them an apple shape, which can lead to higher metabolic and cardiovascular risk.

Women with the same body mass index have 10% higher overall total body fat content compared to men. Significantly, females accumulate more fat in subcutaneous depots prior to menopause, a feature that protects against the negative effects of obesity and gives them a pear shape. After menopause, women tend to accumulate fat in the visceral depot that can lead to increased metabolic risk [105, 106]. In premenopausal women, obesity-related metabolic disorders, such as T2DM, are much lower compared to men, despite the higher level of body fat.

Gender differences in fat accumulation are more pronounced in groups suffering poor socioeconomic conditions, while wealthier environments are associated with smaller variance [106].

Subcutaneous adipose tissue and visceral adipose tissue differ in their sensitivity to insulin, sex hormones, and adrenergic stimulation. Due to a lower sensitivity to insulin's inhibiting effects and higher expression of glucocorticoid and catecholamine β-1, -2, and -3 adrenergic receptors, visceral adipocytes have a higher tendency toward lipolysis, release more FFA, and produce inflammatory cytokines. Furthermore, visceral adipose tissue has a greater number of resident macrophages that produce more pro-inflammatory cytokines than subcutaneous adipose tissue, which is the predominant fat depot in women [107].

In the obese state, both visceral and subcutaneous adipose tissue produce inflammatory cytokines, including TNF-α and IL-6, resulting in increased leptin levels and lower adiponectin levels [51, 108]. Estrogens in women are responsible for the accumulation of subcutaneous fat tissue, which in turn secretes leptin in higher amounts while at the same time adiponectin secretion is decreased [84].

SEX HORMONES AS MODULATORS OF META-INFLAMMATORY RESPONSES IN MEN AND WOMEN

The processes causing sexual dimorphisms in obesity-related T2DM are likely multifactorial and may involve the release of different hormones. Estrogens that have previously been described as female sex hormones are also present in men but at lower levels. Estrogens influence glucose metabolism and may play an important role in the pathogenesis of IFG and IGT. They enhance the accumulation of subcutaneous adipose tissue in women and visceral fat in men. In addition, they enhance the metabolic activity of adipose tissue [106]. Deficits in estrogen in postmenopausal women are associated with an increase in visceral fat. Estrogens suppress appetite and increase energy expenditure, independent of their metabolic effects [109], exerting an important role in preventing body weight gain in women of reproductive age.

The most biologically relevant type of estrogen is 17β-estradiol (E2). Estrogens exert their actions through various receptors: estrogen receptor-α (ERα), estrogen receptor-β (ERβ), and G protein-coupled receptor 30 (GPR30) [110]. By binding to their receptors in pancreatic β cells, estrogens increase insulin production, glucose-dependent insulin secretion (GSIS), and decrease apoptosis (Fig. **3**).

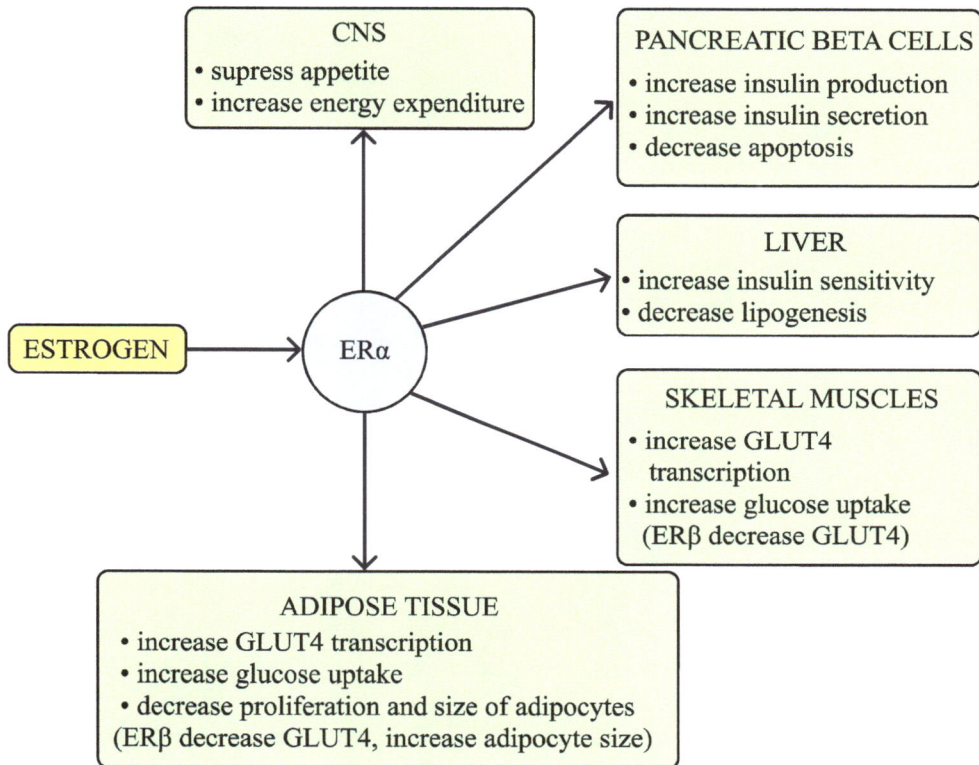

Fig. (3). Metabolic effects of estrogen.
ERα; estrogen receptor-α, ERβ; estrogen receptor-β, GLUT4; glucose transporter protein type-4.

Through the activation of ERα in various cells, estrogens increase transcription of glucose transporter protein type-4 (GLUT4) and inhibit factors responsible for the downregulation of GLUT4, while ERβ activation results in opposite effects [9].

Estrogens in liver cells increase insulin sensitivity and decrease lipogenesis by binding to ERα. Fatty acid oxidation is increased, and the probability of fatty acids accumulating in the liver and skeletal muscle is decreased [111 - 112]. An animal study established that estrogen protects female mice from adipocyte hypertrophy, inflammation, and adipocyte oxidative stress [113]. Many menopausal women with estrogen deficiency have symptoms of metabolic syndrome, including increased visceral obesity, glucose intolerance, and insulin resistance [114].

Progesterone is also a female sex hormone and is synthesized in the gonads, adrenal glands, and in the brain. Unlike estrogen, it does not influence glucose metabolism and it does not affect food intake and adiposity [109].

Androgens, mainly testosterone and androstenedione, are male sex hormones that are also present in women [109]. Androgen receptors are mainly localized in visceral fat. Androgens are involved in regulating energy balance in both men and women. Two metabolic target tissues for androgens are skeletal muscle and adipose tissue. In muscle, androgens enhance protein synthesis, improve insulin sensitivity, and stimulate glucose uptake and lipid oxidation. In adipose tissue, androgens stimulate adipocyte hypertrophy and lipolysis and decrease insulin sensitivity and lipid storage [115]. High testosterone levels have opposite effects on men and women. While high testosterone levels are protective against T2DM in men, in women testosterone is associated with metabolic dysfunction and the development of DM2 (as in women with the polycystic ovarian syndrome) [9]. A strong independent risk factor for the development of T2DM in women is low levels of sex hormone-binding globulin (SHBG), which enhances the free circulating testosterone [77].

Enzyme aromatase can convert androgens to estrogens. This conversion is possible in aromatase-expressing tissues: sex gonads, adipose tissue, muscles, bones, breast, and brain [109]. About 80% of circulating estradiol in men is derived from aromatized testosterone [116]. Estrogens play a protective role in men as they do in women. They regulate body fat and sexual function [105, 116]. Blocking the conversion of androgens to estrogens decreases insulin sensitivity and metabolism [116].

CONCLUDING REMARKS

Gender differences in obesity-related T2DM exist. Our knowledge of these differences is limited due to the fact that most studies have been performed on male subjects. The immunological response is a result of the actions of many factors such as sex hormones, body composition, food intake, energy expenditure, which are different between men and women.

The main source of obesity-related inflammation is white adipose tissue. A different distribution of adipose tissue may contribute to gender differences in meta-inflammation. By secreting many pro- and anti-inflammatory cytokines, adipose tissue could be a modulator of meta-inflammatory responses in men and women. Men accumulate more visceral fat, which is associated with increased insulin resistance and a higher risk of metabolic and cardiovascular disorders.

Sex hormones, estrogens, and androgens, contribute to gender differences in obesity-related T2DM since they regulate not only biological characteristics but also adipose tissue function and metabolism. Estrogens are involved in the distribution of adipose tissue and consequently, in the secretion of cytokines. Moreover, estrogens affect glucose and insulin homeostasis. Androgens are involved in regulating energy balance. Because of the higher level of estrogens, reproductive-aged women are more protected compared to men, but many estrogen-deficient, postmenopausal women accumulate more visceral fat and they have symptoms of obesity-related diseases.

Gender differences have a major impact on the development and progression of obesity-related T2DM and its complications. Future studies should contribute to a better understanding of gender differences in both obesity-related T2DM and inflammatory responses in order to establish prevention and treatment of diabetes in accordance with gender-related guidelines.

CONSENT FOR PUBLICATION

Not applicable.

CONFLICT OF INTEREST

The authors confirm that this chapter content has no conflict of interest.

ACKNOWLEDGEMENTS

The authors would like to express their sincere thanks to the editor and anonymous reviewers for their time and valuable suggestions.

REFERENCES

[1]   Rodríguez-Hernández H, Simental-Mendía LE, Rodríguez-Ramírez G, Reyes-Romero MA. Obesity
        and inflammation: epidemiology, risk factors, and markers of inflammation. Int J Endocrinol 2013;
        2013: 678159.
        [http://dx.doi.org/10.1155/2013/678159] [PMID: 23690772]

[2]   Badawi A, Klip A, Haddad P, *et al.* Type 2 diabetes mellitus and inflammation: Prospects for
        biomarkers of risk and nutritional intervention. Diabetes Metab Syndr Obes 2010; 3: 173-86.
        [http://dx.doi.org/10.2147/DMSO.S9089] [PMID: 21437087]

[3]   Kautzky-Willer A, Harreiter J, Pacini G. Sex and gender differences in risk, pathophysiology and
        complications of type 2 diabetes mellitus. Endocr Rev 2016; 37(3): 278-316.
        [http://dx.doi.org/10.1210/er.2015-1137] [PMID: 27159875]

[4]   Kanter R, Caballero B. Global gender disparities in obesity: a review. Adv Nutr 2012; 3(4): 491-8.
        [http://dx.doi.org/10.3945/an.112.002063] [PMID: 22797984]

[5]   G Duarte F, da Silva Moreira S, Almeida MDCC, *et al.* Sex differences and correlates of poor glycaemic control in type 2 diabetes: a cross-sectional study in Brazil and Venezuela. BMJ Open 2019; 9(3): e023401.
        [http://dx.doi.org/10.1136/bmjopen-2018-023401] [PMID: 30842107]

[6]   Kautzky-Willer A, Harreiter J, Abrahamian H, *et al.* Geschlechtsspezifische Aspekte bei Prädiabetes und Diabetes mellitus – klinische Empfehlungen (Update 2019). Sex and gender-specific aspects in prediabetes and diabetes mellitus—clinical recommendations (Update 2019). Wiener klinische Wochenschrift 2019; 131(Supll 1): 221-8.

[7]   Bhupathiraju SN, Hu FB. Epidemiology of obesity and diabetes and their cardiovascular complications. Circ Res 2016; 118(11): 1723-35.
        [http://dx.doi.org/10.1161/CIRCRESAHA.115.306825] [PMID: 27230638]

[8]   Peters SAE, Woodward M. Sex Differences in the Burden and Complications of Diabetes. Curr Diab Rep 2018; 18(6): 33.
        [http://dx.doi.org/10.1007/s11892-018-1005-5] [PMID: 29671082]

[9]   Franconi F, Campesi I, Occhioni S, Tonolo G. Sex-gender differences in diabetes vascular complications and treatment. Endocr Metab Immune Disord Drug Targets 2012; 12(2): 179-96.
        [http://dx.doi.org/10.2174/187153012800493512] [PMID: 22236023]

[10]   Varì R, Scazzocchio B, D'Amore A, Giovannini C, Gessani S, Masella R. Gender-related differences in lifestyle may affect health status. Ann Ist Super Sanita 2016; 52(2): 158-66.
        [PMID: 27364389]

[11]   World Health Organization. Classification of diabetes mellitus. Geneva: World Health Organization 2019.

[12]   Díaz A, López-Grueso R, Gambini J, *et al.* Sex Differences in Age-Associated Type 2 Diabetes in Rats-Role of Estrogens and Oxidative Stress. Oxid Med Cell Longev 2019; 2019: 6734836.
        [http://dx.doi.org/10.1155/2019/6734836] [PMID: 31089412]

[13]   World Health Organization. Global report on diabetes. Geneva: World Health Organization 2016.

[14]   Zhang P, Zhang X, Brown J, *et al.* Global healthcare expenditure on diabetes for 2010 and 2030. Diabetes Res Clin Pract 2010; 87(3): 293-301.
        [http://dx.doi.org/10.1016/j.diabres.2010.01.026] [PMID: 20171754]

[15]   Zimmet PZ. Diabetes and its drivers: the largest epidemic in human history? Clin Diabetes Endocrinol 2017; 3: 1.
        [http://dx.doi.org/10.1186/s40842-016-0039-3] [PMID: 28702255]

[16]   Kaku K. Pathophysiology of type 2 diabetes and its treatment policy. Japan Med Assoc J 53(1): 41-6.

[17]   Mokdad AH, Bowman BA, Ford ES, Vinicor F, Marks JS, Koplan JP. The continuing epidemics of obesity and diabetes in the United States. JAMA 2001; 286(10): 1195-200.
        [http://dx.doi.org/10.1001/jama.286.10.1195] [PMID: 11559264]

[18]   Lin Y, Sun Z. Current views on type 2 diabetes. J Endocrinol 2010; 204(1): 1-11.
        [http://dx.doi.org/10.1677/JOE-09-0260] [PMID: 19770178]

[19]   Eckel RH, Kahn SE, Ferrannini E, *et al.* Obesity and type 2 diabetes: what can be unified and what needs to be individualized? J Clin Endocrinol Metab 2011; 96(6): 1654-63.
        [http://dx.doi.org/10.1210/jc.2011-0585] [PMID: 21602457]

[20]   Zhao Y, Xu G, Wu W, Yi X. Type 2 diabetes mellitus-disease, diagnosis and treatment. J Diabetes Metab 2015; 6: 533.

[21]   Liu Z, Fu C, Wang W, Xu B. Prevalence of chronic complications of type 2 diabetes mellitus in outpatients - a cross-sectional hospital based survey in urban China. Health Qual Life Outcomes 2010; 8: 62.
        [http://dx.doi.org/10.1186/1477-7525-8-62] [PMID: 20579389]

[22]   Bertoluci MC, Rocha VZ. Cardiovascular risk assessment in patients with diabetes. Diabetol Metab Syndr 2017; 9: 25.
[http://dx.doi.org/10.1186/s13098-017-0225-1] [PMID: 28435446]

[23]   Raghavan S, Vassy JL, Ho YL, *et al.* Diabetes Mellitus-Related All-Cause and Cardiovascular Mortality in a National Cohort of Adults. J Am Heart Assoc 2019; 8(4): e011295.
[http://dx.doi.org/10.1161/JAHA.118.011295] [PMID: 30776949]

[24]   Nickerson HD, Dutta S. Diabetic complications: current challenges and opportunities. J Cardiovasc Transl Res 2012; 5(4): 375-9.
[http://dx.doi.org/10.1007/s12265-012-9388-1] [PMID: 22752737]

[25]   Cornell S. Continual evolution of type 2 diabetes: an update on pathophysiology and emerging treatment options. Ther Clin Risk Manag 2015; 11: 621-32.
[http://dx.doi.org/10.2147/TCRM.S67387] [PMID: 25931824]

[26]   Stumvoll M, Goldstein BJ, van Haeften TW. Type 2 diabetes: principles of pathogenesis and therapy. Lancet 2005; 365(9467): 1333-46.
[http://dx.doi.org/10.1016/S0140-6736(05)61032-X] [PMID: 15823385]

[27]   Kahn SE, Cooper ME, Del Prato S. Pathophysiology and treatment of type 2 diabetes: perspectives on the past, present, and future. Lancet 2014; 383(9922): 1068-83.
[http://dx.doi.org/10.1016/S0140-6736(13)62154-6] [PMID: 24315620]

[28]   Rizza RA. Pathogenesis of fasting and postprandial hyperglycemia in type 2 diabetes: implications for therapy. Diabetes 2010; 59(11): 2697-707.
[http://dx.doi.org/10.2337/db10-1032] [PMID: 20705776]

[29]   Ormazabal V, Nair S, Elfeky O, Aguayo C, Salomon C, Zuñiga FA. Association between insulin resistance and the development of cardiovascular disease. Cardiovasc Diabetol 2018; 17(1): 122.
[http://dx.doi.org/10.1186/s12933-018-0762-4] [PMID: 30170598]

[30]   Dimitriadis G, Mitrou P, Lambadiari V, Maratou E, Raptis SA. Insulin effects in muscle and adipose tissue. Diabetes Res Clin Pract 2011; 93 (Suppl. 1): S52-9.
[http://dx.doi.org/10.1016/S0168-8227(11)70014-6] [PMID: 21864752]

[31]   König M, Bulik S, Holzhütter HG. Quantifying the contribution of the liver to glucose homeostasis: a detailed kinetic model of human hepatic glucose metabolism. PLOS Comput Biol 2012; 8(6): e1002577.
[http://dx.doi.org/10.1371/journal.pcbi.1002577] [PMID: 22761565]

[32]   Leon-Acuña A, Alcala-Diaz JF, Delgado-Lista J, *et al.* Hepatic insulin resistance both in prediabetic and diabetic patients determines postprandial lipoprotein metabolism: from the CORDIOPREV study. Cardiovasc Diabetol 2016; 15: 68.
[http://dx.doi.org/10.1186/s12933-016-0380-y] [PMID: 27095446]

[33]   Ndisang JF, Vannacci A, Rastogi S. Insulin Resistance, Type 1 and Type 2 Diabetes, and Related Complications 2017. J Diabetes Res 2017; 2017: 1478294.
[http://dx.doi.org/10.1155/2017/1478294] [PMID: 29279853]

[34]   Boucher J, Kleinridders A, Kahn CR. Insulin receptor signaling in normal and insulin-resistant states. Cold Spring Harb Perspect Biol 2014; 6(1): a009191.
[http://dx.doi.org/10.1101/cshperspect.a009191] [PMID: 24384568]

[35]   Janochova K, Haluzik M, Buzga M. Visceral fat and insulin resistance - what we know? Biomed Pap Med Fac Univ Palacky Olomouc Czech Repub 2019; 163(1): 19-27.
[http://dx.doi.org/10.5507/bp.2018.062] [PMID: 30398218]

[36]   Purnell JQ. Definitions, Classification, and Epidemiology of Obesity. [Updated 2018 Apr 12]. In: Feingold KR, Anawalt B, Boyce A, Eds. Endotext [Internet]. South Dartmouth (MA): MDText.com, Inc. 2000.

[37]   A Afshin, MH Forouzanfar, MB Reitsma, *et al.* GBD 2015 Obesity Collaborators. Health effects of overweight and obesity in 195 countries over 25 years. N Engl J Med 2017; 377(1): 13-27.

[38]   Lefranc C, Friederich-Persson M, Palacios-Ramirez R, Nguyen Dinh Cat A. Mitochondrial oxidative stress in obesity: role of the mineralocorticoid receptor. J Endocrinol 2018; 238(3): R143-59.
[http://dx.doi.org/10.1530/JOE-18-0163] [PMID: 29875164]

[39]   Chang E, Varghese M, Singer K. Gender and sex differences in adipose tissue. Curr Diab Rep 2018; 18(9): 69.
[http://dx.doi.org/10.1007/s11892-018-1031-3] [PMID: 30058013]

[40]   Saltiel AR, Olefsky JM. Inflammatory mechanisms linking obesity and metabolic disease. J Clin Invest 2017; 127(1): 1-4.
[http://dx.doi.org/10.1172/JCI92035] [PMID: 28045402]

[41]   Ellulu MS, Patimah I, Khaza'ai H, Rahmat A, Abed Y. Obesity and inflammation: the linking mechanism and the complications. Arch Med Sci 2017; 13(4): 851-63.
[http://dx.doi.org/10.5114/aoms.2016.58928] [PMID: 28721154]

[42]   De Lorenzo A, Gratteri S, Gualtieri P, Cammarano A, Bertucci P, Di Renzo L. Why primary obesity is a disease? J Transl Med 2019; 17(1): 169.
[http://dx.doi.org/10.1186/s12967-019-1919-y] [PMID: 31118060]

[43]   Pereira-Lancha LO, Campos-Ferraz PL, Lancha AH Jr. Obesity: considerations about etiology, metabolism, and the use of experimental models. Diabetes Metab Syndr Obes 2012; 5: 75-87.
[http://dx.doi.org/10.2147/DMSO.S25026] [PMID: 22570558]

[44]   Pereira-Lancha LO, Coelho DF, de Campos-Ferraz PL, Lancha AH Jr. Body fat regulation: is it a result of a simple energy balance or a high fat intake? J Am Coll Nutr 2010; 29(4): 343-51.
[http://dx.doi.org/10.1080/07315724.2010.10719850] [PMID: 21041808]

[45]   Houseknecht KL, Baile CA, Matteri RL, Spurlock ME. The biology of leptin: a review. J Anim Sci 1998; 76(5): 1405-20.
[http://dx.doi.org/10.2527/1998.7651405x] [PMID: 9621947]

[46]   Nakaš-Ićindić E, Babić N, Huskić J. Integrativni sistemi ljudskog tijela. Medicinski fakultet Univerzitet u Sarajevu 2015.

[47]   Frankenfield DC, Rowe WA, Cooney RN, Smith JS, Becker D. Limits of body mass index to detect obesity and predict body composition. Nutrition 2001; 17(1): 26-30.
[http://dx.doi.org/10.1016/S0899-9007(00)00471-8] [PMID: 11165884]

[48]   Ahmad N, Adam SI, Nawi AM, Hassan MR, Ghazi HF. Abdominal obesity indicators: waist circumference or waist-to-hip ratio in Malaysian adults population. Int J Prev Med 2016; 7: 82.
[http://dx.doi.org/10.4103/2008-7802.183654] [PMID: 27330688]

[49]   Wildman RP, McGinn AP, Lin J, *et al.* Cardiovascular disease risk of abdominal obesity vs. metabolic abnormalities. Obesity (Silver Spring) 2011; 19(4): 853-60.
[http://dx.doi.org/10.1038/oby.2010.168] [PMID: 20725064]

[50]   Lehr S, Hartwig S, Sell H. Adipokines: a treasure trove for the discovery of biomarkers for metabolic disorders. Proteomics Clin Appl 2012; 6(1-2): 91-101.
[http://dx.doi.org/10.1002/prca.201100052] [PMID: 22213627]

[51]   Terrazas S, Brashear L, Escoto AK, *et al.* Sex differences in obesity-induced inflammation [online first], IntechOpen 2019. Available from: https://www.intechopen.com/online-first/sex-differences-in-obesity-induced-inflammation
[http://dx.doi.org/10.5772/intechopen.84941]

[52]   Cypess AM, Lehman S, Williams G, *et al.* Identification and importance of brown adipose tissue in adult humans. N Engl J Med 2009; 360(15): 1509-17.
[http://dx.doi.org/10.1056/NEJMoa0810780] [PMID: 19357406]

[53] Shuster A, Patlas M, Pinthus JH, Mourtzakis M. The clinical importance of visceral adiposity: a critical review of methods for visceral adipose tissue analysis. Br J Radiol 2012; 85(1009): 1-10.
[http://dx.doi.org/10.1259/bjr/38447238] [PMID: 21937614]

[54] van Greevenbroek MM, Schalkwijk CG, Stehouwer CD. Obesity-associated low-grade inflammation in type 2 diabetes mellitus: causes and consequences. Neth J Med 2013; 71(4): 174-87.
[PMID: 23723111]

[55] Zhang M, Hu T, Zhang S, Zhou L. Associations of different adipose tissue depots with insulin resistance: a systematic review and meta-analysis of observational studies. Sci Rep 2015; 5: 18495.
[http://dx.doi.org/10.1038/srep18495] [PMID: 26686961]

[56] Després JP. Cardiovascular disease under the influence of excess visceral fat. Crit Pathw Cardiol 2007; 6(2): 51-9.
[http://dx.doi.org/10.1097/HPC.0b013e318057d4c9] [PMID: 17667865]

[57] Britton KA, Fox CS. Ectopic fat depots and cardiovascular disease. Circulation 2011; 124(24): e837-41.
[http://dx.doi.org/10.1161/CIRCULATIONAHA.111.077602] [PMID: 22156000]

[58] Han S, Sun HM, Hwang KC, Kim SW. Adipose-derived stromal vascular fraction cells: update on clinical utility and efficacy. Crit Rev Eukaryot Gene Expr 2015; 25(2): 145-52.
[http://dx.doi.org/10.1615/CritRevEukaryotGeneExpr.2015013057] [PMID: 26080608]

[59] Krüger K. Inflammation during obesity – pathophysiological concepts and effects of physical activity. Dtsch Z Sportmed 2017; 68: 163-9.
[http://dx.doi.org/10.5960/dzsm.2017.285]

[60] Ringseis R, Eder K, Mooren FC, Krüger K. Metabolic signals and innate immune activation in obesity and exercise. Exerc Immunol Rev 2015; 21: 58-68.
[PMID: 25825956]

[61] Mraz M, Haluzik M. The role of adipose tissue immune cells in obesity and low-grade inflammation. J Endocrinol 2014; 222(3): R113-27.
[http://dx.doi.org/10.1530/JOE-14-0283] [PMID: 25006217]

[62] Liu R, Nikolajczyk BS. Tissue immune cells fuel obesity-associated inflammation in adipose tissue and beyond. Front Immunol 2019; 10: 1587.
[http://dx.doi.org/10.3389/fimmu.2019.01587] [PMID: 31379820]

[63] Rehman K, Akash MS. Mechanisms of inflammatory responses and development of insulin resistance: how are they interlinked? J Biomed Sci 2016; 23(1): 87.
[http://dx.doi.org/10.1186/s12929-016-0303-y] [PMID: 27912756]

[64] León-Pedroza JI, González-Tapia LA, del Olmo-Gil E, Castellanos-Rodríguez D, Escobedo G, González-Chávez A. Low-grade systemic inflammation and the development of metabolic diseases: from the molecular evidence to the clinical practice. Cir Cir 2015; 83(6): 543-51.
[http://dx.doi.org/10.1016/j.circen.2015.11.008] [PMID: 26159364]

[65] Chan PC, Hsieh PS. The role of adipocyte hypertrophy and hypoxia in the development of obesity-associated adipose tissue inflammation and insulin resistance. In: Gordeladze JO, Ed. Adiposity - Omics and Molecular Understanding. London: IntechOpen 2007; pp. 127-41.
[http://dx.doi.org/10.5772/65458]

[66] Cildir G, Akıncılar SC, Tergaonkar V. Chronic adipose tissue inflammation: all immune cells on the stage. Trends Mol Med 2013; 19(8): 487-500.
[http://dx.doi.org/10.1016/j.molmed.2013.05.001] [PMID: 23746697]

[67] Boutens L, Stienstra R. Adipose tissue macrophages: going off track during obesity. Diabetologia 2016; 59(5): 879-94.
[http://dx.doi.org/10.1007/s00125-016-3904-9] [PMID: 26940592]

[68]   Xu H, Li X, Adams H, Kubena K, Guo S. Etiology of metabolic syndrome and dietary intervention. Int J Mol Sci 2018; 20(1): 128.
[http://dx.doi.org/10.3390/ijms20010128] [PMID: 30602666]

[69]   Weisberg SP, McCann D, Desai M, Rosenbaum M, Leibel RL, Ferrante AW Jr. Obesity is associated with macrophage accumulation in adipose tissue. J Clin Invest 2003; 112(12): 1796-808.
[http://dx.doi.org/10.1172/JCI200319246] [PMID: 14679176]

[70]   Meiliana A, Dewi NM, Wijaya A. Adipose tissue, inflammation (meta-inflammation) and obesity management. Indones Biomed J 2015; 7: 129-46.
[http://dx.doi.org/10.18585/inabj.v7i3.185]

[71]   Li C, Xu MM, Wang K, Adler AJ, Vella AT, Zhou B. Macrophage polarization and meta-inflammation. Transl Res 2018; 191: 29-44.
[http://dx.doi.org/10.1016/j.trsl.2017.10.004] [PMID: 29154757]

[72]   Appari M, Channon KM, McNeill E. Metabolic regulation of adipose tissue macrophage function in obesity and diabetes. Antioxid Redox Signal 2018; 29(3): 297-312.
[http://dx.doi.org/10.1089/ars.2017.7060] [PMID: 28661198]

[73]   Wu H, Ballantyne CM. Skeletal muscle inflammation and insulin resistance in obesity. J Clin Invest 2017; 127(1): 43-54.
[http://dx.doi.org/10.1172/JCI88880] [PMID: 28045398]

[74]   Ely BR, Clayton ZS, McCurdy CE, Pfeiffer J, Minson CT. Meta-inflammation and cardiometabolic disease in obesity: Can heat therapy help? Temperature (Austin) 2017; 5(1): 9-21.
[http://dx.doi.org/10.1080/23328940.2017.1384089] [PMID: 29687041]

[75]   Castro JP, Grune T, Speckmann B. The two faces of reactive oxygen species (ROS) in adipocyte function and dysfunction. Biol Chem 2016; 397(8): 709-24.
[http://dx.doi.org/10.1515/hsz-2015-0305] [PMID: 27031218]

[76]   Horie I, Abiru N, Eto M, *et al.* Sex differences in insulin and glucagon responses for glucose homeostasis in young healthy Japanese adults. J Diabetes Investig 2018; 9(6): 1283-7.
[http://dx.doi.org/10.1111/jdi.12829] [PMID: 29489067]

[77]   Mauvais-Jarvis F. Gender differences in glucose homeostasis and diabetes. Physiol Behav 2018; 187: 20-3.
[http://dx.doi.org/10.1016/j.physbeh.2017.08.016] [PMID: 28843891]

[78]   Peters A, Pellerin L, Dallman MF, *et al.* Causes of obesity: looking beyond the hypothalamus. Prog Neurobiol 2007; 81(2): 61-88.
[http://dx.doi.org/10.1016/j.pneurobio.2006.12.004] [PMID: 17270337]

[79]   Lalitha V, Pal G, Parija S, Pal P, Sathishbabu M, Indumathy J. Effect of gender on food intake, adiposity and immunological responses following lesion of ventromedial hypothalamus in albino Wistar rats Int J Clin. Exp Physiol 2014; 1(1): 44-50.
[PMID: 25557730]

[80]   Park HK, Ahima RS. Physiology of leptin: energy homeostasis, neuroendocrine function and metabolism. Metabolism 2015; 64(1): 24-34.
[http://dx.doi.org/10.1016/j.metabol.2014.08.004] [PMID: 25199978]

[81]   Stern JH, Rutkowski JM, Scherer PE. Adiponectin, leptin, and fatty acids in the maintenance of metabolic homeostasis through adipose tissue crosstalk. Cell Metab 2016; 23(5): 770-84.
[http://dx.doi.org/10.1016/j.cmet.2016.04.011] [PMID: 27166942]

[82]   Choe SS, Huh JY, Hwang IJ, Kim JI, Kim JB. Adipose tissue remodeling: its role in energy metabolism and metabolic disorders. Front Endocrinol (Lausanne) 2016; 7: 30.
[http://dx.doi.org/10.3389/fendo.2016.00030] [PMID: 27148161]

[83]   Choe S-A, Kim JY, Ro YS, Cho S-I. Women are less likely than men to achieve optimal glycemic

control after 1 year of treatment: A multi-level analysis of a Korean primary care cohort. PLoS One 2018; 13(5): e0196719.
[http://dx.doi.org/10.1371/journal.pone.0196719] [PMID: 29718952]

[84] Mauvais-Jarvis F. Sex differences in metabolic homeostasis, diabetes, and obesity. Biol Sex Differ 2015; 6: 14.
[http://dx.doi.org/10.1186/s13293-015-0033-y] [PMID: 26339468]

[85] Schneider AL, Lazo M, Ndumele CE, *et al.* Liver enzymes, race, gender and diabetes risk: the Atherosclerosis Risk in Communities (ARIC) Study. Diabet Med 2013; 30(8): 926-33.
[http://dx.doi.org/10.1111/dme.12187] [PMID: 23510198]

[86] Arnetz L, Ekberg NR, Alvarsson M. Sex differences in type 2 diabetes: focus on disease course and outcomes. Diabetes Metab Syndr Obes 2014; 7: 409-20.
[http://dx.doi.org/10.2147/DMSO.S51301] [PMID: 25258546]

[87] Szalat A, Raz I. Gender-specific care of diabetes mellitus: particular considerations in the management of diabetic women. Diabetes Obes Metab 2008; 10(12): 1135-56.
[PMID: 18494812]

[88] Senthil Kumar SPD, Shi H, Senthil Kumar SPD. Sex differences in obesity-related glucose intolerance and insulin resistance in glucose tolerance. In: Chackrewarthy S, Ed. Glucose Tolerance. London: IntechOpen 2012.
[http://dx.doi.org/10.5772/52972]

[89] Shen L, Song L, Li H, *et al.* Association between earlier age at natural menopause and risk of diabetes in middle-aged and older Chinese women: The Dongfeng-Tongji cohort study. Diabetes Metab 2017; 43(4): 345-50.
[http://dx.doi.org/10.1016/j.diabet.2016.12.011] [PMID: 28129998]

[90] Burhans MS, Hagman DK, Kuzma JN, Schmidt KA, Kratz M. Contribution of adipose tissue inflammation to the development of type 2 diabetes mellitus. Compr Physiol 2018; 9(1): 1-58.
[PMID: 30549014]

[91] Abdullah A, Peeters A, de Courten M, Stoelwinder J. The magnitude of association between overweight and obesity and the risk of diabetes: a meta-analysis of prospective cohort studies. Diabetes Res Clin Pract 2010; 89(3): 309-19.
[PMID: 20493574]

[92] Lalitha V, Pal GK. Gender difference in the neuroimmunomodulation of obesity: A mini review. Int J Clin Exp Physiol 2016; 3: 109-12.

[93] Singer K, Maley N, Mergian T, DelProposto J, Cho KW, Zamarron BF, *et al.* Differences in hematopoietic stem cells contribute to sexually dimorphic inflammatory responses to high fat diet-induced obesity. J Biol Chem 2015; 290(21): 13250-62.

[94] Eaton SA, Sethi JK. Immunometabolic links between estrogen, adipose tissue and female reproductive metabolism. Biology (Basel) 2019; 8(1): 8.
[PMID: 30736459]

[95] Medrikova D, Jilkova ZM, Bardova K, Janovska P, Rossmeisl M, Kopecky J. Sex differences during the course of diet-induced obesity in mice: adipose tissue expandability and glycemic control. Int J Obes 2012; 36(2): 262-72.
[PMID: 21540832]

[96] Crabbe DL, Dipla K, Ambati S, Zafeiridis A, Gaughan JP, Houser SR, *et al.* Gender differences in post-infarction hypertrophy in end-stage failing hearts. J Am Coll Cardiol 2003; 41(2): 300-6.

[97] Qatanani M, Lazar MA. Mechanisms of obesity-associated insulin resistance: many choices on the menu. Genes Dev 2007; 21(12): 1443-55.
[http://dx.doi.org/10.1101/gad.1550907] [PMID: 17575046]

[98] Stolarczyk E. Adipose tissue inflammation in obesity: a metabolic or immune response? Curr Opin

Pharmacol 2017; 37: 35-40.
[http://dx.doi.org/10.1016/j.coph.2017.08.006] [PMID: 28843953]

[99]   Začiragić A, Hasanefendić B, Avdagić N, Lepara O, Babić N, Huskić J, *et al.* Gender comparison of serum asymmetric dimethylarginine and C-reactive protein concentration in patients with diabetes mellitus type 2. Medical Journal 2014; 20(2): 85-90.

[100] Akash MSH, Rehman K, Liaqat A, Numan M, Mahmood Q, Kamal S. Biochemical investigation of gender-specific association between insulin resistance and inflammatory biomarkers in types 2 diabetic patients. Biomed Pharmacother 2018; 106: 285-91.
[http://dx.doi.org/10.1016/j.biopha.2018.06.044] [PMID: 29966972]

[101] Tabassum R, Mia AR, Reza-Ul-Haq KM, Yesmin M, Faruqui JM. C-reactive protein level in type-2 diabetic patients attending Mymensingh medical college hospital, Mymensingh. Mymensingh Med J 2017; 26(1): 56-60.
[PMID: 28260756]

[102] Cozlea DL, Farcas DM, Nagy A, *et al.* The impact of C reactive protein on global cardiovascular risk on patients with coronary artery disease. Curr Health Sci J 2013; 39(4): 225-31.
[PMID: 24778862]

[103] Naila AS, Shaheen S, Sajid S. Association of bio-inflammatory markers (CRP, IL-6) with glucose level in obese T2DM Pakistani patients JOP. J Pancreas (Online) 2018; 19(6): 282-6.

[104] Svensson E, Mor A, Rungby J, *et al.* Lifestyle and clinical factors associated with elevated C-reactive protein among newly diagnosed Type 2 diabetes mellitus patients: a cross-sectional study from the nationwide DD2 cohort. BMC Endocr Disord 2014; 14: 74.
[http://dx.doi.org/10.1186/1472-6823-14-74] [PMID: 25163828]

[105] Palmer BF, Clegg DJ. The sexual dimorphism of obesity. Mol Cell Endocrinol 2015; 402: 113-9.
[http://dx.doi.org/10.1016/j.mce.2014.11.029] [PMID: 25578600]

[106] Griffin C, Lanzetta N, Eter L, Singer K. Sexually dimorphic myeloid inflammatory and metabolic responses to diet-induced obesity. Am J Physiol Regul Integr Comp Physiol 2016; 311(2): R211-6.
[http://dx.doi.org/10.1152/ajpregu.00136.2016] [PMID: 27252473]

[107] Ghigliotti G, Barisione C, Garibaldi S, *et al.* Adipose tissue immune response: novel triggers and consequences for chronic inflammatory conditions. Inflammation 2014; 37(4): 1337-53.
[http://dx.doi.org/10.1007/s10753-014-9914-1] [PMID: 24823865]

[108] Nakamura K, Fuster JJ, Walsh K. Adipokines: a link between obesity and cardiovascular disease. J Cardiol 2014; 63(4): 250-9.
[http://dx.doi.org/10.1016/j.jjcc.2013.11.006] [PMID: 24355497]

[109] Wang C, Xu Y. Mechanisms for sex differences in energy homeostasis. J Mol Endocrinol 2019; 62(2): R129-43.
[http://dx.doi.org/10.1530/JME-18-0165] [PMID: 31130779]

[110] Fuentes N, Silveyra P. Estrogen receptor signaling mechanisms. Adv Protein Chem Struct Biol 2019; 116: 135-70.
[http://dx.doi.org/10.1016/bs.apcsb.2019.01.001] [PMID: 31036290]

[111] Campbell SE, Mehan KA, Tunstall RJ, Febbraio MA, Cameron-Smith D. 17beta-estradiol upregulates the expression of peroxisome proliferator-activated receptor alpha and lipid oxidative genes in skeletal muscle. J Mol Endocrinol 2003; 31(1): 37-45.
[http://dx.doi.org/10.1677/jme.0.0310037] [PMID: 12914523]

[112] Rogers NH, Witczak CA, Hirshman MF, Goodyear LJ, Greenberg AS. Estradiol stimulates Akt, AMP-activated protein kinase (AMPK) and TBC1D1/4, but not glucose uptake in rat soleus. Biochem Biophys Res Commun 2009; 382(4): 646-50.
[http://dx.doi.org/10.1016/j.bbrc.2009.02.154] [PMID: 19265681]

[113] Stubbins RE, Najjar K, Holcomb VB, Hong J, Núñez NP. Oestrogen alters adipocyte biology and

protects female mice from adipocyte inflammation and insulin resistance. Diabetes Obes Metab 2012; 14(1): 58-66.
[http://dx.doi.org/10.1111/j.1463-1326.2011.01488.x] [PMID: 21834845]

[114] Lovre D, Lindsey SH, Mauvais-Jarvis F. Effect of menopausal hormone therapy on components of the metabolic syndrome. Ther Adv Cardiovasc Dis 2016; 11(1): 33-43.
[http://dx.doi.org/10.1177/1753944716649358] [PMID: 27234158]

[115] Gambineri A, Pelusi C. Sex hormones, obesity and type 2 diabetes: is there a link? Endocr Connect 2019; 8(1): R1-9.
[http://dx.doi.org/10.1530/EC-18-0450] [PMID: 30533003]

[116] Finkelstein JS, Lee H, Burnett-Bowie SA, *et al.* Gonadal steroids and body composition, strength, and sexual function in men. N Engl J Med 2013; 369(11): 1011-22.
[http://dx.doi.org/10.1056/NEJMoa1206168] [PMID: 24024838]

CHAPTER 7

Meta-Inflammation, Alzheimer's Disease and Obesity

Almir Fajkić[1,*] and **Lejla Opardija**[2]

[1] *Department of Pathophysiology, Faculty of Medicine, University of Sarajevo, Sarajevo, Bosnia and Herzegovina*

[2] *General Hospital Bugojno, Sarajevo, Bosnia and Herzegovina*

Abstract: Current evidence suggests that obesity, in addition to being a contributing factor for cardiovascular and metabolic disorders, also increases the risk of Alzheimer's disease (AD). It is well-documented fact that the brain is significantly affected by the inflammatory condition of obesity *i.e.* meta-inflammation *via* several pathways. Some systemic inflammatory and metabolic mediators produced by adipose tissue cross the blood-brain barrier in certain conditions. The most essential outcome is the activation of the brain-resident microglia and astrocytes contributing to CNS inflammation. Multiple studies have shown the existence of inflammatory markers in the brain and serum of post-mortem AD. In addition to the role of meta-inflammation, recent research has shown that insulin resistance and impaired insulin signaling can contribute to the development of AD as well as other neurological disorders. With this in mind, a group of scientists has proposed the term brain diabetes, or diabetes type 3, for cognitive impairment in AD patients, to unify the metabolic inflammatory pathways of the development of the disorder. The purpose of this is to show that AD is more than just an aggregation of oligomeric and fibrillar Ab deposits in the brain tissue. The disorder is represented by many pathological alterations, such as a lower degree of metabolism, blood-brain-barrier disturbance, and glial activation. Although not all signaling pathways involved in these processes are known yet, this new name could open a new field in the treatment of neurodegenerative impairments, to either prevent or slow down their development.

Keywords: Alzheimer disease, Antidiabetics, Diabetes type 3, Inflammasomes, Insulin resistance, Meta-inflammation, Obesity, Proinflammatory cytokines, TNF-α.

INTRODUCTION

Obesity, as a global problem, has long been the focus of scientific circles, both because of the systemic consequences it produces in the body and because of the increasing amount of data that speak about the active role of adipose tissue in the

---

[*] **Corresponding author Almir Fajkić:** Department of Pathohysiology, Faculty of Medicine, University of Sarajevo, Sarajevo, Bosnia and Herzegovina; Tel: +387 33 226 478, Ext. 566; E-mail: almir.fajkic@mf.unsa.ba

Asija Začiragić (Ed.)

development of these consequences. At the center of today's research is the role of macrophages infiltrating into the adipose tissue, which, by producing different types of molecules, leads to the development of a chronic inflammatory process. This is thought to be the central mechanism responsible for the development of other obesity-related diseases. Metabolic processes and immune defense are two essential mechanisms for human beings. The appearance of immune cells, such as macrophages, in metabolic tissues, indicates a complex, persistent crosstalk between these important systems.

As a specific endocrine tissue, visceral adipose tissue contains various types of cells, like adipocytes and adipocyte precursors, vascular cells, immune cells, and neuronal cells, which together correspond to the inflammatory state throughout obesity.

This inflammatory state is not fully consistent with the classical definition of acute or chronic inflammation; there is no significant tissue damage and the degree of inflammatory activation is also not large. It is often referred to as low-grade chronic inflammation or meta-inflammation (metabolically induced inflammation) and represents the transient stage between basal and inflammatory states.

Inflammation of the adipose tissue is accompanied by infiltration consisting mainly of macrophages and additional CD8 T lymphocytes, and other immune cell types which may change in numbers and phenotypes in obesity, with little or no appearance of neutrophils. The macrophages, which contribute to the release of cytokines and promote systemic inflammation, are surrounded by adipocytes forming a crown-like structure; a distinctive characteristic of low-grade inflammation in the fat tissue. Th1 cytokines, such as IFN-γ, induce classical activation of M1 macrophages, which produce inflammatory mediators [1, 2].

Even though meta-inflammation is first described in adipose tissue, it can also affect many tissues like the liver, pancreas, or nervous system. Speaking about the nervous system itself, it has been hypothesized that the development of cognitive disorders, like Alzheimer disease (AD) is very closely associated with the development of metabolic disorders such as obesity, metabolic syndrome and diabetes.

AD represents a progressive, degenerative and incurable brain disease, manifested by the progressive decline of cognitive functions and the characteristic appearance of senile plaques, β-amyloid deposits, as well as the formation of neurofibrillary tangles in the cerebral cortex and subcortical gray matter. These changes in the normal process of brain aging occur in small quantities, while in AD they accumulate in large quantities [3].

Although the amyloid cascade hypothesis has long been the basis for interpreting the pathogenesis of AD, many researchers have questioned the importance of this theory in recent decades. It has been consistently shown that Aβ accumulation and deposition do not correlate with neuronal loss and cognitive decline, and that many individuals have significant amyloid plaque without showing symptoms of memory impairment [4].

A review of the available literature reveals a number of theories that seek to explain the pathogenesis of AD. The main assumptions are based on the potential pathophysiological processes that have been identified so far that are considered responsible for the development of AD (Fig. **1**).

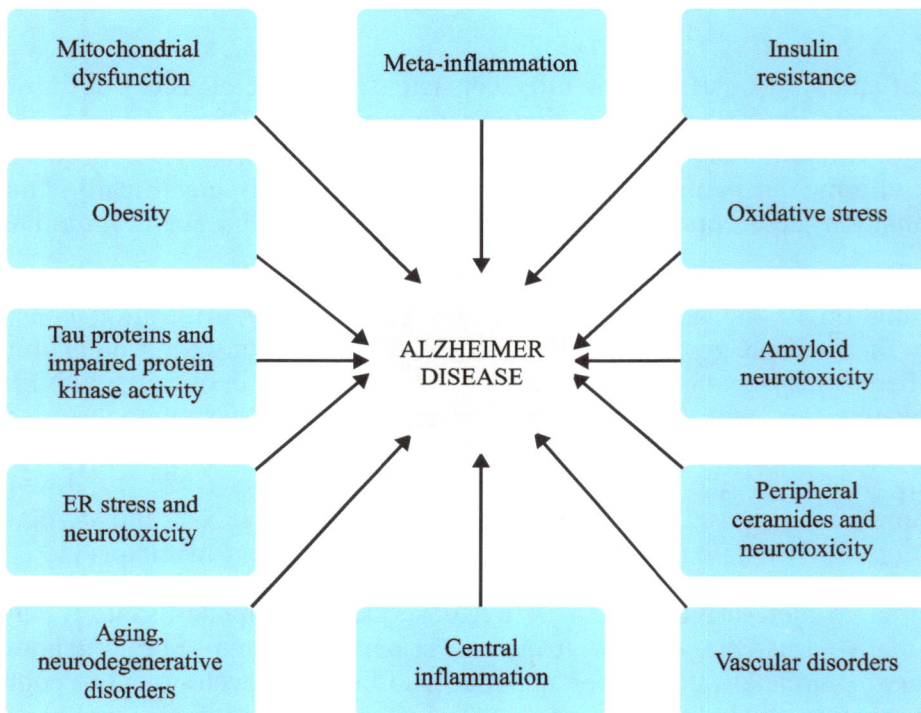

Fig. (1). Potential causes of AD development.
ER-Endoplasmic Reticulum.

Neither of them are strictly exclusive to the others, and it could be that they are all exactly right. The one and only concern could be that we do not have enough information what the primary cause is and what are the harmful effects of the primary disease disorder. However, based on the stated above, it is clear that AD, as we currently understand, is a complex disease.

AD AS A DIABETES TYPE 3

Due to the complexity of the disease, neither of currently existing theories is sufficient to fully explain the pathogenesis of AD, and new hypotheses have emerged that are a combination of the currently known causes of AD. For this reason, a group of scientists proposed the name diabetes type 3 as a counterpart for AD, that is, they tried to hypothesize that AD is a neuroendocrine disease. Their intention was to define the disease as a metabolic disorder characterized by the progressive insulin resistance in brain with consequent damage to the central insulin signaling process, neurotoxin accumulation, neuronal stress, ultimately resulting in neurodegeneration. The concept that AD is "brain diabetes" is based on the following: 1. decreased number or capacity of insulin receptor (IR) binding in the brain of mouse models with AD and DM2, and 2. increased risk of DM2 disease in AD patients [5]. The purpose of this hypothesis was to point out the potential role of obesity in the development of peripheral disorders (diabetes, metabolic syndrome), which would ultimately be a major factor in the development of AD.

The pathways through which obesity raises the risk of AD are unclear, but various theories have been proposed. Two widely discussed and very close connected theories are that AD vulnerability is related to the role of adipose tissue meta-inflammation, and to changes in free fatty acid - glucose metabolism - insulin signaling [6].

Low-grade inflammatory processes in the periphery can affect the nervous system activity, often causing CNS inflammation, especially in the case of prolonged chronic systemic inflammation. This, in turn, causes cognitive decline as a result of neuronal dying, while more severe forms lead to dementia [7].

The mechanism of correlation between meta-inflammation resulting from obesity and the development of AD is very complex and still insufficiently explained. Meta-inflammation in obesity is characterized by the infiltration of macrophages in adipose tissue, which drives to the release of proinflammatory cytokines to promote systemic inflammation and satured free fatty acids (sFFA). Both groups of molecules simultaneously affect the development of central insulin resistance and the development of cognitive dysfunction *via* inflammatory processes. High levels of sFFA trigger an inflammatory cascade initiated by Toll-like receptor 4 (TLR4) and the release of proinflammatory cytokines, Tumor Necrosis Factor-α (TNF-α), IL-1β and IL-6, leading to the development of the neuroinflammation process. In addition, sFFAs cross the blood-brain barrier (BBB) directly, causing neurotoxicity. It is hypothesized that this relates to the development of neuronal insulin resistance [8, 9].

The significant contribution of Amyloid-β peptide (Aβ) should also be stressed here, as it is considered to be the key component of senile plaques that develop in AD brains. Latest data have shown that AβO activities induce pro-inflammatory processes that disrupt neuronal insulin signaling and trigger stress kinase activation, contributing to cognitive disorders in AD models. These conditions are very similar to those in peripheral tissues that affect the metabolism of diabetes and obesity, in the light of the hypothesis that there is a type of metabolic distress in the brain tissue of AD [10].

Another important feature of the metabolic disturbance, chronic hyperglycemia, as a consequence of insulin resistance, activates brain NF-κB and stimulates the release of proinflammatory cytokines. At the same time, the advanced glycation end products (AGEs) resulting from glucose disturbance increase the synthesis of brain NF-κB (nuclear factor kappa light chain enhancer of activated B cells) through their receptors (RAGE) [11, 12].

The net effect of NF-κB-mediated metabolic inflammation is to increase the release of inflammatory mediators in the brain tissue itself. These events, directly or through microglial activation, can affect neuronal function. The released cytokines lead to neuronal damage through various mechanisms, including neurotransmission alteration, apoptosis, and the production of free radicals, glutamate and nitric oxide. Eventually, these events cause the development of neurotoxicity, amyloidogenesis and central inflammation, which is a complex basis for the onset of AD (Fig. **2**).

Experiments on animal models with diabetes and obesity have demonstrated the presence of an inflammatory response in the hypothalamus induced by activation of TNF-α and the IκB kinase (IKK)-β/nuclear factor-KB signaling pathway. This leads to the conclusion that hippocampal dysfunction present in AD and the deregulation of hypothalamus present in obesity may have common inflammatory pathogenic pathways [13].

Finally, one should emphasize the role of adipokines, highly specific molecules produced by adipose cells, in linking meta-inflammation to cognitive impairment.

Adipokines produce multiple effects on various tissues and control many essential physiological processes including appetite, energy consumption, insulin sensitivity and synthesis, body composition, lipid and glucose metabolism, endothelial activity, blood pressure, neuroendocrine function and immunity. Despite reported epidemiological evidence supporting correlations between obesity and AD, the relationship between adipokines and cognitive decline remains widely unknown [14].

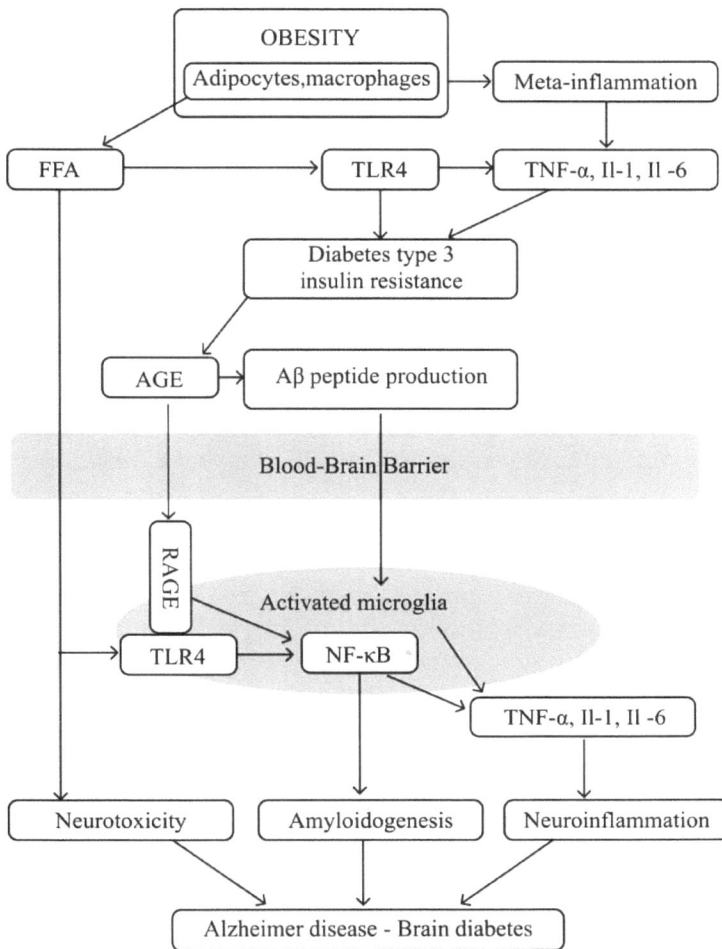

Fig. (2). Basic mechanisms of correlation between meta-inflammation and brain diabetes (AD).
FFA-Free Fatty Acid; TLR4-Toll-like Receptor; AGE-Advanced Glycated End Products; RAGE The receptor for Advanced glycated End Products; NF-kB-Nuclear Factor Kappa B; TNF-α-Tumor Necrosis Factor α; Il- Interleukin

The research to date has given the greatest importance to examining the role of leptin, adiponectin and resistin in the onset of AD, as a response to the inflammatory process in adipose tissue.

Leptin is the most studied adipokine associated with brain structure and function, and has several effects on the brain in relation to cognition and aging. It is an adipocyte-derived hormone and its amount in the blood is positively correlated with the amount of adipose tissue - the larger the adipocyte, the greater the expression of leptin. In addition to serving as a signal to the central nervous system about the amount of energy available, it is involved in the functioning of the immune system, reproduction, bone metabolism, and in the stress response of the body [15].

Receptors for leptin are present in neuronal and non-neuronal cells (astrocytes) in the areas considered to have a high impact on cognition (hypothalamus, cerebral cortex, dental gyrus, and hippocampus) [16].

Although there is plenty of information on the fact that leptin treatment can decrease Aβ levels by targeting all aspects of Aβ metabolism including Aβ production, clearance, degradation, and aggregation which can slow down the development of cognitive impairment, elevated levels of circulating leptin in obese patients contribute significantly to the low-grade inflammatory state that makes obese people more susceptible to develop cardiovascular diseases, type 2 diabetes, neurodegenerative disease like AD. This is based on the fact that leptin provides a contribution to both the innate and adaptive immune response. Specifically, in macrophages, leptin stimulates the expression of CD39, CD69, CD25, CD71 and IL-1Rα, and the production of proinflammatory cytokines IL-6 and TNF-α, which are known to actively participate in the development of AD [17].

Adiponectin (APN), a hormone derived from visceral fat, shows a protective effect against AD and other neurodegenerative diseases. These effects might be attributed to modulation of insulin receptor signaling (APN can sensitize the insulin receptor signaling pathway) and suppression of neuroinflammation by glial cells [18].

Despite these protective effects, some data suggest that an increased concentration of globular form of APN induces a proinflammatory response in human astrocytes, which could facilitate the development of AD. The mechanism by which increased expression of APN in the nervous system, promotes neurodegeneration in AD remains unknown. Increasing evidence indicates that adaptation by APN to an insulin-resistant condition could be associated with AD pathophysiology [19].

Resistin, a type of adipokine that is synthesized by adipocytes, is associated with insulin resistance and has been observed to be involved in inflammation and regulation of several other cytokines. Resistin controls the expression of proinflammatory cytokines and vascular adhesion molecules, suggesting that resistin may play a major role in the host reaction to acute inflammation through the nuclear kappa B-dependent pathway [20].

At present, very little is documented about the effect of resistin on AD. Some researchers have found that the resistin level in cerebrospinal fluid was different in AD patients compared to the healthy subjects with normal cognitive functions, and that resistin levels of patients with AD were significantly higher than healthy controls. Also, levels of resistin were found to be positively correlated with the levels of other proinflammatory cytokines that show a possible connection to the chronic inflammation in AD [21].

THE ROLE OF PROINFLAMMATORY CYTOKINES IN AD DEVELOPMENT

The development of central inflammation, in addition to the action of the above listed factors, is aided by proinflammatory cytokines released as a result of the development of meta-inflammation in the periphery. This was reported in several studies that have identified the presence of inflammatory markers in the brains of patients with AD, such as TNF-α, interleukin (IL) 6, and IL-1β [22].

The CNS has long been considered an immune-privileged tissue in the body, in which inflammation occurs only in the case of direct infection with pathogens or after rupture of BBB. However, it is now known that CNS resident cells can trigger inflammation. The most important players in the CNS inflammatory response are microglial cells and astrocytes, which, triggered by inflammatory cytokines from the periphery, can increase the production of inflammatory cytokines.

Major factors in inflammation in the CNS are microglia cells. Microglia cells begin to enter and "populate" the central nervous system during early embryonic development, as early as week 4 of gestation. Their role is twofold: 1) protecting the brain from pathogens and 2) repairing brain tissue after brain injury. However, microglia cells can alter the usual pattern of activation and thus become harmful to surrounding neurons [23, 24].

Microglia activation has double effects on AD development: on one side microglia activity reduces the deposition of Aβ by raising phagocytosis, removal and degradation, which prevents the production of amyloid plaques in CNS. But on the other side, excessive microglia activation contributes to the production of proinflammatory cytokines, which triggers an inflammatory pathway and then corresponds to neuronal injury and failure [25].

During pathological conditions, an uncontrolled immune response can occur that positively correlates with dysfunction and cell loss during the inflammation process. Similar to peripheral macrophages, several broad classifications of microglia M1, M2a, M2b and M2c have been identified in the literature.

Depending on their environment and what stimulates them, the microglia cells are subject to various activation patterns. They can be in "classic activation", "alternative activation" or "acquired deactivation" states. The most commonly used classification is M1 or proinflammatory phenotype and M2 or regulatory or neuroprotective phenotype, the purpose of which is to "silence" inflammatory processes mediated by the M1 phenotype. Depending on the phenotype, cytokine production and receptor expression on cell surface vary, and this is accompanied by a change in cell morphology, from branched with long extensions during rest to amoeboid during activation [26].

The M1 phenotype is differentiated during "classic activation". It is characterized by the production of proinflammatory cytokines (TNF-α, IL-1β), NO, ROS and protease. The M1 phenotype is activated in response to an injury, infection, or other abnormal phenomena, with the role of defending the tissue and removing pathogen. In response to cytotoxic signals, interferon regulatory factor 5 (IRF5) is activated, which further promotes transcription of proinflammatory cytokine genes (TNF-α, IL-6, IL12 and IL-23) [26, 27].

Previously, all researchers thought that astrocytes had, in addition to structural support, a nutritional role and physical support for neurons. Recent studies have shown that astrocytes play a key role in glutamate neurotransmission and in synaptic transmission. Astrocytes excite and interact with neurons sensitive to the release of neurotransmitters and in turn release their own signaling molecules-transmitters. In addition, astrocytes also associate with the cerebrovascular capillaries *via* the end feet. These formations are located around intra-parenchymal blood vessels of the brain and maintain ionic and osmotic homeostasis and gliovascular signaling. This achieves a close contact between astrocytes and microglia, and there is strong evidence for bidirectional signaling between these two cell types. Astrocyte involvement during brain inflammation is characterized by increased cytokine production and the release of signaling molecules [28].

The events described above, directly or through microglial activation, can affect neuronal function. The NF-κB activated astrocytic pathway releases the complement protein C3, which can bind neuronal C3aR and cause neuronal damage. Another astrocyte signaling molecule, the CD40 ligand, binds with the microglial cell receptor that enhances production and release of TNF-α. The insulin resistance present in brain diabetes can cause changes such as the inflammatory response of astrocytes and microglia, which ultimately causes cortical tissue destruction in AD [29].

The elevated proinflammatory cytokines, as a result of increased microglia activity, also triggered by cytokines released from adipose tissue, can lead to the development of several pathological features of AD. It is believed that some of them could be the main mediators linking meta-inflammation to the development of central neuro-inflammation, that is, the role of obesity in the development of diabetes mellitus and brain diabetes, *i.e.* AD. In this context, the best explained is the role of peripherally and centrally released TNF-α, as a key molecule in the development of both peripheral insulin resistance and central disorders, such as the central insulin resistance and neuro-inflammation, which together lead to the development of AD.

TNF-α is a cytokine released by certain cell types; however, the main sources are monocytic cells, such as macrophages. This cytokine plays a crucial role in stationary or pathological disorders such as infections, injuries, inflammation and tumor development. When released from macrophages TNF- α induces other immune cells and facilitates the synthesis of additional proinflammatory cytokines during inflammatory reactions [30, 31].

The two distinct receptors *i.e.* TNFR1 and TNFR2 *via* TNF-α mediate its biological effect in different tissues. TNF-R1 is universally distributed in the human organisms (except red blood cells), whereas TNF-R2 is limited to myeloid cells, endothelial cells, myocytes, oligodendrocytes, microglia, astrocytes, and neurons. These two receptors are attributed to antagonistic effects with TNF-R1 acting proapoptotic and TNF-R2 providing a protective role [32].

In the development of AD, as a form of brain diabetes, TNF-α helps in two major ways: by promoting central insulin resistance and neuroinflammation.

Although the brain was once considered an insulin-insensitive organ, numerous studies have suggested the presence of insulin and its receptors in different regions of brain tissue. This provided the basis that a signaling disorder, such as that in peripheral tissues, can develop in the brain tissue. TNF-α induces brain insulin resistance in the same way as in peripheral tissues, by activation of the stress kinase c-Jun N terminal kinase (JNK). Activated JNK phosphorylates IRS-1 at serine residues (IRS-1pSer), blocking downstream insulin signaling and causing brain insulin resistance [6].

When considering the role of TNF-α in the onset of neuroinflammation, it is known that TNF-α in brain tissue is significantly increased in AD patients. This increase is primarily the result of peripherally released TNF-α during peripheral tissue meta-inflammation, which crosses BBB easily. Aβ and inflammatory cells, which also cross BBB, further increase the concentration of this inflammatory cytokine [33].

Through its receptors, TNF-α triggers different signaling pathways including NF-κB, activated protein kinase (p38 MPAK), c-jun N-terminal kinase (JNK), extracellular-signal-regulated kinases (ERKs), acid sphingomyelinase (A-SMase), neutral sphingomyelinase (N-SMase) pathways, and the transcription factors AP-1, which stimulates microglia cells to increase the synthesis of pro-inflammatory cytokines, such as Il-2, Il-6, in addition to TNF-α. In this way, the principle of positive feedback causes the development of neuro-inflammation in brain tissue, which, together with the disruption of insulin signaling, leads to the development of cognitive impairment [31].

This shows that TNF-α unites endocrine and inflammatory disorders in the development of brain diabetes, or type 3 diabetes (Fig. **3**).

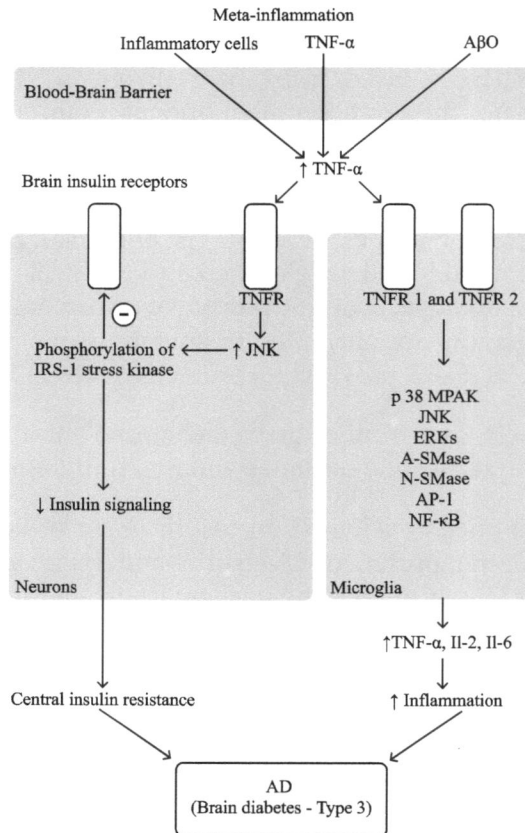

Fig. (3). Role of TNF in the development of brain diabetes.
TNF-α-Tumor Necrosis Factor α; TNFR-Tumor Necrosis Factor Receptor, AβO-Amyloid Beta Oligomers; JNK-c-Jun N-terminal Kinase;IRS-1-Insulin Receptor Substrate-1; p38 MPAK-p38 Mitoge-Activated Protein Kinase; ERKs- Extracellular Signal-Regulated Kinases; A-SMase-Acid Sphingomyelinase; N-ASMase – Neutral Sphingomyelinase;AP-1- Activator Protein 1; NF-kB-Nuclear Factor Kappa B.

In addition to TNF-α, other pro-inflammatory cytokines (IL-1α, IL-1β, IL-6, IL-18) are released during microglia activation, which are also important in the development and maintenance of the neuroinflammatory process.

Scientific data suggest that IL-1α is a reasonable candidate in AD because of its significant role in disease staging. Pathological variations in IL-1α levels are correlated with plaque development and cognitive impairment rates [34].

IL-1β is known to be a significant proinflammatory cytokine in the CNS and plays an important role in the pathogenesis of AD. Numerous studies have shown that over-expression of IL-1β produced by microglia and astrocytes occurs in the AD brain and in animal models of AD [22].

IL-6 is a inflammatory cytokine released primarily by stimulated microglia and astrocytes in different brain locations. IL-6 can induce microglia and astrocytes to generate a cascade of proinflammatory cytokines. A levels of this cytokine have been shown to be significantly increased in the brain, cerebrospinal fluid, and plasma, particularly locally around amyloid plaques in AD patients and experimental models [35].

A various studies have examined the biochemical pathways behind the relationship between IL-18 and AD pathophysiology, because the exact role of IL-18 in AD still requires to be established. Some authors have shown that IL-18 can increase the availability of APP and its phosphorylation in neuron-like differentiated human cells.

It may also rise the amyloidogenic processing of Aβ by inducing the expression of BACE-1 and N-terminal fragment (NTF) of PS-1, part of the functional γ-secretase complex, which indicates that increased or sustained levels of IL-18 may relate to the process of AD through increased Aβ [36].

INFLAMMASOMES AND AD

Although there are abundant data suggesting an association between meta-inflammation and cognitive impairment, the specific immune sensors for the detection of the metabolic stress signals that cause activation of central inflammation are still not sufficiently known.

More recent studies point to the potential role of inflammasomes as the most important control mechanisms in controlling and connecting low-grade inflammation in both periphery and brain tissues.

It is generally recognized that inflammasomes are generated predominantly in immune and inflammatory cells (macrophages, T lymphocytes, and natural killer cells), which lead to the development of anti-pathogenic immune-inflammatory responses. In the relevant literature, several forms of inflammasomes have been described: NLRP 1 (The Nucleotide-Binding Oligomerization Domain, Leucine-Rich Repeat and Pyrin Domain Containing), NLRP2, NLRP3, NLRC4 inflammasome and AIM2 (double-stranded DNA sensors absent from melanoma 2). Among them, NLRP3 is the most described and researched inflammasome, which has been shown to be associated with the pathogenesis and development of different diseases. Strong evidence indicates that the activation of NLRP3 inflammasome plays a central role in inflammation caused by obesity and related consequences: insulin resistance and diabetes type 2. In the case of cognitive disorders, NLRP3 enhances AD and may be involved in synaptic dysfunction, cognitive impairment, and the restriction of microglial clearance functions [37].

NLRP3 inflammasome is a large molecular complex composed of NLRP3, ASC (apoptosis-associated speck-like protein containing a caspase recruitment domain), and a cysteine protease caspase-1. Following activation, The NLRP3 inflammasome complex is integrated to induce caspase-1 to the pro-IL-1β and IL-18 cleaves to the IL-1β and IL-18 and to the IL-1β and cleaves of gasdermine which releases N-gasdermine into the cell surface to generate pores for the secretion of IL-1β and IL-18. These cytokines may further trigger additional astrocytes or microglial cells in the CNS to synthesize more complex inflammatory molecules, and also mobilize other immune cells (monocytes and lymphocytes) to cross BBB and to release more diverse inflammatory molecules. High concentrations IL-1β and IL-18 connect to their receptors on glial cells, neurons, macrophages and endothelial cells, and associate with many other cytokines to initiate the signaling of T-helper cells, inducing a complex cascade of signaling reactions resulting in exacerbation of inflammatory chain reactions inside the central nervous system. All of this results in an increase in amyloidogenesis and neurofibrillary tangles in the neurons [38, 39].

Although inflammasomes are involved in individual inflammatory processes in adipose tissue in obesity, as well as in the development of complications such as diabetes mellitus and cognitive impairment, it is still unclear whether peripheral inflammation can trigger a central production of inflammasomes. Since their production can be triggered not only *via* pathogen associated molecular patterns (PAMPs) and damage associated molecular patterns (DAMPs) but also through the activation of TLR receptors, there is a possibility that certain pro-inflammatory cytokines acting through these receptors may trigger the production of inflammasomes in the brain cells. This primarily applies to TNF-α, which displays affinity for TLR receptors. After the binding of TNF-α to TLR *via* MyD88 activation (the canonical adaptor for inflammatory signaling pathways downstream of members of the Toll-like receptor), the NF-κB synthesis is initiated, which then induces the expression of NLP3 inflammasomes [40].

Recent clinical trials have shown that sFFAs, involved in meta-inflammation in obesity, in addition to the direct neurotoxicity caused by activation of tau hyper-phosphorylation, may also enhance inflammatory processes in the brain tissue by releasing inflammasomes from microglia and astrocytes. As they are involved in the development of metabolic disorders, such as insulin resistance and diabetes, their role in stimulating central inflammation may provide further evidence of the metabolic-inflammatory basis of the development of brain diabetes, or type 3 diabetes (Fig. **4**).

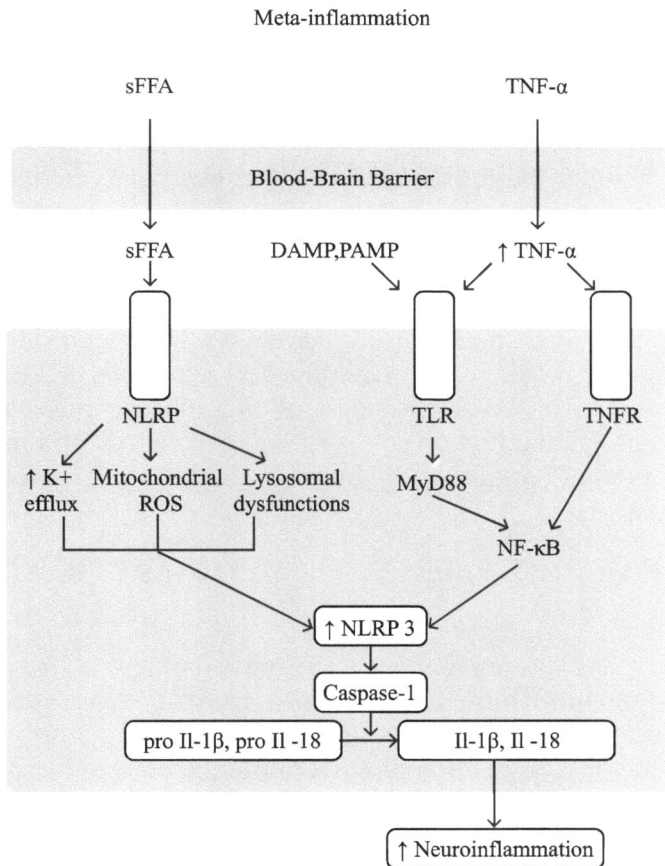

Fig. (4). Impact of meta-inflammation on the synthesis and expression of inflammasomes.
TNF-α-Tumor Necrosis Factor α; TNFR-Tumor Necrosis Factor Receptor, NF-kB-Nuclear Factor Kappa B;sFFA- saturated Free Fatty Acid; TLR-Toll-like Receptor; NF-kB-Nuclear Factor Kappa B; DAMP-Damage Associated Molecular Patterns; PAMP- Pathogen Associated Molecular Patterns; NLRP - The Nucleotide-Binding Oligomerization Domain, Leucine-Rich Repeat And Pyrin Domain Containing; MyD88-Myeloid Differentiation Factor 88; ROS- Reactive Oxygen Species; Il- Interleukin.

Although the precise mechanism through which sFFAs influence the activation of inflammasomes has yet to be fully explained, it is believed that this is accomplished by their binding to NLRP3 (the nucleotide-binding oligomerization domain, leucine-rich repeat and pyrin domain containing 3) and by activation of three possible mechanisms: potassium efflux, production of mitochondrial reactive oxygen species (ROS), and lysosomal dysfunction [41].

From this, it can be concluded that the release of inflamasomes requires two simultaneous and well-coordinated signals in which peripherally released molecules play an important role during meta-inflammation: Signal 1 can be elicited by TLR (Toll-Like Receptor) ligands (TNF-α DAMP, PAMP), whereas numerous molecules can provide signal 2 (*via* NLRP3), including various pore-forming toxins, Aβ, as well as sFFA [42].

Some researchers have pointed out in their studies the importance of inflammasomes in the development of AD. Heneka *et al*. [37] have examined the possible role of the NLRP3 inflammasome in Alzheimer's disease. APP (amyloid precursor protein)/Presenilin-1 (PS1) mice, which develop symptoms similar to AD, were crossed with NLRP3−/− or Casp-1−/− mice. The quantity of cleaved Casp-1 in the brains of the offspring was then measured in comparison to the APP/PS1 mice. APP/PS1 mice exhibited delayed habituation and increased psychomotor agitation, further supporting the fact that the NLRP3 inflammasome plays an important role in the development of cognitive disorders in AD patients. The authors suggest that activation of NLRP3 enhances AD and may be included in synaptic dysfunction, cognitive dysfunction, and the restriction of microglial clearance functions.

ANTI-INFLAMMATORY EFFECTS OF ANTIDIABETIC AGENTS IN AD TREATMENT

Based on a clear association between the development of diabetes and AD through the low-grade inflammation process, it can be concluded that this AD is a complex disease of a neuroendocrine-inflammatory nature and that the introduction of the term type 3 diabetes, or brain diabetes, is justified. Therefore, the development of new therapeutic targets implicated in the maintenance of healthy metabolism will potentially result in innovative clinical applications not only in metabolic disorders but as well as in neuroinflammatory CNS disorders. For this reason, the use of drugs commonly used in the treatment of diabetes has been introduced as possible protocols in the treatment of type 3 diabetes. Drugs, such as GLP-1 agonists and thiazolidinediones, which not only affect insulin resistance but also exhibit a certain degree of anti-inflammatory effect, both in the periphery and centrally, have been highlighted.

Receptors for GLP1 agonists have been shown to exist in the CNS, especially in the hypothalamus, hippocampus, cerebral cortex and olfactory bulb. GLP-1 is assumed to have several beneficial effects within the CNS, where the activation of GLP-1Rs protects against apoptosis, has a neuroprotective effect against various stimuli, and induces neurite growth, especially in the hippocampus. Several preclinical studies have tested the potential neuroprotective effects of GLP-1 analogues in AD, with promising results. Systemic administration of liraglutide for 8 weeks on transgenic mice with AD prevented memory impairment, neuronal loss and deterioration of synaptic plasticity in the hippocampus. Liraglutide was found to be able to reduce the accumulation of amyloid plaques by 40-50% and the inflammatory response, as evidenced by the analysis of activated microglial cells. Similarly, the effect of Aβ-induced impairment of spatial memory and long-term memory was significantly reduced in rats treated with an intrahypocampal injection of Aβ and previously with liraglutide. Other clinical studies have shown that liraglutide promotes neurogenesis, reduces tau hyperphosphorylation and may also have positive effects on cerebral and systemic microvascularization in AD. Importantly, liraglutide not only has preventative properties but can also impact some of the key pathological features of late-stage AD [43, 44].

Among other GLP-1 analogues, exenatide has shown promising results in preclinical studies for its use in neurodegenerative diseases [45].

The inhibitors of DPP4, or gliptins, stabilize GLP-1 levels by inhibiting its degradation and lower fasting and postprandial glucose. Saxagliptin and vildagliptin, drugs approved in the treatment of DM, have also been tested in preclinical studies with induced AD on an animal model. Oral administration of these drugs reduced Aβ accumulation, tau phosphorylation and inflammatory markers, with the improvement of hippocampal GLP-1 levels and memory [46].

The use of PPARγ agonists, especially the class of these drugs known as thiazolidinediones (rosiglitazone and pioglitazone), is based on the fact that peroxisome proliferator-activated receptor-γ (PPARγ) is a key neuromodulator found in larger quantities in the brains of patients with AD. This receptor plays a role in a number of processes thought to be involved in the pathogenesis of diabetes and AD, including inflammatory and metabolic processes and cell growth and differentiation. These drugs act on insulin resistance, cholesterol homeostasis and Ca^{2+} homeostasis in the hippocampus, and reduce cerebral inflammation *via* inhibition of IL-6 and TNF. It is assumed that this is how they control the proliferation of the β-amyloid peptide and improve a cognitive function in patients with AD [47].

Thiazolidinediones (TZDs) help to alleviate some of the symptoms and pathology of AD, improve learning in patients with AD, and reduce amyloid burden and plaque burden in animal models. Through the activation of PPARγ, TZDs have been shown to delay the development of AD using various mechanisms, such as improving insulin sensitivity, reducing inflammation, activating Aβ plaque clearance, enhancing mitochondrial function and preventing tau hyperphosphorylation. PPARγ increases the number of GLUT4 transporters in neural membranes, allowing an increased glucose uptake and facilitating a proper cell function [48].

TZDs reduce inflammation by inhibiting microglia cells with the development of an anti-inflammatory state. When Aβ plaques activate the inflammatory response of macrophages, elevated levels of microglia and macrophages become neurotoxic and damage the brain. Macrophages produce IL-6, which activates multiple macrophages, inflammatory agents, and TNF-α, which induces apoptosis. TZDs have an anti-inflammatory effect by stopping the transcription of a nuclear factor for the activator of Protein 1 (AP-1), and this inhibits microglia activation due to the presence of Aβ plaques [49].

CONCLUDING REMARKS

The findings of various studies provide solid evidence that supports the conclusion that AD is a type of diabetes mellitus that affects the central nervous system. Numerous clinical and basic studies have shown that there are specific pathophysiological modifications with specific signaling pathways, and inflammatory pathways that link the association between the two disorders and are referred to that as T3D diabetes. Although still insufficiently explained, numerous pathways have been discovered through which meta-inflammation, as a consequence of obesity, can stimulate the development of brain diabetes, *i.e.* AD. Complex mechanisms involve numerous signaling molecules that, through a large number of different receptors, can link meta-inflammation with the activation of microglia and astrocytes to produce a state of central inflammation with the consequent prolonged release of pro-inflammatory cytokines. The combined disorder of insulin signaling and the pro-inflammatory state forms the basis for neuronal damage and the development of cognitive impairment.

Some important questions still need to be answered along with how various factors dynamically adjust the triggering of proinflammatory cytokines in brain tissue as well as how the signaling of proinflammatory cytokines is interconnected with metabolic pathways. A deeper understanding of the complex features underlying major disease symptoms, including inflammation and metabolic disorders, may contribute to the development of novel and successful treatments that would not only delay but also stop the development of neurodegenerative brain diseases.

CONSENT FOR PUBLICATION

Not applicable.

CONFLICT OF INTEREST

The authors confirm that this chapter content has no conflict of interest.

ACKNOWLEDGEMENTS

The authors would like to express their sincere thanks to the editor and anonymous reviewers for their time and valuable suggestions.

REFERENCES

[1]   Kalathookunnel Antony A, Lian Z, Wu H. T cells in adipose tissue in aging. Front Immunol 2018; 9: 2945.
[http://dx.doi.org/10.3389/fimmu.2018.02945] [PMID: 30619305]

[2]   Johnson AR, Milner JJ, Makowski L. The inflammation highway: metabolism accelerates inflammatory traffic in obesity. Immunol Rev 2012; 249(1): 218-38.
[http://dx.doi.org/10.1111/j.1600-065X.2012.01151.x] [PMID: 22889225]

[3]   Šimić G, Babić Leko M, Wray S, *et al.* Monoaminergic neuropathology in Alzheimer's disease. Prog Neurobiol 2017; 151: 101-38.
[http://dx.doi.org/10.1016/j.pneurobio.2016.04.001] [PMID: 27084356]

[4]   Mormino EC, Papp KV. Amyloid accumulation and cognitive decline in clinically normal older individuals: implications for aging and early alzheimer's disease. J Alzheimers Dis 2018; 64(s1): S633-46.
[http://dx.doi.org/10.3233/JAD-179928] [PMID: 29782318]

[5]   de la Monte SM, Wands JR. Alzheimer's disease is type 3 diabetes-evidence reviewed. J Diabetes Sci Technol 2008; 2(6): 1101-13.
[http://dx.doi.org/10.1177/193229680800200619] [PMID: 19885299]

[6]   Ferreira LSS, Fernandes CS, Vieira MNN, De Felice FG. Insulin resistance in alzheimer's disease. Front Neurosci 2018; 12: 830.
[http://dx.doi.org/10.3389/fnins.2018.00830] [PMID: 30542257]

[7]   Skaper SD, Facci L, Zusso M, Giusti P. An inflammation-centric view of neurological disease: beyond the neuron. Front Cell Neurosci 2018; 12: 72.
[http://dx.doi.org/10.3389/fncel.2018.00072] [PMID: 29618972]

[8]   Appari M, Channon KM, McNeill E. Metabolic regulation of adipose tissue macrophage function in obesity and diabetes. Antioxid Redox Signal 2018; 29(3): 297-312.
[http://dx.doi.org/10.1089/ars.2017.7060] [PMID: 28661198]

[9]   Diaz B, Fuentes-Mera L, Tovar A, *et al.* Saturated lipids decrease mitofusin 2 leading to endoplasmic reticulum stress activation and insulin resistance in hypothalamic cells. Brain Res 2015; 1627: 80-9.
[http://dx.doi.org/10.1016/j.brainres.2015.09.014] [PMID: 26410780]

[10]   Sergio T. Ferreira, Julia R. Clarke, Theresa R. Bomfim, Fernanda G. De Felice. Inflammation, defective insulin signaling, and neuronal dysfunction in Alzheimer's disease. Alzheimers Dement

2014; 10(1) (Suppl.): 76-83.
[PMID: 23375567]

[11]   Rehman K, Akash MS. Mechanisms of inflammatory responses and development of insulin resistance:
       how are they interlinked? J Biomed Sci 2016; 23(1): 87.
       [http://dx.doi.org/10.1186/s12929-016-0303-y] [PMID: 27912756]

[12]   Fournet M, Bonté F, Desmoulière A. Glycation damage: a possible hub for major pathophysiological
       disorders and aging. Aging Dis 2018; 9(5): 880-900.
       [http://dx.doi.org/10.14336/AD.2017.1121] [PMID: 30271665]

[13]   Benzler J, Ganjam GK, Pretz D, *et al.* Central inhibition of IKKβ/NF-κB signaling attenuates high-fat
       diet-induced obesity and glucose intolerance. Diabetes 2015; 64(6): 2015-27.
       [http://dx.doi.org/10.2337/db14-0093] [PMID: 25626735]

[14]   Bednarska-Makaruk M, Graban A, Wiśniewska A, *et al.* Association of adiponectin, leptin and resistin
       with inflammatory markers and obesity in dementia. Biogerontology 2017; 18(4): 561-80.
       [http://dx.doi.org/10.1007/s10522-017-9701-0] [PMID: 28421328]

[15]   McGuire MJ, Ishii M. Leptin dysfunction and Alzheimer's disease: evidence from cellular, animal,
       and human studies. Cell Mol Neurobiol 2016; 36(2): 203-17.
       [http://dx.doi.org/10.1007/s10571-015-0282-7] [PMID: 26993509]

[16]   Kim JG, Suyama S, Koch M, *et al.* Leptin signaling in astrocytes regulates hypothalamic neuronal
       circuits and feeding. Nat Neurosci 2014; 17(7): 908-10.
       [http://dx.doi.org/10.1038/nn.3725] [PMID: 24880214]

[17]   La Cava A. Leptin in inflammation and autoimmunity. Cytokine 2017; 98: 51-8.
       [http://dx.doi.org/10.1016/j.cyto.2016.10.011] [PMID: 27916613]

[18]   Gilbert T, Roche S, Blond E, *et al.* Association between Peripheral Leptin and Adiponectin Levels and
       Cognitive Decline in Patients with Neurocognitive Disorders ≥65 Years. J Alzheimers Dis 2018;
       66(3): 1255-64.
       [http://dx.doi.org/10.3233/JAD-180533] [PMID: 30400097]

[19]   Waragai M, Ho G, Takamatsu Y, *et al.* Importance of adiponectin activity in the pathogenesis of
       Alzheimer's disease. Ann Clin Transl Neurol 2017; 4(8): 591-600.
       [http://dx.doi.org/10.1002/acn3.436] [PMID: 28812049]

[20]   Kizilarslanoğlu MC, Kara Ö, Yeşil Y, *et al.* Alzheimer disease, inflammation, and novel inflammatory
       marker: resistin. Turk J Med Sci 2015; 45(5): 1040-6.
       [http://dx.doi.org/10.3906/sag-1403-55] [PMID: 26738345]

[21]   Demirci S, Aynalı A, Demirci K, Demirci S, Arıdoğan BC. The serum levels of resistin and its
       relationship with other proinflammatory cytokines in patients with Alzheimer's disease. Clin
       Psychopharmacol Neurosci 2017; 15(1): 59-63.
       [http://dx.doi.org/10.9758/cpn.2017.15.1.59] [PMID: 28138112]

[22]   Wang WY, Tan MS, Yu JT, Tan L. Role of pro-inflammatory cytokines released from microglia in
       Alzheimer's disease. Ann Transl Med 2015; 3(10): 136.
       [PMID: 26207229]

[23]   Ginhoux F, Lim S, Hoeffel G, Low D, Huber T, Cuadros MA. Origin and differentiation of microglia.
       Front Cell Neurosci 2013; 7: 45.
       [http://dx.doi.org/10.3389/fncel.2013.00045] [PMID: 23616747]

[24]   Barrientos RM, Kitt MM, Watkins LR, Maier SF. Neuroinflammation in the normal aging
       hippocampus. Neuroscience 2016; 36: 1011-4.
       [PMID: 25772789]

[25]   Jiang T, Yu JT, Tan L. Novel disease-modifying therapies for Alzheimer's disease. J Alzheimers Dis
       2012; 31(3): 475-92.
       [http://dx.doi.org/10.3233/JAD-2012-120640] [PMID: 22669013]

[26]   Tang Y, Le W. Differential roles of m1 and m2 microglia in neurodegenerative diseases. Mol Neurobiol 2016; 53(2): 1181-94.
[http://dx.doi.org/10.1007/s12035-014-9070-5] [PMID: 25598354]

[27]   von Bernhardi R, Eugenín-von Bernhardi L, Eugenín J. Microglial cell dysregulation in brain aging and neurodegeneration. Front Aging Neurosci 2015; 7: 124.
[http://dx.doi.org/10.3389/fnagi.2015.00124] [PMID: 26257642]

[28]   Harada K, Kamiya T, Tsuboi T. Gliotransmitter release from astrocytes: functional, developmental, and pathological implications in the brain. Front Neurosci 2016; 9: 499.
[http://dx.doi.org/10.3389/fnins.2015.00499] [PMID: 26793048]

[29]   Lian H, Yang L, Cole A, *et al.* NFκB-activated astroglial release of complement C3 compromises neuronal morphology and function associated with Alzheimer's disease. Neuron 2015; 85(1): 101-15.
[http://dx.doi.org/10.1016/j.neuron.2014.11.018] [PMID: 25533482]

[30]   Ruder B, Atreya R, Becker C. Tumour necrosis factor alpha in intestinal homeostasis and gut related diseases. Int J Mol Sci 2019; 20(8): E1887.
[http://dx.doi.org/10.3390/ijms20081887] [PMID: 30995806]

[31]   Cook AD, Christensen AD, Tewari D, McMahon SB, Hamilton JA. Immune cytokines and their receptors in inflammatory pain. Trends Immunol 2018; 39(3): 240-55.
[http://dx.doi.org/10.1016/j.it.2017.12.003] [PMID: 29338939]

[32]   Decourt B, Lahiri DK, Sabbagh MN. Targeting tumor necrosis factor alpha for Alzheimer's disease. Curr Alzheimer Res 2017; 14(4): 412-25.
[PMID: 27697064]

[33]   Chang R, Yee KL, Sumbria RK. Tumor necrosis factor α inhibition for Alzheimer's disease. J Cent Nerv Syst Dis 2017; 9: 1179573517709278.
[http://dx.doi.org/10.1177/1179573517709278] [PMID: 28579870]

[34]   Hu WT, Chen-Plotkin A, Arnold SE, *et al.* Novel CSF biomarkers for Alzheimer's disease and mild cognitive impairment. Acta Neuropathol 2010; 119(6): 669-78.
[http://dx.doi.org/10.1007/s00401-010-0667-0] [PMID: 20232070]

[35]   Wu YY, Hsu JL, Wang HC, Wu SJ, Hong CJ, Cheng IH. Alterations of the neuroinflammatory markers IL-6 and trail in Alzheimer's disease. Dement Geriatr Cogn Disord Extra 2015; 5(3): 424-34.
[http://dx.doi.org/10.1159/000439214] [PMID: 26675645]

[36]   Ojala JO, Sutinen EM. The role of interleukin-18, oxidative stress and metabolic syndrome in Alzheimer's Disease. J Clin Med 2017; 6(5): E55.
[http://dx.doi.org/10.3390/jcm6050055] [PMID: 28531131]

[37]   Heneka MT, Kummer MP, Stutz A, *et al.* NLRP3 is activated in Alzheimer's disease and contributes to pathology in APP/PS1 mice. Nature 2013; 493(7434): 674-8.
[http://dx.doi.org/10.1038/nature11729] [PMID: 23254930]

[38]   Liu L, Chan C. The role of inflammasome in Alzheimer's disease. Ageing Res Rev 2014; 15: 6-15.
[http://dx.doi.org/10.1016/j.arr.2013.12.007] [PMID: 24561250]

[39]   Song L, Pei L, Yao S, Wu Y, Shang Y. NLRP3 inflammasome in neurological diseases, from functions to therapies. Front Cell Neurosci 2017; 11: 63.
[http://dx.doi.org/10.3389/fncel.2017.00063] [PMID: 28337127]

[40]   Kelley N, Jeltema D, Duan Y, He Y. The NLRP3 inflammasome: an overview of mechanisms of activation and regulation. Int J Mol Sci 2019; 20(13): 3328.
[http://dx.doi.org/10.3390/ijms20133328] [PMID: 31284572]

[41]   Karasawa T, Kawashima A, Usui-Kawanishi F, *et al.* Saturated fatty acids undergo intracellular crystallization and activate the NLRP3 inflammasome in macrophages. Arterioscler Thromb Vasc Biol 2018; 38(4): 744-56.

[http://dx.doi.org/10.1161/ATVBAHA.117.310581] [PMID: 29437575]

[42]   Hanamsagar R, Hanke ML, Kielian T. Toll-like receptor (TLR) and inflammasome actions in the central nervous system. Trends Immunol 2012; 33(7): 333-42.
[http://dx.doi.org/10.1016/j.it.2012.03.001] [PMID: 22521509]

[43]   Calsolaro V, Edison P. Novel GLP-1 (glucagon-like peptide-1) analogues and insulin in the treatment for Alzheimer's disease and other neurodegenerative diseases. CNS Drugs 2015; 29(12): 1023-39.
[http://dx.doi.org/10.1007/s40263-015-0301-8] [PMID: 26666230]

[44]   Qi L, Ke L, Liu X, *et al.* Subcutaneous administration of liraglutide ameliorates learning and memory impairment by modulating tau hyperphosphorylation *via* the glycogen synthase kinase-3β pathway in an amyloid β protein induced alzheimer disease mouse model. Eur J Pharmacol 2016; 783: 23-32.
[http://dx.doi.org/10.1016/j.ejphar.2016.04.052] [PMID: 27131827]

[45]   Mullins RJ, Mustapic M, Chia CW, *et al.* A pilot study of exenatide actions in Alzheimer's disease. Curr Alzheimer Res 2019; 16(8): 741-52.
[http://dx.doi.org/10.2174/1567205016666190913155950] [PMID: 31518224]

[46]   Femminella GD, Bencivenga L, Petraglia L, *et al.* Antidiabetic drugs in Alzheimer's disease: mechanisms of action and future perspectives. J Diabetes Res 2017; 2017: 7420796.
[http://dx.doi.org/10.1155/2017/7420796] [PMID: 28656154]

[47]   Fakan B, Szalardy L, Vecsei L. Exploiting the therapeutic potential of endogenous immunomodulatory systems in multiple sclerosis-special focus on the peroxisome proliferator-activated receptors (PPARs) and the kynurenines. Int J Mol Sci 2019; 20(2): 426.
[http://dx.doi.org/10.3390/ijms20020426] [PMID: 30669473]

[48]   Liu J, Wang LN, Jia JP. Peroxisome proliferator-activated receptor-gamma agonists for Alzheimer's disease and amnestic mild cognitive impairment: a systematic review and meta-analysis. Drugs Aging 2015; 32(1): 57-65.
[http://dx.doi.org/10.1007/s40266-014-0228-7] [PMID: 25504005]

[49]   Pérez MJ, Quintanilla RA. Therapeutic actions of the thiazolidinediones in Alzheimer's disease. PPAR Res 2015; 2015: 957248.
[http://dx.doi.org/10.1155/2015/957248] [PMID: 26587016]

CHAPTER 8

Interplay Between Oxidative Stress and Meta-Inflammation in Obesity-Related Neurodegeneration

Orhan Lepara[*]

Department of Human Physiology, University of Sarajevo School of Medicine, Sarajevo, Bosnia and Herzegovina

Abstract: Neurodegeneration refers to the gradual deterioration of neuron structure and function and can lead to debilitating neurological conditions such as Alzheimer's disease (AD), Parkinson's disease (PD), Huntington's disease (HD), and amyotrophic lateral sclerosis (ALS). Common pathogenic mechanisms on which many neurodegenerative disorders (NDDs) are based include abnormal protein dynamics of malfolding, degradation, proteasomal instability, and aggregation; often with molecular chaperone actions and mutations; free radical/reactive oxygen species (ROS) formation and OxS; bioenergetic weakness, mitochondrial dysfunction and damage to DNA, neuronal Golgi system fragmentation, disruption of the movement of cellular/axonal, neurotrophin (NTF) dysfunction and neuroinflammatory/neuroimmune processes. Oxidative stress is a phenomenon caused by an imbalance between production and accumulation of ROS/reactive nitrogen species (RNS) and/or a deficiency of enzymatic and nonenzymatic antioxidants. Oxidative stress can be a result, but also an obesity trigger. It has shown that obesity is coupled with an altered redox state and increased metabolic risk. Antioxidant defenses in obese patients are decreased compared to the control group, and their concentrations correlate inversely with core adiposity. Moreover, obesity is also defined by increased concentrations of reactive oxygen or nitrogen species. Metabolic changes caused by weight are associated with damage to the central nervous system (CNS), which can result in neuronal death, either through apoptosis or cell necrosis, or by modifying the neuron's synaptic plasticity. Adipose tissue dysfunction associated with obesity has been correlated with abnormal brain metabolism, neuroinflammation, brain atrophy, neural impairment, diminished mood, and cognitive decline. Due to their high metabolic rate, visceral fat tissues function as endocrine organs, which secrete adipokines (leptin, adiponectin, visfatin, resistin, apelin, and plasminogen activator inhibitor type 1) and cytokines (TNF-α, IL-6, IL-1β). Inflammatory cytokines bind to their receptors by activating the pathway of the nuclear factor-kappaB, which induces a pro-inflammatory state. Inflammatory pathways and DNA damage may also be triggered by nutritional imbalance, adversely affecting redox control [*via* glutathione peroxidase (GPx); glutathione (GSH), and oxidized glutathione

---

[*] **Corresponding author Orhan Lepara:** Department of Human Physiology, Faculty of Medicine University of Sarajevo, Bosnia and Herzegovina; Tel: +387 33 226 478, Ext. 527; E-mail: orhan.lepara@mf.unsa.ba

Asija Začiragić (Ed.)

(GSSG) levels] and thus fostering oxidative stress. Obesity also impacts the glucose and energy metabolism of brain cells, and by secreting pro-inflammatory agents causes neuroinflammation primarily in the brain's hypothalamic area. The general effect is the loss of neuronal activity and its internal molecular machinery, resulting in intracellular or extracellular or both aberrant protein deposition, contributing to neurodegeneration.

Keywords: Adipokines, Cytokines, Metainflammation, Neuroinflammation, Neurodegeneration, Neurodegenerative disease, Oxidative stress, Obesity.

INTRODUCTION

Oxidants and antioxidants play a significant role in controlling free radical equilibrium in the body generated during active metabolism in living organisms. A troubled endogenous antioxidant mechanism favors shifting to more manufacturing of pro-oxidants. This state is called "oxidative stress" (OxS) [1].

OxS is a phenomenon caused by an imbalance between production and accumulation of Reactive oxygen species (ROS)/Reactive nitrogen species (RNS) and/or a deficiency of enzymatic and nonenzymatic antioxidants. The terms ROS and RNS refer, respectively, to reactive oxygen and nitrogen radicals and non-radical derivatives [2].

ROS are tiny molecules obtained from oxygen molecules, including free oxygen radicals such as superoxide ($O_2^{·-}$), hydroxyl (•OH), peroxyl (ROO•), alkoxyl (RO•), non-radical hypochlorous acid (HOCl), ozone (O_3), single oxygen ($1O_2$), and hydrogen peroxide (H_2O_2). Oxidants containing nitrogen such as peroxynitrite ($ONOO^-$), nitric oxide (NO), nitrogen dioxide (NO2•), as well as non-radicals such as nitrous acid (HNO_2) and dinitrogen tetroxide (N_2O_4) are referred to as RNS [3, 4].

All aerobic cells produce reactive oxygen and nitrogen species (RONS) and play a significant role in both aging and age-related diseases [2].

Endogenous or exogenous sources can produce ROS. The endogenous ROS sources include various cellular organs such as mitochondria, peroxisomes, and endoplasmic reticulum, where oxygen consumption is high [5]. Exogenous sources of ROS and RNS are caused by air and water pollution, alcohol consumption, smoking, certain drugs, heavy metals, certain medications (tacrolimus and cyclosporine), radiation, cooking, and benzene solvents [6] (Fig. **1**).

ROS are now recognized as signaling molecules, which control a broad range of physiological functions. They play key roles in the activation of genes, cell growth, and the modulation of chemical cell responses. They also engage in the control of blood pressure, are mediators in prostaglandin biosynthesis, operate in embryonic development, and act as signaling molecules in the individual cells and cells during their lifetime [7].

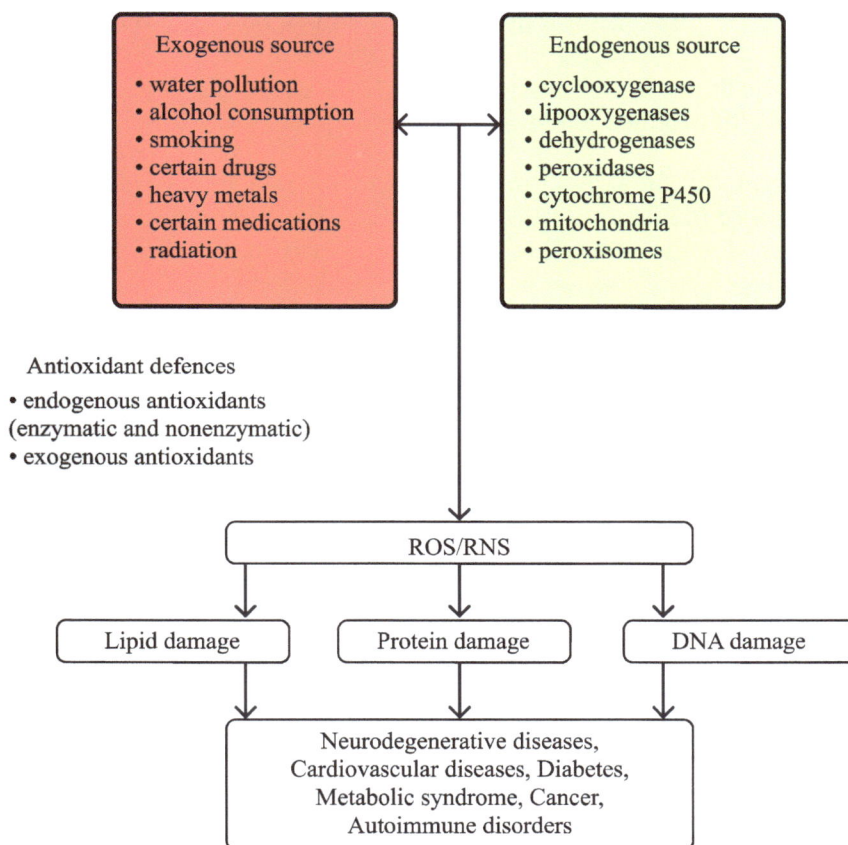

Fig. (1). Reactive oxygen species (ROS) and Reactive nitrogen species (RNS) and their role in the development of disease.
ROS - Reactive oxygen species; RNS - Reactive nitrogen species.

Reactive oxygen and nitrogen species produced *in vivo* result in either physiological levels needed for ordinary cell function or excessive amounts causing nucleic acids, proteins, lipids, and other biomolecules to be damaged [8].

Antioxidant defense protects biological systems and involves both endogenous and exogenous molecules from free radical toxicity [2]. Antioxidants can operate against distinct kinds of free radicals and reactive species synergistically [9].

The natural antioxidant defense consists of endogenous antioxidants, enzymatic and non-enzymatic antioxidants generated by our bodies, and exogenous antioxidants that can be incorporated by diet or dietary supplements [10]. SOD, catalase (CAT), glutathione peroxidase (GPx), glutathione reductase (GRx), and peroxiredoxins are the main antioxidant enzymes. GPx, CAT, and SOD are the most effective enzymatic antioxidants. GPx and SOD (in two forms: CuZnSOD and MnSOD) are discovered in mitochondria and cytosol, while catalases are found in peroxisomes. O_2 is transformed to H_2O_2 by SOD, while GPx and catalase react with H_2O_2 to produce water and oxygen [9].

The non-enzymatic substances involved in the first line of defense belong to preventive antioxidants and are represented by reduced glutathione (GSH), ceruloplasmin, ferritin, transferrin, bilirubin, uric acid and albumin in blood plasma [2, 11].

Exogenous antioxidants include ascorbic acid (vitamin C), α-tocopherol (vitamin E), carotenoids, antioxidants in stilbene, phenolic acids, lecithins in oil, flavonoids, acetylcysteine, zinc, selenium, magnesium and copper [12] (Fig. **1**).

OxS involves the pathogenesis of several diseases, such as Alzheimer's disease (AD), Parkinson's disease (PD), amyotrophic lateral sclerosis (ALS), arthritis, atherosclerosis, hypertension, cancer, autoimmune disorders, osteoporosis, diabetes, and metabolic syndrome [13, 14] (Fig. **1**).

OXIDATIVE STRESS, OBESITY, AND INFLAMMATION

OxS is also involved in the pathological processes of obesity. Obesity is a complex medical condition characterized by excessive, abnormal accumulation of fat due to increased intake of high-energy foods and reduced physical activity. It has become a truly global epidemic that affects all ages, all populations, and countries of all levels of income [15].

Adipose tissue is an endocrine and energy homeostasis storage organ [16]. It consists of two subtypes: adipose white tissue (WAT) and brown adipose tissue (BAT). WAT is renowned for its ability to store lipids and its endocrine function, while BAT is defined by energy expenditure to generate heat (nonshivering thermogenesis) [17]. This tissue, which consists mainly of adipocytes, includes other cells, such as fibroblasts, fibroblastic pre-adipocytes, endothelial and immune cells [16].

Obesity is strongly associated with an increased risk of developing diabetes mellitus, hypertension, dyslipidemia, heart disease, central nervous system, respiratory, gastrointestinal and kidney diseases, osteoarthritis, gynecological and obstetric complications, malignancies and psychological disorders [18].

Diseases evolve from obesity through various processes, including ROS-induced OxS, because hypertrophied adipocytes have been recorded as an important source of ROS [16, 19].

OxS can be a result, but also an obesity trigger. Evidence indicates that the mechanical connection between obesity and associated problems may be OxS. Epidemiological, clinical, and animal studies have shown that obesity is coupled with altered redox state and increased metabolic risk. Antioxidant defenses in obese patients are decreased compared to the control group, and their concentrations correlate inversely with core adiposity. Obesity is also defined by increased concentrations of reactive oxygen or nitrogen species [20].

For instance, in obese people, there is an inverse relationship between body fat, visceral obesity, and antioxidant defense markers. Evidence of obesity-induced OxS is obtained from several clinical studies with proven correlations between end-products of free OxS (lipid peroxidation or protein carbonylation products) and body mass index (BMI) [16].

There are several mechanisms engaged in the obesity OxS generation [21]. Mitochondria ROS derived from ROS may be derived from mitochondria. As a consequence, increased nutrient uptake into adipocytes will boost the mitochondrial substrate load, resulting in increased $O2\bullet-$by-products due to increased ETC activity. The mitochondrial metabolic flux as a basis for enhanced adipocyte ROS manufacturing is controversy concerning the use of adipocyte substrate. Free fatty acids (FFA) entering adipocytes are transformed quickly to fatty acyl-CoA and eventually stored as triglycerides (TGs) without significant mitochondrial oxidation [16].

Excess production of mitochondrial-derived ROS is correlated with the aggravation of inflammation and growth of insulin resistance in adipocytes by the activation of NF-κB [22].

NADPH oxidase is an essential regulatory enzyme in adipose tissue that, in reaction to agonist stimuli, generates superoxide and/or H_2O_2. Nox4 is the significant adipocyte-specific Nox isotype that is activated by high-fat diets. Nox4 is important because it produces H_2O_2 as compared to superoxide anion produced by the other members of the NADPH oxidase family [23].

Adipose tissue, which consists mainly of adipocytes, also includes other cells (*e.g.*, fibroblasts, fibroblastic pre-adipocytes, endothelial and immune cells), which secrete hormones and cytokines (adipokines or adipocytokines) that exert endocrine, paracrine and autocrine actions throughout the body. In physiological and pathological circumstances, adipokines also stimulate the development of ROS, producing OxS and, in turn, the development of other adipokines [21].

Hypertrophied adipocytes have been reported as an important source of ROS [16].

It has been shown that adipose tissue expresses pro-inflammatory mediators, both by macrophages and adipocytes, which cause inflammation of low intensity in adipose tissue. The deposition of triglycerides in adipocytes results in macrophage activation and overproduction of pro-inflammatory cytokines, as well as dysregulation of adipocytokines [24].

The presence of excessive adipose tissue was recognized as a source of pro-inflammatory cytokines, including tumor necrosis factor-alpha (TNF-α), interleukin-6 (IL-6) and IL-1β [21].

ROS generation was reported to involve both cell survival and cell death after TNF-α binding, and mitochondrion is the primary cause of ROS generation contributing to TNF-α-induced cell death. The usually accepted hypothesis is that TNF-induced ROS suppresses NF-kB activation, reducing the signaling of NF-kB-mediated survival and accounting for the cell death associated with elevated ROS [25].

TNF-induced NF-kB signaling also drives gene encoding iNOS. iNOS generates NO/RNS in reaction to multiple stimuli, which provides huge flexibility to the immune system when faced with multiple challenges. For instance, NO can cause BAX/BAK-dependent cell death involving cytochrome c and caspase 9 [25].

IL-6 is a potent cytokine that plays a major role in insulin resistance and type 2 diabetes pathogenesis. In patients with obesity and type 2 diabetes, as well as patients with metabolic syndrome, an increase of IL-6 was documented in adipose tissue [26].

Emerging proof indicates inflammatory cytokines, such as IL-6, influence the expression and activity of eNOS and NADPH oxidase, and thus impact the contribution of NO and superoxide concentration onOxS [27].

IL-6 has an immediate effect on the activity and expression of endothelial nitric oxide synthase and on increased vascular superoxide, which inactivates NO quickly and limits NO bioavailability. In fact, IL-6 mediated NO bioavailability reductions and enhanced OxSare linked with enhanced endothelial production of MCP-1. IL-6 can stimulate the endothelial expression of adhesive molecules, including ICAM-1, VCAM-1, and E-selectin, thereby increasing immune cell adhesion and extravasation in the vascular wall. NADPH oxidase antioxidants or inhibitors are very efficient in reducing IL-6 expression [27]. IL-6 also induces ROS production in rheumatoid arthritis (RA) synovial fibroblastic cells [28].

IL-1β is a canonical IL-1 family member consisting of two IL-1α and IL-1β agonists. IL-1β is a true pleiotropic cytokine that impacts both innate and acquired immune systems.IL-1β is an instigator of the pro-inflammatory reaction in obesity through the production of other pro-inflammatory cytokines, such as IL-6 [21]. IL-1β stimulates the development of ROS in different cell types. Yang *et al.* [29] have shown that IL-1β, TNF-α, and IFN-γ increase mitochondrial- and NADPH oxidase-generated ROS in human retinal pigment epithelial cells. It is shown that IL-1β significantly increased intracellular ROS levels in annulus fibrosus cells [30].

It has been shown that excessive superoxide anion production could lead to NF-kB activation, which would eventually lead to a rise in pro-inflammatory cytokines such as IL-1β and IL-6 [31].

During inflammation, ROS stimulates the activation of mediator signaling molecules such as the NF-kB, which up-regulates the development of inflammatory cytokines such as IL-1β, TNF-α, and other mediators as iNOS or cyclooxygenase-2 (COX-2). ROS can harm cellular lipids, lipid peroxidation products, and lipid aldehydes such as MDA, HNE, and acrolein that are involved in various inflammatory diseases with damaging consequences caused by OxS.ROS may also harm proteins and DNA. DNA damage may trigger mutations and is involved in the initiation and/or advancement of inflammation-mediated carcinogenesis. NF-kB is triggered by a significant form of membrane receptor associated with OxS and inflammation, regulating the action mechanism of certain antioxidant molecules to inhibit the inflammatory process [32].

Adipose tissue is also a source of bioactive adipokines, including leptin, adiponectin, visfatin, resistin, apelin, and plasminogen activator inhibitor type 1 (PAI-1), which are involved in the homeostasis of OxS physiological and pathological processes [21].

Leptin is a circulating protein belonging to the pro-inflammatory cytokine family of IL-6. It is secreted from white adipocytes and has been involved in food intake regulation, energy expenditure, immune and inflammatory reactions, and energy equilibrium [31].

Studies have shown that high leptin induces OxS in both human endothelial cells and the endothelium of obese animals (*e.g.*, reduced NO and enhanced O2•–and

ONOO−). Leptin in microvascular endothelial cells can boost intracellular ROS generation. Two possible mechanisms for leptin-induced OxS have been proposed to date: (i) stimulation of mitochondrial fatty acid oxidation and (ii) elevation of pro-inflammatory cytokines [33].

Studies have shown that leptin also promotes OxS, increases macrophage phagocytic activity, induces pro-inflammatory cytokine synthesis (TNF-α, IL-6, IL-2) and interferon-gamma (IFN-γ), exerts its impact on several organs (*e.g.*, T-cells, monocytes, neutrophils, and endothelial cells), resulting with endothelial dysfunction, and activation of markers [21].

Leptin has been shown to cause ROS in both phagocytic and nonphagocytic cells. It has also been noted that elevated concentrations of leptin can cause ROS generation primarily owing to NADPH oxidase activation. Also, leptin production was boosted by endogenous antioxidant enzyme overexpression, catalase catabolizing hydrogen peroxide generated by superoxide dismutation, and associated with enhanced energy expenditure and reduced inflammatory and OxS markers in ob/ob mice [34].

Other studies have shown that leptin increases the amount of natural antioxidant enzymes and reduces the expression of inflammatory factors in cells, thereby inhibiting OxS cell damage. Results of an *in vitro* model of PD have shown that leptin can also safeguard cultivated dopaminergic cells from 6-hydroxydopamine (6-OHDA)-induced apoptosis. There is evidence that leptin can improve PC12 cells' viability, at least partly, by attenuating OxS and apoptosis caused by hyperglycemia [35].

Adiponectin (APN) is a circulating hormone generated mainly by adipose tissue. Experimental findings have suggested that APN has insulin-sensitizing properties, anti-atherogenic, and anti-inflammatory properties and can have a modulatory impact on OxS [36].

APN concentrations were negatively associated with OxS in patients with hyperglycemic crises, both pre- and post-treatment. It could be because OxS reduces the output of adiponectin by inhibiting peroxisome proliferator-activated receptor gamma (PPAR-γ) mRNA expression, reduces nuclear PPAR-γ content, increases NADPH oxidase activity and reduces antioxidant enzyme action [37]. Ren *et al.* [36] have shown that adiponectin attenuated growth inhibition caused by H2O2 and displayed scavenging activity against H2O2-induced intracellular reactive oxygen species. Gradinaru *et al.* [38] have shown that adiponectin is inversely associated with serum lipid peroxidation and positively associated with the antioxidant capacity. Furthermore, adiponectin level was shown to be negatively correlated with the SOD and GPx activity [39].

Visfatin, a relatively newly identified adipokine, is expressed primarily in human visceral fat, although it is synthesized in bone marrow, liver, brain, heart, lungs, pancreas, peripheral blood lymphocytes, and skeletal muscle. Studies have shown that visfatin, whose serum levels in patients with inflammatory disease, including obesity, were higher than in healthy subjects, induced human leukocytes and the development of pro-inflammatory cytokines and chemokines [TNF-α, IL-1β, IL-6, stromal cell-derived factor 1 (SDF-1) or C-X-C motif chemokine 12 (CXCL12)], vascular endothelial growth factor (VEGF) and matrix metallo-proteinase (MMP)-2/9 [21, 40].

Visfatin produces ROS, which includes both O2•–and H2O2 as well as OxS development. Nevertheless, visfatin-induced OxS occurs irrespective of activation of protein kinases MAPKs triggered by mitogen. NF-kB pathway phosphorylation is associated with visfatin-mediated ROS generation and blocking this pathway by selective IkB kinase (IKK) inhibition leading to partial OxS reduction [21].

Resistin is also known as an adipocyte-secreted factor. WAT is the primary source of resistin in rodents, whereas in humans, it is mainly expressed in macrophages. Resistin levels have been shown to increase in multiple chronic inflammatory conditions such as diabetic retinopathy, atherosclerosis, rheumatoid arthritis, chronic kidney disease, and coronary heart disease [41, 42]. Resistin encourages the activation of endothelial cells and upregulates multiple adhesion molecules and vascular pro-inflammatory cytokines [12].

There is a body of evidence that indicates that resistin has a pro-oxidant role. In porcine coronary arteries, resistin evokes an increase in superoxide radical production. In contrast, in rats, long-term resistin overexpression in cardiomyocytes *in vivo* results in higher amounts of TNFα release along with increased phosphorylation of IkBα and intracellular content of ROS [43].

A rise in the concentration of resistin significantly decreases the expression of endothelial nitric oxide synthase (NOS), and NO formation in cultivated human coronary artery endothelial cells, indicating that resistin effects can be mediated through OxS [21].

Human apelin is a peptide that has numerous biological functions in several molecular forms. The apelin signaling pathway plays a role in the cardiovascular system's central and peripheral control, such as blood pressure and blood flow, energy metabolism, water and food intake, and immune function. Apelin induces vasorelaxation based on the endothelium by causing NO release and increases myocardial contractility [44].

Than *et al*. have reported that apelin attenuates OxS in human adipocytes. Authors have shown that apelin suppresses the development and release of ROS in adipocyte by interacting with the APJ. Their findings showed that apelin promotes the expression of antioxidant enzymes *via* MAPK kinase/ERK and AMPK pathways and suppresses pro-oxidant enzyme expression through the AMPK pathway [45]. Previous studies have documented that apelin and its structural comparison involve increasing the generation of short-lived ROS and improving the antioxidant state under OxS-related conditions [21].

PAI-1 can be synthesized in adipocytes, liver, hepatocytes, spleen, platelets, macrophages, megakaryocytes, smooth muscle cells, placenta, and endothelial cells. This protein has procoagulant, inflammatory, and profibrotic properties [46].

PAI-1 can play a significant role in controlling adipose tissue, increasing the fatty acid blood flow, and the risk of insulin resistance [33].

PAI-1 is causally correlated with inflammatory signaling pathways and OxS activation. Furthermore, although the additive activation of PAI-1 gene transcription by OxS may explain the increase in PAI-1 circulation, it is not well understood how OxS mediates PAI-1 development. Hypertrophic adipocytes might lead to the existence of local hypoxic areas that enhance the expression of many pro-inflammatory cytokines (TNF-α, IL-6) and ROS through the hypoxia-inducible factor (HIF)-1α, leading to higher PAI-1 expression in adipocytes [33].

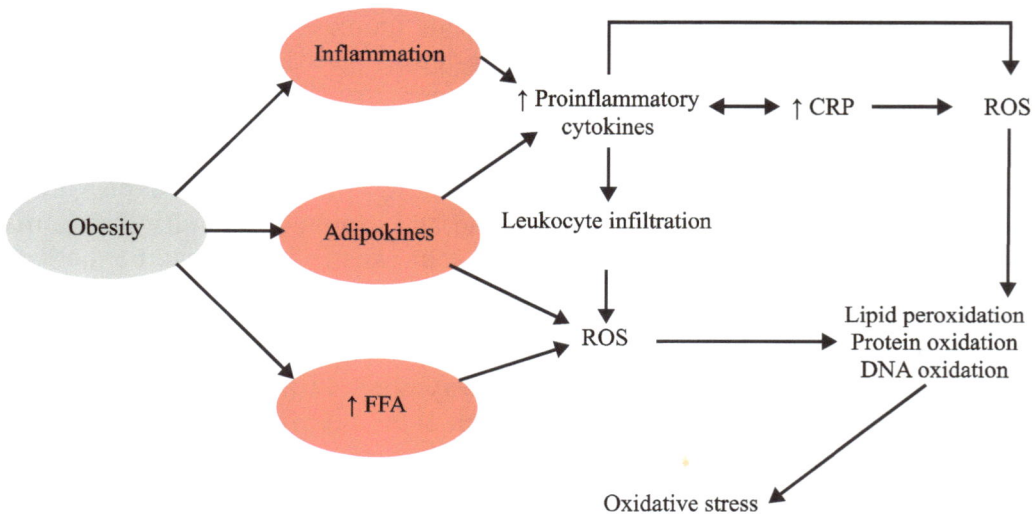

Fig. (2). The link between obesity and oxidative stress.
ROS - Reactive oxygen species; FFA - free fatty acid; CRP – C-reactive protein.

Excessive accumulation of fat in obese patients results in a pathological rise in serum FFA levels, which in effect impairs the metabolism of glucose, hepatic, muscular, and adipose production of energy substrates. This status results in a major synthesis of free radicals, OxS, mitochondrial DNA damage, adenosine triphosphate degradation, and eventually lipotoxicity with various negative effects of fatty acids on cellular structures (Fig. **2**). Cell damage results in high cytokine development, such as TNF-α, which generates additional ROS in tissues and increases the level of lipid peroxidation [33].

OXIDATIVE STRESS, OBESITY, AND NEURODEGENERATION

Neurodegeneration refers to the gradual deterioration of neuron structure and function and can lead to debilitating neurological conditions such as Alzheimer's disease (AD), Parkinson's disease (PD), Huntington's disease (HD), and amyotrophic lateral sclerosis (ALS). OxS, proteasomal damage, mitochondrial dysfunction, and accumulation of irregular protein aggregates are primary pathological features of neurodegenerative diseases [47].

The key fundamental mechanisms contributing to neurodegeneration (ND) are considered multifactorial due to aging-related genetic, environmental, and endogenous factors, but their pathogenic function and essential molecular mechanisms are not fully understood. However, common pathogenic mechanisms on which many neurodegenerative disorders (NDDs) are based include abnormal protein dynamics of malfolding, degradation, proteasomal instability, and aggregation, often with molecular chaperone actions and mutations; free radical/ROS formation and OxS, bioenergetic weakness, mitochondrial dysfunction and damage to DNA, neuronal Golgi system fragmentation; disruption of movement on cellular/axonal level, neurotrophin (NTF) dysfunction and neuroinflammatory/neuroimmune processes [48].

AD's key histopathological characteristic is the formation of extracellular plaques consisting mainly of amyloid-beta (Aβ) aggregates produced by the proteolytic processing of the amyloid precursor protein (APP) C-terminus by different proteases, β-secretase, and γ-secretase. In contrast, intracellular protein aggregates, the so-called neurofibrillary tangles consisting mainly of hyperphosphorylated and misfolded tau protein, are present in AD patients ' neurons [49].

PD is caused by a decrease in brain dopamine (DA) levels. The death of neuron-producing DA in substantia nigra is caused by the intracellular accumulation of α-synuclein protein linked to the ubiquitin complex. Such protein aggregates form cytoplasmic inclusions, commonly known as Lewy's bodies, which play an important role in the family and intermittent PD events [50].

HD is caused by intracellular aggregation of Huntington's mutant protein aggregates, leading to brain cell apoptosis predominantly in the striatum [50].

ALS is characterized by partial and progressive loss of motor cortex upper motor neurons and lower brain and spinal cord motor neurons [51]. ALS is divided into two types. The most common form is sporadic, which has no apparent genetically inherited component (90–95 percent). The remaining 5–10% of cases were family-type ALS (FALS) because of their associated genetic dominant heritage factor [52]. This disease is a complex disease that has many pathological causes, including OxS, mitochondrial dysfunction, axonal injury, microglial activation, inflammation, excitotoxicity, and protein aggregation [53].

Increasing numbers of researchers indicate a correlation between obesity and NDD pathology, marked by a progressive loss of memory and cognition that can eventually lead to death. Although there is little knowledge between obesity and NDDs genetic links, much is now understood about the functional changes and the reciprocal effects of the two diseases [54].

Adipose tissue dysfunction associated with obesity has been correlated with abnormal brain metabolism, neuroinflammation, brain atrophy, neural impairment, diminished mood, and cognitive decline [55]. Obesity was related to the accelerated process of aging. Specific physiological changes are found in obese patients. Insulin resistance leads to deficiency within homeostasis of insulin, central obesity, dyslipidemia, the latter being called metabolic syndrome (MS). Such two structural changes are also due to obesity and MS, *i.e.*, oxidative damage to cellular components and enhanced secretion of pro-inflammatory factors such as cytokines and interleukins [54] (Fig. **3**).

A major cause of insulin resistance is visceral adiposity. Visceral fat tissues serve as endocrine organs that secrete adipokines and cytokines due to their high metabolic rate. Pro-inflammatory activation and cytokine production contribute to insulin resistance [54].

Insulin resistance, described as an inadequate cell response to a given hormone dose, decreases the cell's ability to maintain homeostasis of energy [55]. Insulin deficiency and resistance in the brain causes neuronal death due to the removal of trophic factor, energy metabolism deficiencies, and the suppression of insulin-responsive gene expression [56].

It has been shown that an increase in insulin resistance and diminished brain activity leads to the accumulation of amyloid-β within the cell, one of the first factors that could cause neurodegeneration in AD. Also, in animal models, it has been shown that the increased insulin levels lead to Erk activation, resulting in tau phosphorylation at Ser202 and an increased number of neurofibrillary tangles [57].

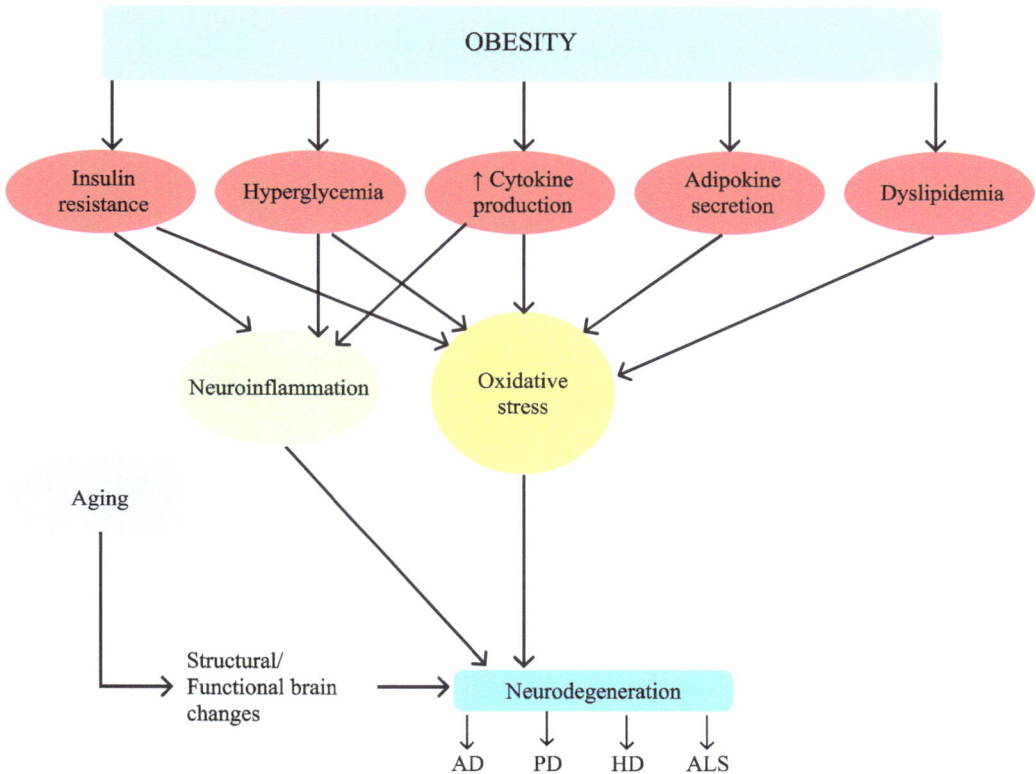

Fig. (3). Schematic illustrating the key roles of obesity and oxidative stress in the development of neurodegenerative disease.
AD - Alzheimer's disease; PD - Parkinson's disease; HD - Huntington's disease; ALS - Amyotrophic lateral sclerosis

Insulin adversely controls brain dopaminergic function in the case of PD. Insulin inhibits the firing of dopamine-containing neurons located in the substantia nigra and stops or reverses the rise in dopaminergic cell discharge rates usually induced by the haloperidol dopamine-receptor antagonist. A mechanism underlying dopaminergic cell loss in hyperglycemic animals may also be the ROS created by chronic hyperglycemia. Chronic hyperglycemia, however, is only a mild risk factor for human PD [54].

Hyperglycemia and resistance to insulin are likely to affect the brain's OxS pathways and neuroinflammatory signals, linking diabetes with neurodegeneration. Four pathological-free radical sources in the brain have also been identified that feed OxS in diabetes: mitochondrial dysfunction, inflammation, AGEs, and high cytosolic ionic-calcium levels. Redox-dysregulation is a particular issue with regard to OxS, a critical disorder that needs further focus. However, hyperglycemia and resistance to insulin produce free radicals that cause damage to the tissue. The primary source of free radicals are mitochondrial dysfunction, cytosolic-free Ca^{2+}, the vicious cycle between inflammation and OxS, and advance glycation end products that stimulate innate immune reaction through their receptors. Such factors create a large pool of free radicals that are sufficient to cause OxS in the brain. Excessive amounts of ROS/RNS disrupt the delicate regulation of key signals and effector proteins needed to keep homeostasis in the brain [58].

Previous studies have been carried out to investigate the function of ROS in neurodegenerative progression. While ROS may not cause neurodegenerative diseases, the disease's progression is likely to be accelerated by oxidative damage and association with mitochondria. Many neurodegenerative diseases, such as AD and PD, are associated with the accumulation of misfolded proteins. In effect, aggregating these modified proteins can cause an inflammatory response in the brain, leading to the marked release of ROS and subsequent OxS. Also, neural inflammation or abnormal mitochondrial function can disrupt the redox balance. Moreover, mitochondrial dysfunction is closely linked to neurodegenerative disorders, which often accompany aberrant ROS development [59].

Oxidative damage is a significant characteristic of AD pathophysiology. ROS-induced OxS is one of the major factors in AD pathogenesis as ROS overproduction is believed to play a critical role in Aβ peptide aggregation and deposition in AD [60].

Aβ plaques in the endoplasmic reticulum (ER) can reduce calcium ions (Ca^{2+}) storage, leading in cytosolic Ca^{2+} overload. In addition to the rise in cytosolic Ca^{2+}, endogenous GSH levels are decreased, and ROS can be over accumulated within the cells [59].

Aβ-mediated source of ROS production involves microglia activated in the brain during an inflammatory response to extracellular amyloid plaque deposition. Increased Aβ levels can speed up ROS development by binding directly to mitochondrial membranes, altering mitochondrial dynamics and function, resulting in abnormal energy metabolism and loss of synaptic function. Aβ peptide-induced membrane-associated OxS disrupts ceramide and cholesterol metabolism, which in effect activates a neurodegenerative cascade leading to further Aβ accumulation, tau phosphorylation, and clinical disease [61].

Studies support the hypothesis that HD reduces energy levels as decreased use of glucose and increased lactate levels are found in HD patients. Recent research shows that oxidative damage is associated with reduced glucose transporter (GLUT)-3 expression, resulting in impaired glucose absorption and lactate accumulation. The underlying cause of Huntington's disease is a mutation in a gene HTT and mHtt was shown to play a key role in mitochondrial dysfunction [59].

On the other hand, the catalytic activity of glyceraldehyde-3-phosphate dehydrogenase (GAPDH) could be inactivated by mitochondrial damage and OxS. As a result, weakened mitochondria can not be swallowed up by lysosome and accumulate unfavorably in the mHtt-expressed cells, leading to cell death [59].

OxS plays an important role in PD degeneration of dopaminergic neurons. Disruptions in neuronal redox potential physiological maintenance interact with several biological processes, ultimately leading to cell death. In the PD, oxidative and nitrative damage has been observed within substantia nigra [62]. Mitochondrial dysfunction associated with PD pathogenesis may result from impairment of mitochondrial biogenesis, increased ROS production, insufficient mitophagy, variations in mitochondrial dynamics, dysfunction of the ETC, impaired trafficking, calcium imbalance or its combinations. Evidence suggests that a key factor in PD pathophysiology is mitochondrial dysfunction [63].

Increased OxS can cause dysfunction of the ubiquitin-proteasome network, exacerbating the vulnerability of PD nigral dopaminergic neurons. The ubiquitin-proteasome (UPS) process is the main route through which cells degrade and extract damaged and unwanted proteins [62].

It was confirmed that OxS is involved in the initiation and progression of ALS [64]. Nerve terminals are responsive to ROS in ALS mouse models, indicating that OxS, along with impaired mitochondria and increased intracellular $Ca2+$ amplifies the decline in presynaptic neuromuscular junctions [65]. Studies have shown that the gene encoding SOD1 has mutations in patients with ALS; these mutations are also present in exon regions, indicating that their toxic effects result from protein instability with increased OxS [66].

A mechanistic correlation between obesity, diabetes, and dementia could be low peripheral inflammation due to chronically high levels of circulating free fatty acids and insulin resistance [56]. Obesity is correlated with dyslipidemia and fatty acid imbalance and cholesterol metabolism, which can impair various neuronal functions and has been involved in neurodegenerative disorders such as AD. Fatty acids, such as palmitic and stearic acids, have been shown to promote astrocyte-mediated amyloidogenesis and tau hyperphosphorylation in primary rat cortical neurons through the metabolism of FFA in astrocytes [67].

FFAs have a lipotoxic effect on peripheral and nervous tissues, and they are responsible for the development of the metabolic syndrome and the development of neurological diseases. They can affect both the central nervous system (CNS) and the peripheral nervous system (PNS), resulting in cognitive impairment, and other CNS and peripheral neuropathies [68].

The production of free fatty acids, frequent in obesity, leads to the development of insulin resistance. Changes in insulin signaling can lead to cognitive deficits as they affect neuronal excitability regulation, metabolism of nerve cells, and cell survival. Changes in insulin-like signals for growth factor 1 (IGF-1) also contribute to a progressive neural loss [69].

Obese patients show low-grade chronic inflammation in the adipose tissue characterized by inflammatory cell infiltration and increased production and discharge of pro-inflammatory factors. High dietary levels of FFA can cause an inflammatory cascade and the release of pro-inflammatory cytokines such as TNF-α and IL-1β and IL-6 interleukins [56].

Hypertrophied adipocytes and immune cells of adipose tissue induce elevated proliferation levels of pro-inflammatory cytokines such as TNF-α, IL-6, IL-1β, *etc*. from which IL-6 and IL-1β can damage cognitive and memory-involved neuronal circuits [54].

Increased inflammatory signals also lead to increased development of ROS. In the brain, ROS production includes synaptic signaling and long-term potency and memory retention mechanisms. An imbalance between ROS production and antioxidant defenses can lead to OxS and increased oxidized lipids, proteins, and nucleic acids [56].

Peripheral inflammation impedes the blood-brain barrier (BBB) and may hinder the hippocampus synaptic plasticity and neurogenesis. Cytokines such as interleukin-6 can lead to a decreased volume of hippocampal gray matter [70].

Obesity influences the brain cells' insulin and energy metabolism and causes neuroinflammation primarily in the hypothalamic region of the brain through the secretion of pro-inflammatory agents such as TNF-α, IL-1, IL-6 [54].

Neuroinflammation has been known to occur in AD for many years. Glial cell activation is observed in the vicinity of brain lesions. Moreover, preclinical genetic data have shown that immune system activation contributes to the pathogenesis of AD [56].

Neuroinflammation is characterized within the brain or spinal cord as an inflammatory response. The development of cytokines, chemokines, ROS, and secondary messengers mediate this inflammation. Such mediators are provided by resident CNS glial cells (microglia and astrocytes), endothelial cells, and immune cells derived from the periphery. These neuroinflammatory reactions have immune, physiological, biochemical, and psychological effects [71].

Neuroinflammation plays an important role in the progression of neurodegenerative diseases and can be responsible for the degeneration of susceptible regions such as the hippocampus [69]. The fact that cytokines secreted by immune cells can have strong neurotoxic effects is now well recognized [72].

Cytokines are triggered by glial cells when the microenvironment in the CNS is compromised by damages such as injury, infection, or ischemic attack. Uncontrolled and sustained inflammatory changes have adverse effects and exacerbate neuronal injury further [73].

TNF-α can play either neuroprotective or neurotoxic roles depending on the expression of other factors including NO, the timing of exposure of damaged neurons to TNF, upregulation of NF-κB, and the existence of excess NMDA receptor agonists. TNF-α can have neurotoxic effects when growth factors such as IGF are inhibited [72].

Previous studies indicated that tumor necrosis factor receptor-1 (TNFR-1), containing an intracellular 'death domain,' has a negative impact on adult hippocampal neurogenesis [73].

In the rat brain, IL-1β caused enhanced neuronal cell death and edema at the time of experimental ischemia and traumatic injury. These results are inhibited by over-expression of IL-1 receptor antagonists in the CNS. IL-1 *in vitro* results in neuronal apoptosis and its neurotoxic effects seem to depend on the expression of iNOS. IL-1 can be an important factor in neuronal and axonal damage in the CNS alone or in conjunction with iNOS [72].

IL-1β was consistently associated with neurogenesis in the brain, mainly in the hippocampal region. IL-1β is also active in the suppression of neurogenesis caused by IFN-γ. IL-1β inhibition blocked the decline in neurogenesis caused by acute stress and chronic anhedonic and anti-neurogenic effects. Continuous expression of hippocampal IL-1β affects adult neurogenesis [73]. In neurodegenerative dementia disorders associated with neuroinflammation, IL-6 secretion was found to be altered [74].

IL-6-mediated neuronal degeneration is based on trans-signaling in CNS, while classical signaling has a regenerative function in neural tissue. It highlights the importance of differentiating between the two pathways when developing medications for neurological disease treatment [75].

Overexpression of IL-6 in the CNS is involved in neurodegenerative pathology with dendritic vacuolization [72]. Post-mortem brain tissue tests in patients with AD showed activated glial cells as well as increased expression of IL-6 adjacent to amyloid-β (Aβ)1–42 forming senile plaques, a characteristic of AD pathology [74].

Obesity is also associated with increased C-reactive protein (CRP) in the blood, a well-known acute phase protein [76].

High-sensitivity (hs)-CRP is a systemic marker for exquisitely sensitive inflammation, disease, and tissue damage. There is a strong association between increased levels of hs-CRP and inflammatory reactions. Several previous studies have suggested that high levels of hs-CRP are associated with increased risk of cerebrovascular and neurodegenerative diseases because hs-CRP enhances BBB paracellular permeability when its concentration reaches the threshold to impair BBB function [77].

Elevated serum levels of CRP have been observed in patients with Alzheimer's disease [78]. By promoting the neurodegenerative cycle, CRP levels in medically non-inflammatory conditions may influence long-term prognosis. CRP has been associated with Alzheimer's disease progression. High CRP enhances the permeability of the blood-brain barrier by binding to the Fcγ receptor, resulting in microglial activation. Impacted brain areas were found to contain activated microglia and CRP in patients with AD [79].

Adipokines have autocrine, paracrine, and endocrine action pathways, and many adipokines influence peripheral and CNS processes [80].

Leptin is an important hormone that controls the consumption of food and energy expenditure *via* behavior regulated by its hypothalamus receptor that is also present in other brain regions, such as the hippocampus associated with cognitive functions, which indicates that the hormone also plays a critical role in learning and memory. As the circulating levels of leptin increase in obesity, the hormone resistance increases rapidly, making it a characteristic of the disease [69].

However, there is strong evidence that leptin signaling has beneficial effects on neural networks, and therefore it can only be helpful to implement preventive approaches to people who are affected by this. Leptin manifests its beneficial properties on the nervous system from neuronal survival to synaptic plasticity at multiple levels, indicating that it may help AD patients in several ways [81].

Many pathways associated with AD pathophysiology have been shown to interfere with leptin signaling. Aβ disrupts leptin signaling leading to hippocampal leptin and LepR expression being down-regulated. In comparison, by suppressing Aβ accumulation and toxicity and attenuating tau pathology, leptin was reported to be neuroprotective in AD models. Leptin's anti-amyloidogenic activity includes inhibiting APP production by decreasing the β-APP cleaving enzyme Beta-secretase 1 (BACE1) and increasing the APOE-dependent Aβ uptake, which appears to be mediated by activating AMP-activated protein kinase [55].

Many studies have found that, in different disease models, an obese phenotype exacerbates neurodegeneration. For example, leptin-deficient ob/ob mice treated with both methamphetamine or kainic acid show significantly higher mortality and neurotoxic damage levels than lean control mice - nonetheless, transgenic mice α-synuclein A53 T, the family PD template, exhibit metabolic abnormalities, and hypoleptinemia. This means that leptin deficiency leads to disease progression and that the leptin mechanism can be a new target for other neurodegenerative diseases [82].

Adiponectin appears to induce a pro-inflammatory response in human astrocytes, especially through IL-6 and MCP-1 *via* NF-πB, p38MAPK, and ERK1/2 pathways. On the other hand, adiponectin was identified to inhibit pro-inflammatory signals, notably by suppressing the release of IL-6 from endothelial cells of the BBB. It shows that, by negatively modulating the release of IL-6and TNF-α, adiponectin indirectly modulates inflammatory signals across the BBB. In vitro study of hippocampal neurons shows that adiponectin has neuroprotective effects [83].

While current literature has shown that resistin has different effects on different disease states, the relationship between resistin and AD remains obscure. High levels of plasma resistin observed in AD patients indicate that cytokine release activity during monocyte-macrophage differentiation plays a key role in the inflammation cycle [84].

Resistin gene expression is reported in the mouse brain cortex along the side ventricle walls and the hippocampus as well. Studies have shown that cortical and hypothalamic resistance expression can inactivate neurons. Resistin may be involved in acute cerebral injury responses, possibly through inflammatory mechanisms [83].

Serum resistin levels in AD patients have been significantly increased and associated with certain inflammatory markers, indicating that resistin may play a role in the inflammatory AD cycle [85].

CONCLUDING REMARKS

Oxidative stress can be a result, but also an obesity trigger. Obesity is coupled with an altered redox state and increased metabolic risk. Adipose tissue secretes adipokines (leptin, adiponectin, visfatin, resistin, apelin, and plasminogen activator inhibitor type 1) and cytokines (TNF-α, IL-6, IL-1β) that are connected to oxidative stress. Metabolic changes caused by overweight are associated with damage to the central nervous system (CNS), which can result in neuronal death, either through apoptosis or cell necrosis or by modifying the neuron's synaptic plasticity, contributing to neurodegeneration.

CONSENT FOR PUBLICATION

Not applicable.

CONFLICT OF INTEREST

The authors confirm that this chapter content has no conflict of interest.

ACKNOWLEDGEMENTS

The authors would like to express their sincere thanks to the editor and anonymous reviewers for their time and valuable suggestions.

REFERENCES

[1]   Ahmad W, Ijaz B, Shabbiri K, Ahmed F, Rehman S. Oxidative toxicity in diabetes and Alzheimer's disease: mechanisms behind ROS/ RNS generation. J Biomed Sci 2017; 24(1): 76.
        [http://dx.doi.org/10.1186/s12929-017-0379-z] [PMID: 28927401]

[2]   Liguori I, Russo G, Curcio F, *et al.* Oxidative stress, aging, and diseases. Clin Interv Aging 2018; 13: 757-72.
        [http://dx.doi.org/10.2147/CIA.S158513] [PMID: 29731617]

[3]   Kasten D, Mithöfer A, Georgii E, Lang H, Durner J, Gaupels F. Nitrite is the driver, phytohormones are modulators while NO and H2O2 act as promoters of NO2-induced cell death. J Exp Bot 2016; 67(22): 6337-49.
        [http://dx.doi.org/10.1093/jxb/erw401] [PMID: 27811003]

[4]   Del Río LA. ROS and RNS in plant physiology: an overview. J Exp Bot 2015; 66(10): 2827-37.
        [http://dx.doi.org/10.1093/jxb/erv099] [PMID: 25873662]

[5]   Phaniendra A, Jestadi DB, Periyasamy L. Free radicals: properties, sources, targets, and their implication in various diseases. Indian J Clin Biochem 2015; 30(1): 11-26.
        [http://dx.doi.org/10.1007/s12291-014-0446-0] [PMID: 25646037]

[6]   Adwas AA, Elsayed ASI, Azab AE, Quwaydir FA. Oxidative stress and antioxidant mechanisms in human body. J Appl Biotechnol Bioeng 2019; 6(1): 43-7.
        [PMID: 1245049]

[7]   Di Meo S, Reed TT, Venditti P, Victor VM. Role of ROS and RNS Sources in Physiological and Pathological Conditions. Oxid Med Cell Longev 2016; 2016: 1245049.
        [http://dx.doi.org/10.1155/2016/1245049] [PMID: 27478531]

[8]   Joshi P, Kumar A, Arora N. Study of effect of examination stress on lipid peroxidation and superoxide dismutase level. Natl J Physiol Pharm Pharmacol 2018; 8(8): 1084-7.
        [http://dx.doi.org/10.5455/njppp.2018.8.0308630032018]

[9]   Nimalaratne C, Wu J. Hen egg as an antioxidant food commodity: a review. Nutrients 2015; 7(10): 8274-93.
        [http://dx.doi.org/10.3390/nu7105394] [PMID: 26404361]

[10]   Mut-Salud N, Álvarez PJ, Garrido JM, Carrasco E, Aránega A, Rodríguez-Serrano F. Antioxidant intake and antitumor therapy: toward nutritional recommendations for optimal results. Oxid Med Cell Longev 2016; 2016: 6719534.
        [http://dx.doi.org/10.1155/2016/6719534] [PMID: 26682013]

[11]   Mirończuk-Chodakowska I, Witkowska AM, Zujko ME. Endogenous non-enzymatic antioxidants in the human body. Adv Med Sci 2018; 63(1): 68-78.
        [http://dx.doi.org/10.1016/j.advms.2017.05.005] [PMID: 28822266]

[12]   Ozsurekci Y, Aykac K. Oxidative stress related diseases in newborns. Oxid Med Cell Longev 2016; 2016: 2768365.
        [http://dx.doi.org/10.1155/2016/2768365] [PMID: 27403229]

[13]   Tan BL, Norhaizan ME, Liew WP, Sulaiman Rahman H. Antioxidant and oxidative stress: a mutual interplay in age-related diseases. Front Pharmacol 2018; 9: 1162.
        [http://dx.doi.org/10.3389/fphar.2018.01162] [PMID: 30405405]

[14]   Kreuz S, Fischle W. Oxidative stress signaling to chromatin in health and disease. Epigenomics 2016; 8(6): 843-62.
        [http://dx.doi.org/10.2217/epi-2016-0002] [PMID: 27319358]

[15]   Narayanaswami V, Dwoskin LP. Obesity: Current and potential pharmacotherapeutics and targets. Pharmacol Ther 2017; 170: 116-47.
        [http://dx.doi.org/10.1016/j.pharmthera.2016.10.015] [PMID: 27773782]

[16]   Le Lay S, Simard G, Martinez MC, Andriantsitohaina R. Oxidative stress and metabolic pathologies: from an adipocentric point of view. Oxid Med Cell Longev 2014; 2014: 908539.
        [http://dx.doi.org/10.1155/2014/908539] [PMID: 25143800]

[17]   Friederich-Persson M, Nguyen Dinh Cat A, Persson P, Montezano AC, Touyz RM. Brown adipose tissue regulates small artery function through nadph oxidase 4-derived hydrogen peroxide and redox-sensitive protein kinase G-1α. Arterioscler Thromb Vasc Biol 2017; 37(3): 455-65.
        [http://dx.doi.org/10.1161/ATVBAHA.116.308659] [PMID: 28062507]

[18]   Al-Mulhim AS, Al-Hussaini HA, Al-Jalal BA, Al-Moagal RO, Al-Najjar SA. Obesity disease and surgery. Int J Chronic Dis 2014; 2014: 652341.
        [http://dx.doi.org/10.1155/2014/652341] [PMID: 26464861]

[19]   Togo M, Konari N, Tsukamoto M, *et al.* Effects of a high-fat diet on superoxide anion generation and membrane fluidity in liver mitochondria in rats. J Int Soc Sports Nutr 2018; 15: 13.
        [http://dx.doi.org/10.1186/s12970-018-0217-z] [PMID: 29568243]

[20]　Han YH, Buffolo M, Pires KM, Pei S, Scherer PE, Boudina S. Adipocyte-specific deletion of manganese superoxide dismutase protects from diet-induced obesity through increased mitochondrial uncoupling and biogenesis. Diabetes 2016; 65(9): 2639-51.
[http://dx.doi.org/10.2337/db16-0283] [PMID: 27284109]

[21]　Marseglia L, Manti S, D'Angelo G, *et al.* Oxidative stress in obesity: a critical component in human diseases. Int J Mol Sci 2014; 16(1): 378-400.
[http://dx.doi.org/10.3390/ijms16010378] [PMID: 25548896]

[22]　Dludla PV, Nkambule BB, Jack B, *et al.* Inflammation and oxidative stress in an obese state and the protective effects of gallic acid. Nutrients 2018; 11(1): E23.
[http://dx.doi.org/10.3390/nu11010023] [PMID: 30577684]

[23]　Ivanov VV, Shakhristova EV, Stepovaya EA, *et al.* Oxidative stress in the pathogenesis of type 1 diabetes: the role of adipocyte xanthine oxidase. Bulletin of Siberian Medicine 2017; 16(4): 134-43.
[http://dx.doi.org/10.20538/1682-0363-2017-4-134-143]

[24]　Khaybullina ZR. Inflammation and oxidative stress: critical role for metabolic syndrome. J Vasc Med Surg 2017; 5: 302.
[http://dx.doi.org/10.4172/2329-6925.1000302]

[25]　Blaser H, Dostert C, Mak TW, Brenner D. TNF and ROS crosstalk in inflammation. Trends Cell Biol 2016; 26(4): 249-61.
[http://dx.doi.org/10.1016/j.tcb.2015.12.002] [PMID: 26791157]

[26]　Alicka M, Marycz K. The effect of chronic inflammation and oxidative and endoplasmic reticulum stress in the course of metabolic syndrome and its therapy. Stem Cells Int 2018; 2018: 4274361.
[http://dx.doi.org/10.1155/2018/4274361] [PMID: 30425746]

[27]　Didion SP. Cellular and oxidative mechanisms associated with interleukin-6 signaling in the vasculature. Int J Mol Sci 2017; 18(12): E2563.
[http://dx.doi.org/10.3390/ijms18122563] [PMID: 29186034]

[28]　Hirao M, Yamasaki N, Oze H, *et al.* Serum level of oxidative stress marker is dramatically low in patients with rheumatoid arthritis treated with tocilizumab. Rheumatol Int 2012; 32(12): 4041-5.
[http://dx.doi.org/10.1007/s00296-011-2135-0] [PMID: 21909945]

[29]　Yang D, Elner SG, Bian ZM, Till GO, Petty HR, Elner VM. Pro-inflammatory cytokines increase reactive oxygen species through mitochondria and NADPH oxidase in cultured RPE cells. Exp Eye Res 2007; 85(4): 462-72.
[http://dx.doi.org/10.1016/j.exer.2007.06.013] [PMID: 17765224]

[30]　Yang X, Wang L, Yuan ZQ, *et al.* Interleukin-1β induces apoptosis in annulus fibrosus cells through the extracellular signal-regulated kinase pathway. Connect Tissue Res 2018; 59(6): 593-600.
[http://dx.doi.org/10.1080/03008207.2018.1442445] [PMID: 29457525]

[31]　Blanca AJ, Ruiz-Armenta MV, Zambrano S, *et al.* Leptin induces oxidative stress through activation of nadph oxidase in renal tubular cells: antioxidant effect of L-carnitine. J Cell Biochem 2016; 117(10): 2281-8.
[http://dx.doi.org/10.1002/jcb.25526] [PMID: 26918530]

[32]　Sánchez A, Calpena AC, Clares B. Evaluating the oxidative stress in inflammation: role of melatonin. Int J Mol Sci 2015; 16(8): 16981-7004.
[http://dx.doi.org/10.3390/ijms160816981] [PMID: 26225957]

[33]　Huang CJ, McAllister MJ, Slusher AL, Webb HE, Mock JT, Acevedo EO. Obesity-related oxidative stress: the impact of physical activity and diet manipulation. Sports Med Open 2015; 1(1): 32.
[http://dx.doi.org/10.1186/s40798-015-0031-y] [PMID: 26435910]

[34]　Berger S, Polotsky VY. Leptin and leptin resistance in the pathogenesis of obstructive sleep apnea: a possible link to oxidative stress and cardiovascular complications. Oxid Med Cell Longev 2018; 2018: 5137947.

[http://dx.doi.org/10.1155/2018/5137947] [PMID: 29675134]

[35] Kaeidi A, Hajializadeh Z, Jahandari F, Fatemi I. Leptin attenuates oxidative stress and neuronal apoptosis in hyperglycemic condition. Fundam Clin Pharmacol 2019; 33(1): 75-83.
[http://dx.doi.org/10.1111/fcp.12411] [PMID: 30203422]

[36] Ren Y, Li Y, Yan J, *et al.* Adiponectin modulates oxidative stress-induced mitophagy and protects C2C12 myoblasts against apoptosis. Sci Rep 2017; 7(1): 3209.
[http://dx.doi.org/10.1038/s41598-017-03319-2] [PMID: 28600493]

[37] Ouedraogo R, Wu X, Xu SQ, *et al.* Adiponectin suppression of high-glucose-induced reactive oxygen species in vascular endothelial cells: evidence for involvement of a cAMP signaling pathway. Diabetes 2006; 55(6): 1840-6.
[http://dx.doi.org/10.2337/db05-1174] [PMID: 16731851]

[38] Gradinaru D, Margina D, Borsa C, *et al.* Adiponectin: possible link between metabolic stress and oxidative stress in the elderly. Aging Clin Exp Res 2017; 29(4): 621-9.
[http://dx.doi.org/10.1007/s40520-016-0629-z] [PMID: 27688246]

[39] Chen SJ, Yen CH, Huang YC, Lee BJ, Hsia S, Lin PT. Relationships between inflammation, adiponectin, and oxidative stress in metabolic syndrome. PLoS One 2012; 7(9): e45693.
[http://dx.doi.org/10.1371/journal.pone.0045693] [PMID: 23029185]

[40] Azamar-Llamas D, Hernández-Molina G, Ramos-Ávalos B, Furuzawa-Carballeda J. Adipokine contribution to the pathogenesis of osteoarthritis. Mediators Inflamm 2017; 2017: 5468023.
[http://dx.doi.org/10.1155/2017/5468023] [PMID: 28490838]

[41] Abella V, Scotece M, Conde J, *et al.* Adipokines, metabolic syndrome and rheumatic diseases. J Immunol Res 2014; 2014: 343746.
[http://dx.doi.org/10.1155/2014/343746] [PMID: 24741591]

[42] Devanoorkar A, Kathariya R, Guttiganur N, Gopalakrishnan D, Bagchi P. Resistin: a potential biomarker for periodontitis influenced diabetes mellitus and diabetes induced periodontitis. Dis Markers 2014; 2014: 930206.
[http://dx.doi.org/10.1155/2014/930206] [PMID: 24692844]

[43] Fantuzzi G, Braunschweig C. Adipose tissue and adipokines in health and disease. 2014.
[http://dx.doi.org/10.1007/978-1-62703-770-9]

[44] Kurowska P, Barbe A, Różycka M, Chmielińska J, Dupont J, Rak A. Apelin in reproductive physiology and pathology of different species: a critical review. Int J Endocrinol 2018; 2018: 9170480.
[http://dx.doi.org/10.1155/2018/9170480] [PMID: 29977292]

[45] Tan EK, Srivastava AK, Arnold WD, Singh MP, Zhang Y. Neurodegeneration: etiologies and new therapies. BioMed Res Int 2015; 2015: 272630.
[http://dx.doi.org/10.1155/2015/272630] [PMID: 25685777]

[46] Yasar Yildiz S, Kuru P, Toksoy Oner E, Agirbasli M. Functional stability of plasminogen activator inhibitor-1. ScientificWorldJournal 2014; 2014: 858293.
[http://dx.doi.org/10.1155/2014/858293] [PMID: 25386620]

[47] Johri A, Beal MF. Mitochondrial dysfunction in neurodegenerative diseases. J Pharmacol Exp Ther 2012; 342(3): 619-30.
[http://dx.doi.org/10.1124/jpet.112.192138] [PMID: 22700435]

[48] Jellinger KA. Basic mechanisms of neurodegeneration: a critical update. J Cell Mol Med 2010; 14(3): 457-87.
[http://dx.doi.org/10.1111/j.1582-4934.2010.01010.x] [PMID: 20070435]

[49] Fischer R, Maier O. Interrelation of oxidative stress and inflammation in neurodegenerative disease: role of TNF. Oxid Med Cell Longev 2015; 2015: 610813.
[http://dx.doi.org/10.1155/2015/610813] [PMID: 25834699]

[50]   Hussain R, Zubair H, Pursell S, Shahab M. Neurodegenerative diseases: regenerative mechanisms and novel therapeutic approaches. Brain Sci 2018; 8(9): E177.
[http://dx.doi.org/10.3390/brainsci8090177] [PMID: 30223579]

[51]   Meininger V, Pradat PF, Corse A, *et al.* Safety, pharmacokinetic, and functional effects of the nogo-a monoclonal antibody in amyotrophic lateral sclerosis: a randomized, first-in-human clinical trial. PLoS One 2014; 9(5): e97803.
[http://dx.doi.org/10.1371/journal.pone.0097803] [PMID: 24841795]

[52]   Zarei S, Carr K, Reiley L, *et al.* A comprehensive review of amyotrophic lateral sclerosis. Surg Neurol Int 2015; 6: 171.
[http://dx.doi.org/10.4103/2152-7806.169561] [PMID: 26629397]

[53]   Vu LT, Bowser R. Fluid-based biomarkers for amyotrophic lateral sclerosis. Neurotherapeutics 2017; 14(1): 119-34.
[http://dx.doi.org/10.1007/s13311-016-0503-x] [PMID: 27933485]

[54]   Gupta R, Sawhney P. K Ambasta R, Kumar P. Obesity and neurodegeneration. Adv Obes Weight Manag Control 2015; 2(5): 96-101.

[55]   Forny-Germano L, De Felice FG, Vieira MNDN. The role of leptin and adiponectin in obesity-associated cognitive decline and Alzheimer's disease. Front Neurosci 2019; 12: 1027.
[http://dx.doi.org/10.3389/fnins.2018.01027] [PMID: 30692905]

[56]   Rigotto G, Basso E. Mitochondrial dysfunctions: a thread sewing together Alzheimer's disease, diabetes, and obesity. Oxid Med Cell Longev 2019; 2019: 7210892.
[http://dx.doi.org/10.1155/2019/7210892] [PMID: 31316720]

[57]   Schuh AF, Rieder CM, Rizzi L, Chaves M, Roriz-Cruz M. Mechanisms of brain aging regulation by insulin: implications for neurodegeneration in late-onset Alzheimer's disease. ISRN Neurol 2011; 2011: 306905.
[http://dx.doi.org/10.5402/2011/306905] [PMID: 22389813]

[58]   Rosales-Corral S, Tan DX, Manchester L, Reiter RJ. Diabetes and Alzheimer disease, two overlapping pathologies with the same background: oxidative stress. Oxid Med Cell Longev 2015; 2015: 985845.
[http://dx.doi.org/10.1155/2015/985845] [PMID: 25815110]

[59]   Liu Z, Zhou T, Ziegler AC, Dimitrion P, Zuo L. Oxidative stress in neurodegenerative diseases: from molecular mechanisms to clinical applications. Oxid Med Cell Longev 2017; 2017: 2525967.
[http://dx.doi.org/10.1155/2017/2525967] [PMID: 28785371]

[60]   Cenini G, Lloret A, Cascella R. Oxidative stress in neurodegenerative diseases: from a mitochondrial point of view. Oxid Med Cell Longev 2019; 2019: 2105607.
[http://dx.doi.org/10.1155/2019/2105607] [PMID: 31210837]

[61]   Tönnies E, Trushina E. Oxidative stress, synaptic dysfunction, and Alzheimer's disease. J Alzheimers Dis 2017; 57(4): 1105-21.
[http://dx.doi.org/10.3233/JAD-161088] [PMID: 28059794]

[62]   Dias V, Junn E, Mouradian MM. The role of oxidative stress in Parkinson's disease. J Parkinsons Dis 2013; 3(4): 461-91.
[http://dx.doi.org/10.3233/JPD-130230] [PMID: 24252804]

[63]   Park JS, Davis RL, Sue CM. Mitochondrial dysfunction in Parkinson's disease: new mechanistic insights and therapeutic perspectives. Curr Neurol Neurosci Rep 2018; 18(5): 21.
[http://dx.doi.org/10.1007/s11910-018-0829-3] [PMID: 29616350]

[64]   Wang Z, Bai Z, Qin X, Cheng Y. Aberrations in oxidative stress markers in amyotrophic lateral sclerosis: a systematic review and meta-analysis. Oxid Med Cell Longev 2019; 2019: 1712323.
[http://dx.doi.org/10.1155/2019/1712323] [PMID: 31281567]

[65]   Pollari E, Goldsteins G, Bart G, Koistinaho J, Giniatullin R. The role of oxidative stress in

degeneration of the neuromuscular junction in amyotrophic lateral sclerosis. Front Cell Neurosci 2014; 8: 131.
[http://dx.doi.org/10.3389/fncel.2014.00131] [PMID: 24860432]

[66] Pansarasa O, Bordoni M, Diamanti L, Sproviero D, Gagliardi S, Cereda C. SOD1 in amyotrophic lateral sclerosis: "Ambivalent" behavior connected to the disease. Int J Mol Sci 2018; 19(5): E1345.
[http://dx.doi.org/10.3390/ijms19051345] [PMID: 29751510]

[67] Ashrafian H, Harling L, Darzi A, Athanasiou T. Neurodegenerative disease and obesity: what is the role of weight loss and bariatric interventions? Metab Brain Dis 2013; 28(3): 341-53.
[http://dx.doi.org/10.1007/s11011-013-9412-4] [PMID: 23653255]

[68] Niccolai E, Boem F, Russo E, Amedei A. The Gut-Brain axis in the neuropsychological disease model of obesity: a classical movie revised by the emerging director "microbiome". Nutrients 2019; 11(1): E156.
[http://dx.doi.org/10.3390/nu11010156] [PMID: 30642052]

[69] Mazon JN, de Mello AH, Ferreira GK, Rezin GT. The impact of obesity on neurodegenerative diseases. Life Sci 2017; 182: 22-8.
[http://dx.doi.org/10.1016/j.lfs.2017.06.002] [PMID: 28583368]

[70] Shalev D, Arbuckle MR. Metabolism and memory: obesity, diabetes, and dementia. Biol Psychiatry 2017; 82(11): e81-3.
[http://dx.doi.org/10.1016/j.biopsych.2017.09.025] [PMID: 29110819]

[71] DiSabato DJ, Quan N, Godbout JP. Neuroinflammation: the devil is in the details. J Neurochem 2016; 139 (Suppl. 2): 136-53.
[http://dx.doi.org/10.1111/jnc.13607] [PMID: 26990767]

[72] Chitnis T, Weiner HL. CNS inflammation and neurodegeneration. J Clin Invest 2017; 127(10): 3577-87.
[http://dx.doi.org/10.1172/JCI90609] [PMID: 28872464]

[73] Kim YK, Na KS, Myint AM, Leonard BE. The role of pro-inflammatory cytokines in neuroinflammation, neurogenesis and the neuroendocrine system in major depression. Prog Neuropsychopharmacol Biol Psychiatry 2016; 64: 277-84.
[http://dx.doi.org/10.1016/j.pnpbp.2015.06.008] [PMID: 26111720]

[74] Wennström M, Hall S, Nägga K, Londos E, Minthon L, Hansson O. Cerebrospinal fluid levels of IL-6 are decreased and correlate with cognitive status in DLB patients. Alzheimers Res Ther 2015; 7(1): 63.
[http://dx.doi.org/10.1186/s13195-015-0145-y] [PMID: 26434635]

[75] Rothaug M, Becker-Pauly C, Rose-John S. The role of interleukin-6 signaling in nervous tissue. Biochim Biophys Acta 2016; 1863 (6 Pt A): 1218-27.
[http://dx.doi.org/10.1016/j.bbamcr.2016.03.018] [PMID: 27016501]

[76] Paepegaey AC, Genser L, Bouillot JL, Oppert JM, Clément K, Poitou C. High levels of CRP in morbid obesity: the central role of adipose tissue and lessons for clinical practice before and after bariatric surgery. Surg Obes Relat Dis 2015; 11(1): 148-54.
[http://dx.doi.org/10.1016/j.soard.2014.06.010] [PMID: 25393045]

[77] Song IU, Chung SW, Kim YD, Maeng LS. Relationship between the hs-CRP as non-specific biomarker and Alzheimer's disease according to aging process. Int J Med Sci 2015; 12(8): 613-7.
[http://dx.doi.org/10.7150/ijms.12742] [PMID: 26283879]

[78] Zaciragic A, Lepara O, Valjevac A, *et al.* Elevated serum C-reactive protein concentration in Bosnian patients with probable Alzheimer's disease. J Alzheimers Dis 2007; 12(2): 151-6.
[http://dx.doi.org/10.3233/JAD-2007-12204] [PMID: 17917159]

[79] Umemura A, Oeda T, Yamamoto K, *et al.* Baseline plasma c-reactive protein concentrations and motor prognosis in parkinson disease. PLoS One 2015; 10(8): e0136722.
[http://dx.doi.org/10.1371/journal.pone.0136722] [PMID: 26308525]

[80] Kiliaan AJ, Arnoldussen IA, Gustafson DR. Adipokines: a link between obesity and dementia? Lancet Neurol 2014; 13(9): 913-23.
[http://dx.doi.org/10.1016/S1474-4422(14)70085-7] [PMID: 25142458]

[81] Doherty GH. Obesity and the ageing brain: could leptin play a role in neurodegeneration? Curr Gerontol Geriatr Res 2011; 2011: 708154.
[http://dx.doi.org/10.1155/2011/708154] [PMID: 22013440]

[82] McGregor G, Harvey J. Regulation of hippocampal synaptic function by the metabolic hormone, leptin: implications for health and neurodegenerative disease. Front Cell Neurosci 2018; 12: 340.
[http://dx.doi.org/10.3389/fncel.2018.00340] [PMID: 30386207]

[83] Parimisetty A, Dorsemans AC, Awada R, Ravanan P, Diotel N, Lefebvre d'Hellencourt C. Secret talk between adipose tissue and central nervous system *via* secreted factors-an emerging frontier in the neurodegenerative research. J Neuroinflammation 2016; 13(1): 67.
[http://dx.doi.org/10.1186/s12974-016-0530-x] [PMID: 27012931]

[84] Kizilarslanoğlu MC, Kara Ö, Yeşil Y, *et al.* Alzheimer disease, inflammation, and novel inflammatory marker: resistin. Turk J Med Sci 2015; 45(5): 1040-6.
[http://dx.doi.org/10.3906/sag-1403-55] [PMID: 26738345]

[85] Demirci S, Aynalı A, Demirci K, Demirci S, Arıdoğan BC. The Serum Levels of Resistin and Its Relationship with Other Proinflammatory Cytokines in Patients with Alzheimer's Disease. Clin Psychopharmacol Neurosci 2017; 15(1): 59-63.
[http://dx.doi.org/10.9758/cpn.2017.15.1.59] [PMID: 28138112]

CHAPTER 9

Inflammaging and Obesity

Asija Začiragić[*]

Department of Human Physiology, Faculty of Medicine University of Sarajevo, Bosnia and Herzegovina

Abstract: The term inflammaging refers to chronic, low-grade systemic inflammation that can be conceptualized as a basis for human aging. Although the importance of inflammaging in the aging process is now well recognized, its etiology remains largely unknown. In this chapter, several possible mechanisms underlying chronic systemic low-grade inflammation are discussed in addition to several pillars of geroscience that attempt to explain the association between aging and age-related diseases. Health preservation strategies that restrict or prevent inflammaging and serve to boost anti-inflammaging mechanisms are also discussed. Moreover, this chapter presents an overview of obesity and obesity-related diseases in the elderly. The relationship between inflammaging and obesity in the elderly is explored as well as a potential explanation of the "obesity survival paradox". The chapter also briefly presents the most common obesity-related complications in older individuals as well as treatment options in aging populations. The final part of the chapter links inflammation with obesity in more detail. The potential of obesity to accelerate the aging process is also discussed, as well as features of dysfunctional, aged adipose tissue. Given that in the last two decades, the role of chronic systemic low-grade inflammation has gained significant attention as the key player in pathophysiology of obesity- and aging-associated diseases, future studies should unravel whether inflammatory processes are the cause or consequence of obesity and aging. Furthermore, although some therapeutic interventions alleviate obesity, it seems that they are not sufficient alone and should be reinforced with the use of medications and other therapeutic modalities proven to decrease inflammatory processes.

Keywords: Aging, Aging-related diseases, Geroscience, Inflammaging, Low-grade systemic inflammation, Obesity, Obesity-related diseases.

INTRODUCTION

The term inflammaging refers to chronic, low-grade systemic inflammation that can be conceptualized as a basis for human aging. Obesity and cardio-metabolic diseases, as well as other age-related diseases, result in inflammation that can

---

[*] **Corresponding author Asija Začiragić:** Department of Human Physiology, Faculty of Medicine University of Sarajevo, Bosnia and Herzegovina; Tel: +387 33 226 478, Ext. 525; E-mail: zarias@lol.ba

accelerate aging. Hence, inflammaging should be regarded as a highly significant risk factor for both morbidity and mortality in the elderly. The introduction and explanation of inflammaging as scientific concepts are laid out nicely in Franceschi *et al*. [1]. Numerous epidemiological studies point to a significant role played by inflammatory markers, such as C-reactive protein and Interleukin-6 (IL-6), in aging. Elevated levels of these markers have been associated with varying aging phenotypes, such as metabolic homeostasis, changes in body composition and energy production, neuronal health, and immunosenescence.

Although the importance of inflammaging in the aging process is now well recognized, its etiology remains largely unknown. In an attempt to explain the role of inflammatory processes in the development of aging, it is crucial to distinguish between acute and chronic inflammation. As an acute, transient immune response to damaging conditions, such as infections or tissue injury, inflammation can be beneficial. This physiological inflammation represents the basic mechanism of coping with and neutralizing numerous kinds of stressors [2]. However, persistent and chronic low-grade inflammation may lead to tissue degeneration. A persistent, systemic, and low-grade type of inflammation might be explained by several possible mechanisms, including cellular damage by reactive molecules produced by infiltrating leukocytes combatting pathogens. Moreover, chronic, low-grade inflammation may be a result of cytokines that amplify the inflammatory response. Finally, chronic, systemic, low-grade inflammation may be a consequence of "anabolic signaling" that is, for example, manifested in down-regulation of insulin, insulin-like growth factor-1, and erythropoietin signaling and protein synthesis by pro-inflammatory cytokines, such as tumor necrosis factor-α (TNF- α) or IL-6 [3].

A possible role played by chronic inflammation in the aging process may also be explained by the accumulation of damaged cells and macromolecules that occurs with advancing age and leads to activation of the innate immune system. Although the innate immune system attempts to remove damaged cells and macromolecules, the products of chronic inflammation, in fact, accumulate. The ability of the immune system to achieve physiological repair is insufficient and results in the progression of aging [2].

Novel evidence from the literature points to yet another possible explanation of inflammaging. According to a recent hypothesis, the gut's ability to destroy microorganisms (the microbiota) invading or residing in the gut declines with age and it is plausible that microbiota trigger inflammaging. The hypothesis that gut microbiota has a significant impact on inflammaging strongly relies on the role of mitochondrial activation of the Nlrp3 inflammasome. A multiprotein complex, the Nlrp3 inflammasome plays a pivotal role in inducing the secretion of numerous pro-inflammatory cytokines. According to a number of recent articles, the activation of the inflammasome is a key event in inflammaging and plays a significant role in the pathogenesis of numerous age-related diseases, such as atherosclerosis, Alzheimer's disease, degenerative arthritis, and macular degeneration, among others [4].

In the process of aging, mitochondria become dysfunctional and activate not only the Nlrp3 inflammasome but also the innate immune system as well. Moreover, studies have shown that mitochondria contain cardiolipin, which is also present in bacteria. With mitochondrial dysfunction, cardiolipin can act as an endogenous pathogen-associated molecular pattern that is capable of inducing accelerated aging caused by chronic, low-grade inflammation [5, 6].

Results of recent longitudinal studies have reported that gut microbiota may modulate human longevity by affecting host metabolism, since results have shown an association between the distinct metabolomic signatures and longevity in humans [7]. Moreover, data from the literature point to the possible use of calorie restriction (CR) and diet intervention in manipulating the gut microbiota as potential therapies aimed at achieving healthy aging [8, 9].

It is important to emphasize that inflammaging might also be a consequence of cellular senescence. Under conditions of stress and various forms of damage, cells tend to respond with senescence. This process is accompanied by the formation of senescent cells that secrete potent pro-inflammatory signals and lead to the development of the senescence-associated secretory phenotype (SASP) [10, 11]. It is of note that these types of cells tend to accumulate in adipose tissue where they secrete pro-inflammatory cytokines together with cytokines produced by non-senescent adipose tissue. In obesity, pro-inflammatory cytokines secreted both by senescent and adipose tissue cells lead to the development of chronic low-grade inflammation and consequent age-related diseases [12, 13].

Blood hypercoagulability is present in advanced age and certain authors attempt to explain inflammaging as a consequence of this condition. The link between inflammation and coagulation is well-established and often each follows the other. In the elderly, increased inflammation and hypercoagulability may lead to the development of numerous cardio-vascular diseases. However, earlier studies have shown that even in centenarians high plasma levels of coagulation activation markers do not always reflect a high risk of arterial or venous thrombosis, which represents a paradox in the aging process [14]. However, based on novel research, this paradox is explained by anti-inflammatory responses that are more prominent in certain centenarians than in the general population. Also, studies have shown that in these elderly inflammaging progresses more slowly and thus anti-inflammatory responses can balance or restrict inflammaging [15].

Furthermore, inflammaging can be a consequence of immune system maladaptation with advanced age. Studies have shown that with aging the ability of the adaptive immune system to combat pathogens declines, whereas the innate immune system becomes hypersensitive possibly as a way to compensate for its decreased function. These changes are known as immunesenescence and they are frequently accompanied by low-grade systemic inflammation [16 - 18].

Chronic inflammation involves several cytokines, tissue responses, effector cells, and molecular pathways that seem to be shared across numerous age-related diseases. Our understanding of these processes in inflammaging and their role in the development of age-related diseases continues to grow. Still, it is largely unknown if a difference between inflammatory pathways and components exists that would enable us to distinguish one age-related disease from another. Inflammaging is regulated by transcriptional pathways and intracellular signaling cascades. These regulatory processes include regulated secretion (including processing by the inflammasome), regulation by micro-RNAs, posttranslational modifications, as well as regulation at the level of transcription and translation [19]. However, whether or not these regulatory processes are the same or distinct among age-related diseases remains to be elucidated.

There are numerous inflammatory markers, which include different types of cytokines, acute-phase proteins and chemokines. Those best described include TNF-α, IL-6, IL-18, IL-8, IL-12, monocyte chemoattractant protein (MCP), as well as high-sensitivity C-reactive protein (hs-CRP). All of these inflammatory molecules have been associated with age-related chronic disease and overall mortality in the elderly population [20].

An important role in the etiology of inflammaging is played by epigenetic mechanisms. Epigenetics was first described as an interaction between environmental factors and genes that results in the production of a certain phenotype. Epigenetics studies are concerned primarily with two factors: 1) the influence of surroundings, diet, lifestyle, *etc.* as environmental factors that influence the genome and 2) the results of the interactions between environment and the genome that manifest as heritable molecular variations in gene expression without perturbation of the underlying DNA sequence. During aging, diet is regarded as a pivotal factor in provoking epigenetic changes. Epigenetic changes on immune system inflammatory processes lead to disease [21].

The best described epigenetic mechanisms are DNA methylation and reversible post-translational modification of histone tail residues [22 - 26]. Epigenetic mechanisms are thought to be responsible for the development and differentiation of several immune cells related to inflammation [27]. Moreover, epigenetic mechanisms play a crucial role in the regulation of numerous genes that directly influence the inflammatory response [28].

Although current evidence points to complex interactions between epigenetic modifications of the genome and inflammaging, the nature of these interactions is less clear. It seems that inflammaging can cause epigenetic changes but epigenetic changes can also cause age-related chronic inflammatory processes [29]. Studies evaluating the interactions between inflammaging and epigenetic modifications are still limited and are mainly based on an assessment of the association between pro- and anti-inflammatory cytokines on one side and DNA methylation on the other in the elderly [30, 31]. A causal relationship between epigenetic modifications and inflammaging is beginning to be recognized by scientists around the globe and will likely soon lead to the development of epigenetic drugs to treat inflammaging.

Studies thus far have demonstrated that epigenetic variations resulting from environmental factors may affect the immune response leading to inflammation and the consequent development of chronic diseases. During aging, epigenetic and immune system changes increase the risk of infection, inflammation, reactivity to self-antigens, and may lead to the development of cancer [32]. Accordingly, DNA hypomethylation that arises as a consequence of aging process has been shown to cause chronic inflammation and cancer [33].

The results of a recent systematic review aimed at assessing the role of epigenetic changes in the development of neurodegenerative diseases such as Alzheimer disease (AD) and Parkinson disease (PD) have demonstrated that there was no consistent association between epigenetic modifications of the genome and neurodegenerative diseases. However, studies included in this systematic review did report epigenetic regulation of 31 genes (including apoptosis, cell communication, and neurogenesis genes in brain and blood tissue) related to AD and PD. Methylation at the brain-derived neurotrophic factor (BDNF), APP, and SORBS3 genes in AD were the most frequently found associations. Moreover, association between PD and methylation of the α-synuclein gene (SNCA) was also reported and data suggest histone protein alterations in both PD and AD. The authors concluded that larger longitudinal and cohort studies are needed in order to fully assess clinically significant epigenetic variations in neurodegenerative diseases that may lead to the introduction of interventional strategies to treat AD and PD [34]. The role of epigenetic mechanisms has also been reported in the development of autoimmune inflammatory diseases such as systemic lupus erythematosus (SLE) and rheumatoid arthritis (RA) that occur with aging [35 - 38].

The onset of chronic diseases that adversely affect longevity and health span, such as cardiovascular (CVD) and neurodegenerative diseases, type 2 diabetes mellitus (T2DM), cancer, frailty, arthritis, sarcopenia, and chronic obstructive pulmonary disease, among others, is often the consequence of local and systemic inflammation combined with additional determinants, including genetics, early events that promote an unhealthy lifestyle, and the development of inflammation in later stages of life [39].

Although many diseases are related to inflammaging, CVDs are the most important given their prevalence in the aging population. The majority of studies thus far point to a causal link between cardio-metabolic diseases and inflammaging. However, it remains to be elucidated whether increased levels of pro-inflammatory markers are a cause or consequence of pathological processes in the elderly with CVD. Based on our current understanding, numerous mechanisms modulate the role of inflammation in atherogenesis. Accordingly, vascular endothelial dysfunction and inflammation participate in the formation of atherosclerotic plaques, and atherosclerosis, on the other hand, produces antigens that lead to inflammatory processes [40].

One of the best-studied inflammatory markers in CVD in middle-aged and elderly subjects is hs-CRP. Studies conducted on endothelial cells have shown that CRP directly contributes to CVD by elevating oxidative stress [41]. However, Mendelian randomization analyses and mechanistic studies in large populations have reported that CRP is not causally associated with atherosclerotic processes but is only a prognostic biomarker of CVD [42]. The role of CRP in inflammaging has been investigated less. Studies thus far have shown, however, an increased concentration of CRP in multiple age-related diseases [43].

Inflammaging has been shown to be a risk factor not only for age-related diseases but also for global indicators of poor health status, such as a disability in activities of daily living, multimorbidity, mobility disability, and premature death [40]. Many authors propose that inflammaging might be a marker of accelerated aging and should be regarded as one of the cornerstones of the biology of aging [44].

Based on these notions, an increase in the elderly population as well as in age-related diseases has led to the development of a new scientific discipline known as geroscience. Geroscience is founded on seven basic principles/mechanisms or "pillars" that attempt to explain the association between aging and age-related diseases. These pillars include epigenetics, inflammation, stress adaptations, metabolism, proteostasis, regeneration, macromolecular damage, and stem cells (Fig. **1**). It is crucial to understand that these mechanisms do not operate independently but are interconnected and significantly influence each other, and in doing so, form interwoven networks [45 - 47]. One of the main postulates of geroscience is that age-related diseases should not be investigated and treated without treating the aging process itself. Moreover, the importance of the aging process as a factor in the development of age-related disease, as well as the role played by age-related disease in the acceleration of aging, should not be overlooked.

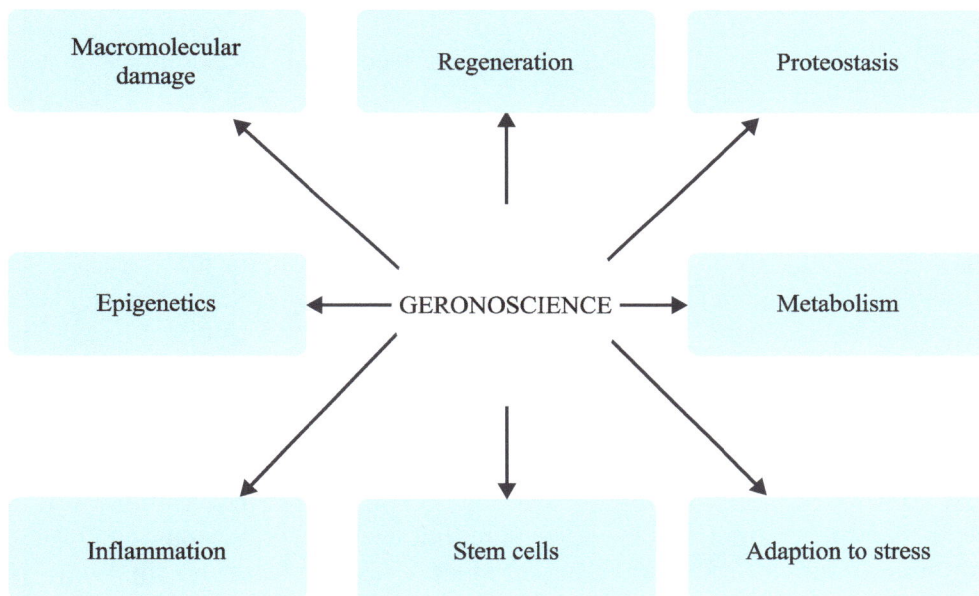

Fig. (1). The pillars of geroscience.

Many authors agree that the common denominator of all geroscience pillars included in the aging process is chronic low-grade inflammation or inflammaging. As mentioned above, the possible mechanisms underlying inflammaging are mitochondrial dysfunction, cellular senescence, activation of the inflammasome, dysbiosis (changes in the composition of the host microbiota), but also activation of the DNA damage response, dysregulation of the ubiquitin-proteasome system as well as defective autophagy and mitophagy [48].

A novel concept related to aging and inflammaging known as "garb-aging" was introduced in 2017. According to this new concept, not yet quantitatively measured, accumulation of cellular "self-garbage" molecules, which include misplaced and/or misfolded proteins, cell debris, apoptotic and senescent cells contribute to the development of inflammaging. Namely, it is thought that formation of pro-inflammatory molecules starts within the cells as a response to malfunction of various cell organelles, especially mitochondria, together with defective disposal of cellular structures by autophagy and mitophagy. This malfunctioning together with endoplasmic reticulum stress, inflammasome activation, accumulation of misplaced and/or misfolded proteins as a consequence of dysfunctional ubiquitin/proteasome, induction of cell senescence, and the DNA damage response eventually leads to inflammaging. Based on these assumptions, inflammaging is a consequence of accumulation of self-garbage and, as such, might be thought of as an autoinflammatory and autoimmune process [39].

Recently, a review discussed commonalities and differences between inflammaging and meta-inflammation. Notably, the authors argued that, although the stressors underlying inflammatory processes in these two conditions differ, the mechanisms that sustain persistent low-grade inflammation are the same. Meta-inflammation, metabolic inflammation caused by an excess of nutrients, plays an important role in the development of T2DM and obesity. As such, meta-inflammation presents a specific form of chronic inflammation that results from overnutrition and shares the same molecular mechanisms as inflammaging. Based on the authors' point of view, the gut microbiota plays a dominant role in the pathogenesis of inflammaging and meta-inflammation, which release pro-inflammatory products that lead to the development of chronic low-grade inflammation with consequent detrimental effects on the human body. Gut microbiota are thought to be important since they represent a common ground for metabolism, diet, and the innate immune response [45]. In addition to gut microbiota, other stimuli that have the potential to cause inflammaging and meta-inflammation include persistent bacterial and viral infections, misfolded and oxidized proteins, misplaced self-molecules, and cell debris [49].

More importantly, inflammaging and meta-inflammation influence each other, since it has been reported that meta-inflammation can lead to inflammaging. Overnutrition can accelerate aging, which results in the development of age-related diseases [50]. This implies that meta-inflammation and inflammaging are interconnected and that inflammaging can follow meta-inflammation and vice versa. Based on this assumption, cardio-metabolic age-related diseases might be regarded as indicators of accelerated aging.

Aging can be best described as a deterioration of homeostasis of all body systems, including the immune system. On a macromolecular level, aging is characterized by disturbed signal transduction pathways, organelle dysfunction, and inflammation leading to cell death. On a systemic level, aging leads to organ failure, an increase in disease incidence, and finally results in death. Although the underlying mechanisms that lead to aging are still not fully elucidated, telomere theory holds promising potential. Telomeres are present at the ends of eukaryotic chromosomes and play a pivotal role in the determination of the rate of biological aging. In higher mammals, they are one of the most important determinants of longevity and aging. Accordingly, predictions of longevity and healthspan can be calculated by measuring average telomere length in animals as well as in humans in all but the oldest subpopulations [51].

Telomeres have numerous functions but one of the most important is maintaining a balance between genome integrity and metabolic dysfunction. Data from the literature point to the possible influence of positive and negative health factors on the length of telomeres. Telomere length is strongly influenced by inflammation and shortening of telomeres has been associated with adiposity and adiposity indices. Earlier study conducted on animals found an inverse relationship between CRP and telomere length. Although studies have shown that chronic systemic inflammation caused by obesity can influence the length of telomeres, in general, research that has evaluated the impact of obesity on telomere length have yielded conflicting results [52]. Namely, cancer incidence, DNA damage, and short telomere length were found to be associated with high BMI values in numerous studies [53]. Higher total and abdominal obesity have also been associated with shorter telomeres [54]. Moreover, shorter telomeres have been reported as a risk factor for increased obesity [55]. It is of note that the impact of obesity on telomere length is gender-specific and more pronounced in women [56]. Results of Valdes *et al.* [57] conducted on a total of 1122 Caucasian women have shown that obese women had shorter telomeres compared with their lean counterparts. However, the association between shorter telomeres and obesity has not been confirmed in a number of studies [55]. Results of a recent systematic review and meta-analysis aimed at assessing the impact of obesity on telomere length have demonstrated that although there was a weak to moderate association between telomere length and obesity, the relationship between these two variables remains questionable and additional controlled longitudinal studies assessing this topic are necessary [58].

PREVENTION AND RESTRICTION OF INFLAMMAGING

Keeping in mind the rapidly aging population worldwide and the established role of chronic, low-grade inflammation in the aging process, it is crucial to discover and implement health-preservation strategies in order to restrict or prevent inflammaging. These strategies serve to boost anti-inflammaging mechanisms. In order to achieve healthy aging, a lifelong balance between inflammatory and anti-inflammatory processes in our body must be maintained. Studies thus far have shown that the use of aspirin and statins as well as physical activity potentially reduce chronic inflammation. Moreover, since obesity has significant pro-inflammatory potential, weight reduction interventions, and well-balanced diets together with calorie restriction, are important in the prevention of inflammaging [59].

Calorie restriction is of special importance since studies have shown that calorie intake reduction or intermittent fasting have protective effects in almost all tissues and organs and lead to lifespan extension [60]. Restriction of calorie intake has favorable effects on pathways that activate autophagy, stress defense mechanisms, and survival, and attenuates the pro-inflammatory response [61]. Although calorie restriction encompasses different types of macronutrients, a reduction in dietary amino acids and proteins has demonstrated the best longevity-promoting potential. For example, restriction of tryptophan intake has been shown to have beneficial effects in neurodegenerative diseases and generally promotes longevity [62, 63]. A novel study by Zapata *et al.* [64] demonstrated that severe restriction of tryptophan (40TRP, 10TRP) decreased circulating glucose, insulin, C□peptide, and leptin, together with a reciprocal increase in plasma glucagon, PP, and glucagon-like peptide-1 in obesity-prone rats. Moreover, the results of the above study have shown that severe dietary tryptophan restriction dose-dependently modulates energy balance, leading to hypophagia and weight loss, while moderate restriction promotes thermogenesis as well as concurrent changes in gut microbiota and hormone levels.

More importantly, calorie restriction has been shown to combat inflammatory processes in the human body and, as such, has favorable actions on different mechanisms proven to influence aging, such as insulin resistance, mitochondrial biogenesis, autophagy, as well as adult neurogenesis and neuronal plasticity. It is believed that the restriction of calorie intake increases lifespan because cells respond to diminished nutrients availability by promoting protective immune and a variety of other metabolic reactions [45]. Accordingly, nutritional interventions, such as the Mediterranean diet (MedDiet), have been found to be anti-inflammatory. Moreover, MedDiet has been shown to affect the modification of epigenetic enzymatic activity [65]. Results of the PREDIMED study have reported beneficial effects of MedDiet on genome-wide DNA methylation [66].

Another nutritional intervention that may have promising effects on inflammaging and epigenetic mechanisms is zinc supplementation since zinc is known for its anti-inflammatory and anti-oxidant properties [67]. Although these findings are still not fully supported clinically, zinc deficiency is one of the numerous consequences of old age. Studies have shown that zinc deficiency has pro-inflammatory actions modulated by epigenetic mechanisms [29]. It remains to be fully assessed whether dietary zinc supplementation will lead to the improvement of inflammatory processes in the elderly.

Novel findings point to the possible use of drugs that eliminate senescent cells or reduce the activity of Nlrp3 inflammasome-dependent pro-inflammatory cascades in the reduction of chronic inflammation in numerous age-related degenerative diseases [4]. Furthermore, the use of local and/or systemic neutralization of pro-inflammatory cytokines and thymic replacement are being explored in the reduction of immunosenescence, a potent inducer of inflammaging. Finally, one should not overlook the potential of healthy lifestyle strategies in the prevention and restriction of inflammaging and age-related disorders.

It should be noted that if the concept of garb-aging, as an explanation for the development of inflammaging, is fully proven, then interventions that increase the removal of self-garbage molecules in our body (*e.g.*, autophagy) will most certainly benefit the aging population and promote healthy aging. Accordingly, studies so far have demonstrated that autophagy decreases with age with a consequent accumulation of undisposed cellular components [68, 69]. The autophagic process is boosted by calorie restriction, fasting-mimicking diets, as well as by drugs, such as rapamycin and its analogs. In general, all autophagy-stimulating interventions include, not only well-balanced, but, if necessary, even restrictive diets together with good stress management strategies, age-appropriate physical activity, and potentially drugs, such as rapamycin, should be used in combination to prevent or restrict inflammaging and its harmful effects and to promote healthy aging and longevity. The implementation of this kind of comprehensive and integrative approach should, in the future, be fully individualized and personalized.

OBESITY IN THE ELDERLY INDIVIDUALS

The prevalence of elderly adults and obesity is rising worldwide. This combination will certainly have significant societal and financial impacts in the future [70, 71]. A majority of studies on obesity thus far have been focused on children and adults, whereas data on obesity in elderly populations are still insufficient. Moreover, treatment modalities for obese elderly individuals are different from those proscribed for children and adults [71, 72]. Bearing this in mind, studies that have evaluated obesity in older individuals, conducted both in Europe and in the USA, have reported an increase of obesity prevalence in the elderly, predominately in elderly women [73]. Furthermore, results from the Scottish Health Survey have shown that, even though the increase in BMI in persons aged 50-70 years was small, the increase was due primarily to waist circumference, which suggests weight gain in visceral fat and loss of lean body mass may detrimentally affect the health of older individuals [74]. Rising obesity prevalence is also seen in nursing homes, and a multisite study reported that 30% of nursing home habitants aged 65 and older had BMIs >35 [75].

It is well known that visceral and central obesity are more pro-inflammatory than global obesity [76]. This pro-inflammatory profile of obesity is linked to a rise in pro-inflammatory cytokines such as TNF-α, IL-6, and CRP as well as with reduced immune function, cognitive decline, insulin resistance, and decreased lean body mass. As a person ages, the distribution of body fat changes. Fat from subcutaneous regions is redistributed to intra-hepatic, intra-abdominal, and intra-muscular regions. Elderly individuals often have sarcopenic adiposity, which manifests as an increase in adiposity and age-related muscle atrophy. Peak total body fat occurs when a person reaches 70 years of age and, subsequently, total body fat begins to decline [77]. An increase of total body fat is the result of normal hormonal changes accompanied by a decrease in total energy expenditure. As previously mentioned, muscle tissue goes through atrophy as individuals age and muscle atrophy is coupled with a decline in physical activity and basal metabolic rate. Hormonal changes that occur with aging include decreased responsiveness to leptin and thyroid hormone, as well as diminished production of growth hormone and testosterone [78 - 80]. Endocrine changes also seen in the elderly include decreased levels of insulin-like growth factor-1, downregulation of ghrelin, and insulin resistance. Studies have shown that hormonal changes are more prominent if insulin resistance and abdominal obesity are also present in older individuals [73].

According to a recent paper by Moyarles *et al.* [81], there are several different subtypes of obesity including, among others, metabolically healthy obesity, metabolically abnormal obesity, as well as sarcopenic obesity. Sarcopenic obesity in elderly individuals is characterized by reduced lean mass and is linked to increased age as well as other predictive factors such as decreased physical activity, low socio-economic status, atherosclerosis, pulmonary disease, and smoking [82]. The predicting factors in sarcopenic obesity are associated with accumulation of an unhealthy profile of body fat as well as with a decline in muscle strength and skeletal muscle mass. It is of note that IL-6 and TNF-α exert a catabolic effect on muscle strength and are involved in sarcopenic obesity [83].

Currently, obesity has reached pandemic proportions and its relationship with inflammaging is the focus of numerous scientific studies. This comes as no surprise given an aging population and increasing obesity prevalence. Many authors recognize obesity as the most frequent age-related disease. If obesity is present among elderly, it significantly increases the level of low-grade systemic inflammation with all its detrimental effects. In those cases, inflammaging serves as a link between obesity and age-related diseases such as atherosclerosis, insulin resistance, diabetes mellitus, cognitive decline, or cancer. Studies thus far have shown that the combination of obesity and inflammaging is characterized by infiltration of adipose tissue by both innate and adaptive immune cells, which leads to the production of pro-inflammatory cytokines together with the conversion of a metabolically normal phenotype to decreased insulin sensitivity and cardio-metabolic syndrome. Accordingly, obesity in aging individuals is followed by increased levels of glucose, free fatty acids, and lipids, as well as by reactive oxygen species. Moreover, therapeutic interventions are less effective in aging individuals with obesity [84].

An interesting proposition has recently been proposed by Alam *et al*. [85]. According to their view, it is inflammation and more precisely inflammaging that determines whether obesity is metabolically healthy or unhealthy in the elderly. Since aging individuals often present with varying etiopathogeneses of obesity, it is of pivotal importance to make clear the distinction between health and unhealthy obesity. Thus far, the relationship between obesity and aging remains controversial. Elderly have more diverse variations in body fat distribution and body weight. Sarcopenia and frailty are also frequently present in this age group. Results from the literature point to a necessity of taking into account the amount of excess fat rather than BMI as a variable in assessing any increased health risk in the elderly [86]. A majority of studies conducted thus far have used BMI as an indicator of body weight and did not fully assess whether obesity found in the elderly was metabolically healthy or unhealthy. This line of research has led to many misconceptions and misleading conclusions in terms of a proper definition of obesity and its consequences in the aging population. Accordingly, the majority of authors agree that in the elderly, the best indicator for obesity has yet to be found. This view is based on a fact that older individuals have a greater amount of body fat compared to younger individuals, even though they might have similar BMIs. In practice, there is no clinical consensus concerning which method is best to use when measuring body fat in the elderly. Thus, the prognostic significance of BMI in measuring obesity in the elderly remains elusive.

It is of note that in elderly obese individuals, there is an inverse association between BMI and relative mortality risk. This "obesity survival paradox" is seen in adults aged 60 to 75 years and is described as a lack of association between elevated mortality risk and obesity, unlike the risk seen in young and middle-aged adults [77]. As for a relationship between cardiovascular mortality and BMI in individuals less than 75 years of age, data from the literature are conflicting. Moreover, in those studies that reported an association between cardiovascular mortality and BMI in the elderly, the association was weak [87].

A potential explanation for the "obesity survival paradox" is the fact that the majority of studies investigating this phenomenon were cross-sectional studies and did not allow for any cause-effect conclusions. One of the reasons why these types of studies have shown improved survivability in obese older individuals might be that BMI is not an appropriate measure of total body fat in this age group. On the other hand, it may be possible that obesity in elderly individuals provides a certain degree of protection, which is also seen in heart failure, cancer, hemodialysis, and HIV [80]. Obese elderly individuals with good survival are, according to many authors, referred to as metabolically healthy obese individuals. The elderly that belong to this group are characterized by an increased BMI, less abdominal fat, and smaller waist circumference. Furthermore, metabolically healthy obese elderly have favorable immune and hormone profiles, alongside with fewer inflammatory markers and greater insulin sensitivity [88]. Finally, as compared to younger individuals, metabolically healthy obese elderly may not have the same level of cardiovascular risk factors, such as elevated blood pressure and low-density lipoprotein [87].

The majority of studies conducted thus far have investigated obesity-related complications in middle-aged populations [80, 89]. Aging and obesity are independent risk factors for numerous disease states. Body mass index greater than 25 kg/m^2 in elderly individuals is linked with osteoarthritis, diabetes, and physical disability. Moreover, studies have shown that as BMI rises in this age group, the risk for CVD and certain types of cancer increases. Interestingly, in these cases, although the risk for CVD and certain types of cancer is elevated, rates of CVD mortality do not increase [90]. For this line of evidence are data that show that in elderly obese individuals, the metabolic syndrome does not carry the same prognostic value, even though metabolic syndrome is inversely related to visceral adiposity [80, 89]. According to numerous authors, both aging and obesity develop as a result of chronic low-grade inflammation and are accompanied with decreased quality of life, mobility impairment, disability institutionalization, and increased costs [91 - 93]. Obesity in later stages of life is linked with a variety of consequences, as stated earlier, that lead to a decrease in physical function, endurance, and strength, followed by increased risk for injuries, higher fall rates, chronic pain, as well as cognitive impairment [94].

In general, obesity complications seen in the elderly are mainly of cardiometabolic nature and include hypertension, glucose intolerance, cardiovascular disease, and dyslipidemia. Obesity in older individuals can also be a risk factor for stroke, Alzheimer's disease, and vascular dementia. Furthermore, obstructive sleep apnea syndrome, obesity hypoventilation, reduced cognitive skills, urinary incontinence, and decreased sexual function may be the consequences of obesity in the elderly [73].

When it comes to weight loss interventions that might be prescribed in the obese elderly, no strict recommendations are implemented since there are conflicting reports from investigating these interventions. Obese elderly have been shown to gain weight easily after weight loss and in the majority of cases, weight loss has been characterized by loss in lean mass, including both muscle strength and bone mineral density [95]. Hence, recommendations for weight loss in elderly obese individuals must be personalized and should respect and recognize an individual's quality of life, physical function, and goals of care [79].

Studies that have evaluated the benefits of lifestyle interventions as weight loss therapy in obese elderly have shown that this type of intervention leads to improvement in muscle quality and physical function, as well as in cardiometabolic outcomes [72, 79] and should be prescribed as first line treatment for the elderly. In order to prevent loss of bone mineral density and muscle mass, patients are advised to take calcium and vitamin D supplements as well as to eat higher-protein diets [72, 95 - 97]. Physical activity such as resistance training, balance activities, and aerobic activities should also be prescribed for older obese individuals, especially for those that have decreased lean body mass [72, 80, 89, 98]. These types of weight loss interventions can significantly improve physical function and quality of life in elderly individuals even though weight loss may not be achieved.

Thus far, studies that specifically evaluated drugs for the treatment of obesity in the elderly are scarce and limited. Polypharmacy is a major concern in this age group as well as are any potential side effects. In general, weight loss drugs should be used with extreme caution in elderly obese individuals [90]. Use of bariatric surgery is also not recommended in older obese individuals because of secondary complications and surgical risk [71]. These types of surgical procedures are linked with significant weight loss that may represent an overwhelming disruption to older individuals. Currently, there is no clear consensus on whether bariatric treatments should be used in elderly patients and, if they are used, there is no consensus concerning preferred procedures, safety, and age cut offs.

LINKING INFLAMMAGING AND OBESITY

Studies have shown that aging *per se* increases the pro-inflammatory response to overnutrition [99]. By now, it is well known that both aging and obesity are associated with chronic systemic low-grade inflammation [100]. Data from the literature point to the negative health impacts of inflammation. Chronic obesity-associated inflammation is characterized by infiltration and activation of macrophages and T-cells in adipose tissue, elevated circulating values of pro-inflammatory markers, and increased pro-inflammatory gene expression in insulin target tissues [101 - 103] (Fig. **2**).

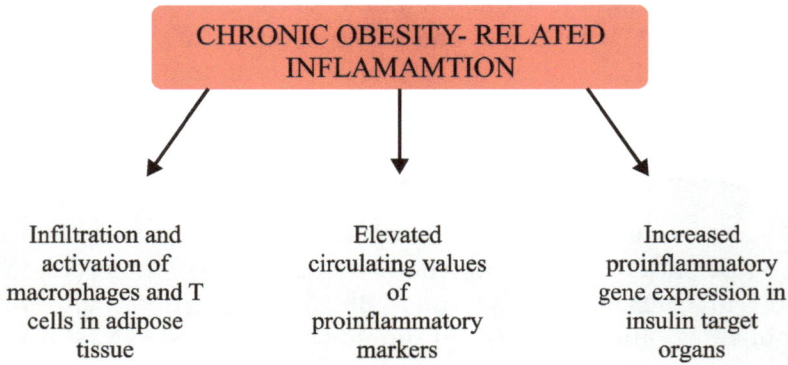

Fig. (**2**).   Characteristics of chronic obesity-associated inflammation.

Cytokines and chemokines jointly named adipokines secreted by adipose tissue modulate chronic low-grade inflammation in obesity both in adipose tissue and in the whole body. This chronic low-grade inflammation exerts predominantly pro-inflammatory effects [104]. Macrophages, originating from the circulation, migrate into adipose tissue and are thought to be the primary source of pro-inflammatory cytokines. These macrophages, together with T-cells, spread the inflammatory response within adipose tissue. In obesity, local inflammation within adipose tissue is regarded as a pivotal controller of chronic systemic inflammation [105].

As stated before, there is a clear distinction between acute inflammation and chronic low-grade systemic inflammation. Acute inflammation is characterized by signs such as swelling, redness, pain, heat, and loss of function. All of the cardinal signs of acute inflammation are absent in chronic systemic low-grade inflammation. Obesity-related low-grade inflammation seen in elderly individuals and in general, is primarily characterized by increased circulating levels of inflammatory cytokines such as IL-6, IL-8, IL-1β, as well as TNF-α [106, 107]. Moreover, levels of acute-phase proteins such as CRP and serum amyloid A are also increased to a certain degree [103, 108], as well as a soluble adhesion molecule (P-selectin, E-selectin), chemokines such as monocyte chemotactic protein 1 (MCP-1) [106], and multifunctional proteins such as osteopontin or leptin [109, 110].

In obese older persons, mediators secreted from visceral adipose tissue are transported in the circulation to the liver. Studies have shown that IL-6 in the liver stimulates the production of CRP, which has been shown as a contributing factor in the development of both cardiovascular diseases and diabetes mellitus [111, 112]. Furthermore, the association between chemokines secreted from visceral adipose tissue and BMI in older obese individuals has been reported [103, 113]. Studies have also shown that osteopontin is upregulated in obesity and might be an important mediator of cell adhesion and migration, macrophage activation, fibrosis, and inflammation [114].

An interesting connection between inflammaging and obesity has recently been proposed by Perez *et al.* [115]. They have introduced a new concept named "adipaging", which posits that obese individuals are prone to aging prematurely. Based on this concept, adipose tissue during aging undergoes significant changes, including not only redistribution of fat to ectopic fat reservoirs, but also intrusion of adipose tissue by senescent cells. This increased intrusion of senescent cells into adipose tissue during aging is driven by metabolic stress, cytokines, as well as decreased removal of these cells. Other features of aged adipose tissue include decreased angiogenic capacity and revascularization, endothelial dysfunction, decreased adipocyte size, as well as tissue fibrosis [116]. Moreover, in aged adipose tissue, altered lipolysis, and enhanced insulin resistance are present [117]. (Fig. **3**).

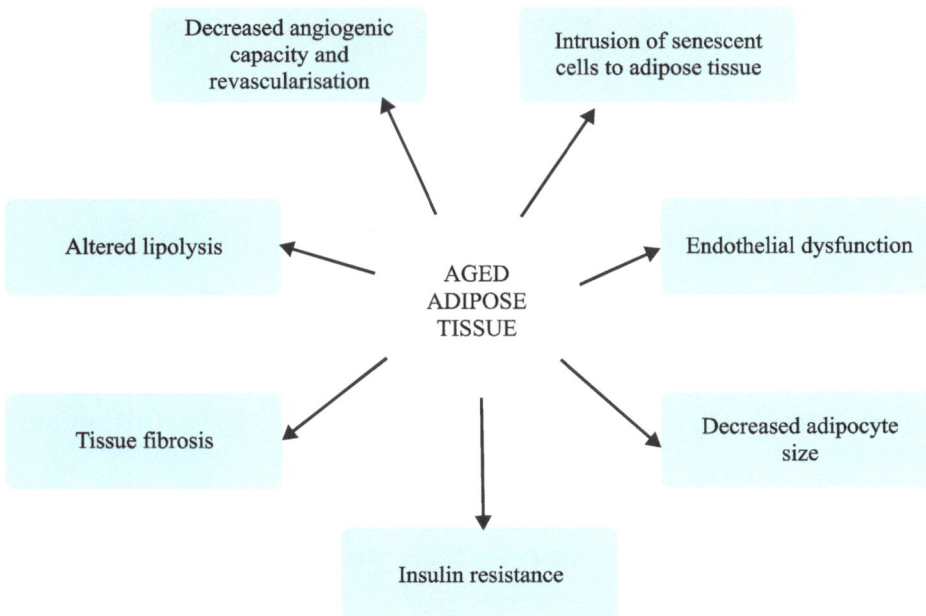

Fig. (3). Features of aged adipose tissue.

Studies have also shown that obesity accelerates the aging process. Accordingly, Ahima *et al.* [118], in an earlier study, have reported that obesity in mice shortens telomeres and increases the formation of reactive oxygen species resulting in inflammation, insulin resistance, and activation of tumor suppressor p53. As stated by Perez *et al.* [115], dysfunctional adipose tissue as a hallmark of 'adipaging' is characterized by mechanisms equally shared by aging and obesity, such as endocrine and metabolic disturbances, multi-organ perturbations, chronic low-grade systemic inflammation, and impaired immune function.

CONCLUDING REMARKS

In the last two decades, the role of chronic systemic low-grade inflammation has gained significant attention as the key player in the pathophysiology of obesity- and aging-associated diseases. However, whether inflammatory processes are the cause or consequence of obesity and aging still needs to be fully elucidated. Although the relationship between inflammaging and obesity remains largely unknown, scientific breakthroughs in this regard will have a significant impact on aging populations. The focus of future research in this area should unravel the molecular mechanisms through which obesity makes obese individuals prone to premature aging. Although therapeutic interventions that alleviate obesity exist, it seems that they are not sufficient and should be reinforced with the use of medications as well as other therapeutic modalities that decrease inflammatory processes.

CONSENT FOR PUBLICATION

Not applicable.

CONFLICT OF INTEREST

The authors confirm that this chapter content has no conflict of interest.

ACKNOWLEDGEMENTS

The authors would like to express their sincere thanks to the editor and anonymous reviewers for their time and valuable suggestions.

REFERENCES

[1]   Franceschi C, Campisi J. Chronic inflammation (inflammaging) and its potential contribution to age-associated diseases. J Gerontol A Biol Sci Med Sci 2014; 69 (Suppl. 1): S4-9.
      [http://dx.doi.org/10.1093/gerona/glu057] [PMID: 24833586]

[2]   Franceschi C, Valensin S, Bonafè M, *et al.* The network and the remodeling theories of aging: historical background and new perspectives. Exp Gerontol 2000; 35(6-7): 879-96.
      [http://dx.doi.org/10.1016/S0531-5565(00)00172-8] [PMID: 11053678]

[3]   Dall'Olio F, Vanhooren V, Chen CC, Slagboom PE, Wuhrer M, Franceschi C. N-glycomic biomarkers of biological aging and longevity: a link with inflammaging. Ageing Res Rev 2013; 12(2): 685-98.
[http://dx.doi.org/10.1016/j.arr.2012.02.002] [PMID: 22353383]

[4]   Youm YH, Grant RW, McCabe LR, *et al.* Canonical Nlrp3 inflammasome links systemic low-grade inflammation to functional decline in aging. Cell Metab 2013; 18(4): 519-32.
[http://dx.doi.org/10.1016/j.cmet.2013.09.010] [PMID: 24093676]

[5]   Zhang Q, Raoof M, Chen Y, *et al.* Circulating mitochondrial DAMPs cause inflammatory responses to injury. Nature 2010; 464(7285): 104-7.
[http://dx.doi.org/10.1038/nature08780] [PMID: 20203610]

[6]   Iyer SS, He Q, Janczy JR, *et al.* Mitochondrial cardiolipin is required for Nlrp3 inflammasome activation. Immunity 2013; 39(2): 311-23.
[http://dx.doi.org/10.1016/j.immuni.2013.08.001] [PMID: 23954133]

[7]   Cheng S, Larson MG, McCabe EL, *et al.* Distinct metabolomic signatures are associated with longevity in humans. Nat Commun 2015; 6: 6791.
[http://dx.doi.org/10.1038/ncomms7791] [PMID: 25864806]

[8]   Cai D, Zhao S, Li D, *et al.* Nutrient intake is associated with longevity characterization by metabolites and element profiles of healthy centenarians. Nutrients 2016; 8(9): 564.
[http://dx.doi.org/10.3390/nu8090564] [PMID: 27657115]

[9]   Fontana L, Partridge L. Promoting health and longevity through diet: from model organisms to humans. Cell 2015; 161(1): 106-18.
[http://dx.doi.org/10.1016/j.cell.2015.02.020] [PMID: 25815989]

[10]   Campisi J, d'Adda di Fagagna F. Cellular senescence: when bad things happen to good cells. Nat Rev Mol Cell Biol 2007; 8(9): 729-40.
[http://dx.doi.org/10.1038/nrm2233] [PMID: 17667954]

[11]   Baker DJ, Wijshake T, Tchkonia T, *et al.* Clearance of p16Ink4a-positive senescent cells delays ageing-associated disorders. Nature 2011; 479(7372): 232-6.
[http://dx.doi.org/10.1038/nature10600] [PMID: 22048312]

[12]   Tchkonia T, Morbeck DE, Von Zglinicki T, *et al.* Fat tissue, aging, and cellular senescence. Aging Cell 2010; 9(5): 667-84.
[http://dx.doi.org/10.1111/j.1474-9726.2010.00608.x] [PMID: 20701600]

[13]   Grant RW, Dixit VD. Mechanisms of disease: inflammasome activation and the development of type 2 diabetes. Front Immunol 2013; 4: 50.
[http://dx.doi.org/10.3389/fimmu.2013.00050] [PMID: 23483669]

[14]   Mari D, Mannucci PM, Coppola R, Bottasso B, Bauer KA, Rosenberg RD. Hypercoagulability in centenarians: the paradox of successful aging. Blood 1995; 85(11): 3144-9.
[http://dx.doi.org/10.1182/blood.V85.11.3144.bloodjournal85113144] [PMID: 7756646]

[15]   Franceschi C, Capri M, Monti D, *et al.* Inflammaging and anti-inflammaging: a systemic perspective on aging and longevity emerged from studies in humans. Mech Ageing Dev 2007; 128(1): 92-105.
[http://dx.doi.org/10.1016/j.mad.2006.11.016] [PMID: 17116321]

[16]   Franceschi C, Bonafè M, Valensin S. Human immunosenescence: the prevailing of innate immunity, the failing of clonotypic immunity, and the filling of immunological space. Vaccine 2000; 18(16): 1717-20.
[http://dx.doi.org/10.1016/S0264-410X(99)00513-7] [PMID: 10689155]

[17]   McElhaney JE, Effros RB. Immunosenescence: what does it mean to health outcomes in older adults? Curr Opin Immunol 2009; 21(4): 418-24.
[http://dx.doi.org/10.1016/j.coi.2009.05.023] [PMID: 19570667]

[18]   Shaw AC, Joshi S, Greenwood H, Panda A, Lord JM. Aging of the innate immune system. Curr Opin

Immunol 2010; 22(4): 507-13.
[http://dx.doi.org/10.1016/j.coi.2010.05.003] [PMID: 20667703]

[19]   Olivieri F, Rippo MR, Monsurrò V, *et al.* MicroRNAs linking inflamm-aging, cellular senescence and cancer. Ageing Res Rev 2013; 12(4): 1056-68.
[http://dx.doi.org/10.1016/j.arr.2013.05.001] [PMID: 23688930]

[20]   Morrisette-Thomas V, Cohen AA, Fülöp T, *et al.* Inflamm-aging does not simply reflect increases in pro-inflammatory markers. Mech Ageing Dev 2014; 139: 49-57.
[http://dx.doi.org/10.1016/j.mad.2014.06.005] [PMID: 25011077]

[21]   Jones PA. Moving AHEAD with an international human epigenome project. Nature 2008; 454(7205): 711-5.
[http://dx.doi.org/10.1038/454711a] [PMID: 18685699]

[22]   Eckhardt F, Lewin J, Cortese R, *et al.* DNA methylation profiling of human chromosomes 6, 20 and 22. Nat Genet 2006; 38(12): 1378-85.
[http://dx.doi.org/10.1038/ng1909] [PMID: 17072317]

[23]   Rollins RA, Haghighi F, Edwards JR, *et al.* Large-scale structure of genomic methylation patterns. Genome Res 2006; 16(2): 157-63.
[http://dx.doi.org/10.1101/gr.4362006] [PMID: 16365381]

[24]   Kouzarides T. Chromatin modifications and their function. Cell 2007; 128(4): 693-705.
[http://dx.doi.org/10.1016/j.cell.2007.02.005] [PMID: 17320507]

[25]   Barth TK, Imhof A. Fast signals and slow marks: the dynamics of histone modifications. Trends Biochem Sci 2010; 35(11): 618-26.
[http://dx.doi.org/10.1016/j.tibs.2010.05.006] [PMID: 20685123]

[26]   Strahl BD, Allis CD. The language of covalent histone modifications. Nature 2000; 403(6765): 41-5.
[http://dx.doi.org/10.1038/47412] [PMID: 10638745]

[27]   Mikkelsen TS, Ku M, Jaffe DB, *et al.* Genome-wide maps of chromatin state in pluripotent and lineage-committed cells. Nature 2007; 448(7153): 553-60.
[http://dx.doi.org/10.1038/nature06008] [PMID: 17603471]

[28]   Bernstein BE, Mikkelsen TS, Xie X, *et al.* A bivalent chromatin structure marks key developmental genes in embryonic stem cells. Cell 2006; 125(2): 315-26.
[http://dx.doi.org/10.1016/j.cell.2006.02.041] [PMID: 16630819]

[29]   Nardini C, Moreau JF, Gensous N, Ravaioli F, Garagnani P, Bacalini MG. The epigenetics of inflammaging: The contribution of age-related heterochromatin loss and locus-specific remodelling and the modulation by environmental stimuli. Semin Immunol 2018; 40: 49-60.
[http://dx.doi.org/10.1016/j.smim.2018.10.009] [PMID: 30396810]

[30]   Sun YV, Lazarus A, Smith JA, *et al.* Gene-specific DNA methylation association with serum levels of C-reactive protein in African Americans. PLoS One 2013; 8(8): e73480.
[http://dx.doi.org/10.1371/journal.pone.0073480] [PMID: 23977389]

[31]   Verschoor CP, McEwen LM, Kohli V, *et al.* The relation between DNA methylation patterns and serum cytokine levels in community-dwelling adults: a preliminary study. BMC Genet 2017; 18(1): 57.
[http://dx.doi.org/10.1186/s12863-017-0525-3] [PMID: 28637423]

[32]   Bayarsaihan D. Epigenetic mechanisms in inflammation. J Dent Res 2011; 90(1): 9-17.
[http://dx.doi.org/10.1177/0022034510378683] [PMID: 21178119]

[33]   Agrawal A, Tay J, Yang GE, Agrawal S, Gupta S. Age-associated epigenetic modifications in human DNA increase its immunogenicity. Aging (Albany NY) 2010; 2(2): 93-100.
[http://dx.doi.org/10.18632/aging.100121] [PMID: 20354270]

[34]   Wen KX, Miliç J, El-Khodor B, *et al.* The Role of DNA Methylation and Histone Modifications in

Neurodegenerative Diseases: A Systematic Review. PLoS One 2016; 11(12): e0167201.
[http://dx.doi.org/10.1371/journal.pone.0167201] [PMID: 27973581]

[35] Javierre BM, Fernandez AF, Richter J, *et al.* Changes in the pattern of DNA methylation associate with twin discordance in systemic lupus erythematosus. Genome Res 2010; 20(2): 170-9.
[http://dx.doi.org/10.1101/gr.100289.109] [PMID: 20028698]

[36] Brooks WH, Le Dantec C, Pers JO, Youinou P, Renaudineau Y. Epigenetics and autoimmunity. J Autoimmun 2010; 34(3): J207-19.
[http://dx.doi.org/10.1016/j.jaut.2009.12.006] [PMID: 20053532]

[37] Maciejewska Rodrigues H, Jüngel A, Gay RE, Gay S. Innate immunity, epigenetics and autoimmunity in rheumatoid arthritis. Mol Immunol 2009; 47(1): 12-8.
[http://dx.doi.org/10.1016/j.molimm.2009.01.010] [PMID: 19232437]

[38] Strietholt S, Maurer B, Peters MA, Pap T, Gay S. Epigenetic modifications in rheumatoid arthritis. Arthritis Res Ther 2008; 10(5): 219.
[http://dx.doi.org/10.1186/ar2500] [PMID: 18947370]

[39] Franceschi C, Garagnani P, Vitale G, Capri M, Salvioli S. Inflammaging and 'Garb-aging'. Trends Endocrinol Metab 2017; 28(3): 199-212.
[http://dx.doi.org/10.1016/j.tem.2016.09.005] [PMID: 27789101]

[40] Ferrucci L, Fabbri E. Inflammageing: chronic inflammation in ageing, cardiovascular disease, and frailty. Nat Rev Cardiol 2018; 15(9): 505-22.
[http://dx.doi.org/10.1038/s41569-018-0064-2] [PMID: 30065258]

[41] Ridker PM. From C-Reactive Protein to Interleukin-6 to Interleukin-1: Moving Upstream To Identify Novel Targets for Atheroprotection. Circ Res 2016; 118(1): 145-56.
[http://dx.doi.org/10.1161/CIRCRESAHA.115.306656] [PMID: 26837745]

[42] Elliott P, Chambers JC, Zhang W, *et al.* Genetic Loci associated with C-reactive protein levels and risk of coronary heart disease. JAMA 2009; 302(1): 37-48.
[http://dx.doi.org/10.1001/jama.2009.954] [PMID: 19567438]

[43] Slevin M, Molins B. Editorial: C-reactive protein in age-related disorders. Front Immunol 2018; 9: 2745.
[http://dx.doi.org/10.3389/fimmu.2018.02745] [PMID: 30524450]

[44] Hodes RJ, Sierra F, Austad SN, *et al.* Disease drivers of aging. Ann N Y Acad Sci 2016; 1386(1): 45-68.
[http://dx.doi.org/10.1111/nyas.13299] [PMID: 27943360]

[45] Franceschi C, Garagnani P, Parini P, Giuliani C, Santoro A. Inflammaging: a new immune-metabolic viewpoint for age-related diseases. Nat Rev Endocrinol 2018; 14(10): 576-90.
[http://dx.doi.org/10.1038/s41574-018-0059-4] [PMID: 30046148]

[46] Kennedy BK, Berger SL, Brunet A, *et al.* Geroscience: linking aging to chronic disease. Cell 2014; 159(4): 709-13.
[http://dx.doi.org/10.1016/j.cell.2014.10.039] [PMID: 25417146]

[47] López-Otín C, Blasco MA, Partridge L, Serrano M, Kroemer G. The hallmarks of aging. Cell 2013; 153(6): 1194-217.
[http://dx.doi.org/10.1016/j.cell.2013.05.039] [PMID: 23746838]

[48] Vitale G, Salvioli S, Franceschi C. Oxidative stress and the ageing endocrine system. Nat Rev Endocrinol 2013; 9(4): 228-40.
[http://dx.doi.org/10.1038/nrendo.2013.29] [PMID: 23438835]

[49] Biagi E, Nylund L, Candela M, *et al.* Through ageing, and beyond: gut microbiota and inflammatory status in seniors and centenarians. PLoS One 2010; 5(5): e10667.
[http://dx.doi.org/10.1371/journal.pone.0010667] [PMID: 20498852]

[50]   Franceschi C, Garagnani P, Morsiani C, *et al.* The continuum of aging and age-related diseases: common mechanisms but different rates. Front Med (Lausanne) 2018; 5: 61.
[http://dx.doi.org/10.3389/fmed.2018.00061] [PMID: 29662881]

[51]   Bär C, Blasco MA. Telomeres and telomerase as therapeutic targets to prevent and treat age-related diseases. F1000Res. 2016; 5: F1000 Faculty Rev-89.

[52]   Abbas G, Salman A, Ur Rahman S, *et al.* Aging mechanisms: linking oxidative stress, obesity and inflammation. Matrix Science Medica 2017; 1(1): 30-3.
[http://dx.doi.org/10.26480/msm.01.2017.30.33]

[53]   Huzen J, Wong LS, van Veldhuisen DJ, *et al.* Telomere length loss due to smoking and metabolic traits. J Intern Med 2014; 275(2): 155-63.
[http://dx.doi.org/10.1111/joim.12149] [PMID: 24118582]

[54]   Lee M, Martin H, Firpo MA, Demerath EW. Inverse association between adiposity and telomere length: The Fels Longitudinal Study. Am J Hum Biol 2011; 23(1): 100-6.
[http://dx.doi.org/10.1002/ajhb.21109] [PMID: 21080476]

[55]   Njajou OT, Cawthon RM, Blackburn EH, *et al.* Shorter telomeres are associated with obesity and weight gain in the elderly. Int J Obes 2012; 36(9): 1176-9.
[http://dx.doi.org/10.1038/ijo.2011.196] [PMID: 22005719]

[56]   Vidacek NS, Nanic L, Ravlic S, *et al.* Telomeres, nutrition, and longevity: can we really navigate our aging? J Gerontol A Biol Sci Med Sci 2017; 73(1): 39-47.
[http://dx.doi.org/10.1093/gerona/glx082] [PMID: 28510637]

[57]   Valdes AM, Andrew T, Gardner JP, *et al.* Obesity, cigarette smoking, and telomere length in women. Lancet 2005; 366(9486): 662-4.
[http://dx.doi.org/10.1016/S0140-6736(05)66630-5] [PMID: 16112303]

[58]   Mundstock E, Sarria EE, Zatti H, *et al.* Effect of obesity on telomere length: Systematic review and meta-analysis. Obesity (Silver Spring) 2015; 23(11): 2165-74.
[http://dx.doi.org/10.1002/oby.21183] [PMID: 26407932]

[59]   Handschin C, Spiegelman BM. The role of exercise and PGC1alpha in inflammation and chronic disease. Nature 2008; 454(7203): 463-9.
[http://dx.doi.org/10.1038/nature07206] [PMID: 18650917]

[60]   Ingram DK, de Cabo R. Calorie restriction in rodents: Caveats to consider. Ageing Res Rev 2017; 39: 15-28.
[http://dx.doi.org/10.1016/j.arr.2017.05.008] [PMID: 28610949]

[61]   Barzilai N, Huffman DM, Muzumdar RH, Bartke A. The critical role of metabolic pathways in aging. Diabetes 2012; 61(6): 1315-22.
[http://dx.doi.org/10.2337/db11-1300] [PMID: 22618766]

[62]   Mirzaei H, Suarez JA, Longo VD. Protein and amino acid restriction, aging and disease: from yeast to humans. Trends Endocrinol Metab 2014; 25(11): 558-66.
[http://dx.doi.org/10.1016/j.tem.2014.07.002] [PMID: 25153840]

[63]   Lee C, Longo V. Dietary restriction with and without caloric restriction for healthy aging. F1000Res 2016; 5 pii: F1000 Faculty Rev-117.

[64]   Zapata RC, Singh A, Ajdari NM, Chelikani PK. Dietary tryptophan restriction dose-dependently modulates energy balance, gut hormones, and microbiota in obesity-prone rats. Obesity (Silver Spring) 2018; 26(4): 730-9.
[http://dx.doi.org/10.1002/oby.22136] [PMID: 29504260]

[65]   Bacalini MG, Friso S, Olivieri F, *et al.* Present and future of anti-ageing epigenetic diets. Mech Ageing Dev 2014; 136-137: 101-15.
[http://dx.doi.org/10.1016/j.mad.2013.12.006] [PMID: 24388875]

[66]   Arpón A, Riezu-Boj JI, Milagro FI, *et al.* Adherence to mediterranean diet is associated with methylation changes in inflammation-related genes in peripheral blood cells. J Physiol Biochem 2016; 73(3): 445-55.
[http://dx.doi.org/10.1007/s13105-017-0552-6] [PMID: 28181167]

[67]   Wessels I, Maywald M, Rink L. Zinc as a gatekeeper of immune function. Nutrients 2017; 9(12): E1286.
[http://dx.doi.org/10.3390/nu9121286] [PMID: 29186856]

[68]   Cuervo AM, Wong E. Chaperone-mediated autophagy: roles in disease and aging. Cell Res 2014; 24(1): 92-104.
[http://dx.doi.org/10.1038/cr.2013.153] [PMID: 24281265]

[69]   Shirakabe A, Ikeda Y, Sciarretta S, Zablocki DK, Sadoshima J. Aging and autophagy in the heart. Circ Res 2016; 118(10): 1563-76.
[http://dx.doi.org/10.1161/CIRCRESAHA.116.307474] [PMID: 27174950]

[70]   Han TS, Wu FC, Lean ME. Obesity and weight management in the elderly: a focus on men. Best Pract Res Clin Endocrinol Metab 2013; 27(4): 509-25.
[http://dx.doi.org/10.1016/j.beem.2013.04.012] [PMID: 24054928]

[71]   Felix HC, West DS. Effectiveness of weight loss interventions for obese older adults. Am J Health Promot 2013; 27(3): 191-9.
[http://dx.doi.org/10.4278/ajhp.110617-LIT-259] [PMID: 23286596]

[72]   Waters DL, Ward AL, Villareal DT. Weight loss in obese adults 65years and older: a review of the controversy. Exp Gerontol 2013; 48(10): 1054-61.
[http://dx.doi.org/10.1016/j.exger.2013.02.005] [PMID: 23403042]

[73]   Mathus-Vliegen EM. Obesity and the elderly. J Clin Gastroenterol 2012; 46(7): 533-44.
[http://dx.doi.org/10.1097/MCG.0b013e31825692ce] [PMID: 22772735]

[74]   Han TS, Tajar A, Lean ME. Obesity and weight management in the elderly. Br Med Bull 2011; 97: 169-96.
[http://dx.doi.org/10.1093/bmb/ldr002] [PMID: 21325341]

[75]   Diouf I, Charles MA, Ducimetière P, Basdevant A, Eschwege E, Heude B. Evolution of obesity prevalence in France: an age-period-cohort analysis. Epidemiology 2010; 21(3): 360-5.
[http://dx.doi.org/10.1097/EDE.0b013e3181d5bff5] [PMID: 20375843]

[76]   Schrager MA, Metter EJ, Simonsick E, *et al.* Sarcopenic obesity and inflammation in the InCHIANTI study. J Appl Physiol 2007; 102(3): 919-25.
[http://dx.doi.org/10.1152/japplphysiol.00627.2006] [PMID: 17095641]

[77]   Oreopoulos A, Kalantar-Zadeh K, Sharma AM, Fonarow GC. The obesity paradox in the elderly: potential mechanisms and clinical implications. Clin Geriatr Med 2009; 25(4): 643-659, viii.
[http://dx.doi.org/10.1016/j.cger.2009.07.005] [PMID: 19944265]

[78]   Waters DL, Baumgartner RN. Sarcopenia and obesity. Clin Geriatr Med 2011; 27(3): 401-21.
[http://dx.doi.org/10.1016/j.cger.2011.03.007] [PMID: 21824555]

[79]   Bales CW, Buhr G. Is obesity bad for older persons? A systematic review of the pros and cons of weight reduction in later life. J Am Med Dir Assoc 2008; 9(5): 302-12.
[PMID: 18519110]

[80]   Villareal DT, Apovian CM, Kushner RF, Klein S. Obesity in older adults: technical review and position statement of the American Society for Nutrition and NAASO, The Obesity Society. Am J Clin Nutr 2005; 82(5): 923-34.
[PMID: 16280421]

[81]   Mayoral LP, Andrade GM, Mayoral EP, *et al.* Obesity subtypes, related biomarkers & heterogeneity. Indian J Med Res 2020; 151(1): 11-21.

[PMID: 32134010]

[82]   Tyrovolas S, Koyanagi A, Olaya B, *et al.* Factors associated with skeletal muscle mass, sarcopenia, and sarcopenic obesity in older adults: a multi-continent study. J Cachexia Sarcopenia Muscle 2016; 7(3): 312-21.
       [PMID: 27239412]

[83]   Florez H, Troen BR. Fat and inflammaging: a dual path to unfitness in elderly people? J Am Geriatr Soc 2008; 56(3): 558-60.
       [http://dx.doi.org/10.1111/j.1532-5415.2007.01584.x] [PMID: 18315667]

[84]   Hotamisligil GS. Inflammation, metaflammation and immunometabolic disorders. Nature 2017; 542: 177-85.
       [http://dx.doi.org/10.1038/nature21363]

[85]   Alam I, Ng TP, Larbi A. Does inflammation determine whether obesity is metabolically healthy or unhealthy? The aging perspective. Mediators Inflamm 2012; 2012: 456456.
       [http://dx.doi.org/10.1155/2012/456456] [PMID: 23091306]

[86]   De Lorenzo A, Del Gobbo V, Premrov MG, Bigioni M, Galvano F, Di Renzo L. Normal-weight obese syndrome: early inflammation? Am J Clin Nutr 2007; 85(1): 40-5.
       [http://dx.doi.org/10.1093/ajcn/85.1.40] [PMID: 17209175]

[87]   Heiat A, Vaccarino V, Krumholz HM. An evidence-based assessment of federal guidelines for overweight and obesity as they apply to elderly persons. Arch Intern Med 2001; 161(9): 1194-203.
       [http://dx.doi.org/10.1001/archinte.161.9.1194] [PMID: 11343442]

[88]   Lang PO, Mahmoudi R, Novella JL, *et al.* Is obesity a marker of robustness in vulnerable hospitalized aged populations? Prospective, multicenter cohort study of 1 306 acutely ill patients. J Nutr Health Aging 2014; 18(1): 66-74.
       [http://dx.doi.org/10.1007/s12603-013-0352-9] [PMID: 24402392]

[89]   Executive summary of the clinical guidelines on the identification, evaluation, and treatment of overweight and obesity in adults. Arch Intern Med 1998; 158(17): 1855-67.
       [http://dx.doi.org/10.1001/archinte.158.17.1855] [PMID: 9759681]

[90]   McTigue KM, Hess R, Ziouras J. Obesity in older adults: a systematic review of the evidence for diagnosis and treatment. Obesity (Silver Spring) 2006; 14(9): 1485-97.
       [http://dx.doi.org/10.1038/oby.2006.171] [PMID: 17030958]

[91]   Donini LM, Savina C, Gennaro E, *et al.* A systematic review of the literature concerning the relationship between obesity and mortality in the elderly. J Nutr Health Aging 2012; 16(1): 89-98.
       [http://dx.doi.org/10.1007/s12603-011-0073-x] [PMID: 22238007]

[92]   Zanandrea V, Barreto de Souto P, Cesari M, Vellas B, Rolland Y. Obesity and nursing home: a review and an update. Clin Nutr 2013; 32(5): 679-85.
       [http://dx.doi.org/10.1016/j.clnu.2013.05.008] [PMID: 23759736]

[93]   Visvanathan R, Haywood C, Piantadosi C, Appleton S. Australian and New Zealand Society for Geriatric Medicine: position statement - obesity and the older person. Australas J Ageing 2012; 31(4): 261-7.
       [http://dx.doi.org/10.1111/j.1741-6612.2012.00652.x] [PMID: 23252986]

[94]   Morley JE, Vellas B, van Kan GA, *et al.* Frailty consensus: a call to action. J Am Med Dir Assoc 2013; 14(6): 392-7.
       [http://dx.doi.org/10.1016/j.jamda.2013.03.022] [PMID: 23764209]

[95]   Mathus-Vliegen L, Toouli J, Fried M, *et al.* World Gastroenterology Organisation global guidelines on obesity. J Clin Gastroenterol 2012; 46(7): 555-61.
       [http://dx.doi.org/10.1097/MCG.0b013e318259bd04] [PMID: 22772737]

[96]   Du YF, Ou HY, Beverly EA, Chiu CJ. Achieving glycemic control in elderly patients with type 2 diabetes: a critical comparison of current options. Clin Interv Aging 2014; 9: 1963-80.

[PMID: 25429208]

[97] Li Z, Heber D. Sarcopenic obesity in the elderly and strategies for weight management. Nutr Rev 2012; 70(1): 57-64.
[http://dx.doi.org/10.1111/j.1753-4887.2011.00453.x] [PMID: 22221216]

[98] Porter Starr KN, McDonald SR, Bales CW. Obesity and physical frailty in older adults: a scoping review of lifestyle intervention trials. J Am Med Dir Assoc 2014; 15(4): 240-50.
[http://dx.doi.org/10.1016/j.jamda.2013.11.008] [PMID: 24445063]

[99] Einstein FH, Huffman DM, Fishman S, *et al.* Aging per se increases the susceptibility to free fatty acid-induced insulin resistance. J Gerontol A Biol Sci Med Sci 2010; 65(8): 800-8.
[http://dx.doi.org/10.1093/gerona/glq078] [PMID: 20504893]

[100] Zeyda M, Stulnig TM. Obesity, inflammation, and insulin resistance--a mini-review. Gerontology 2009; 55(4): 379-86.
[http://dx.doi.org/10.1159/000212758] [PMID: 19365105]

[101] Gregor MF, Hotamisligil GS. Inflammatory mechanisms in obesity. Annu Rev Immunol 2011; 29: 415-45.
[http://dx.doi.org/10.1146/annurev-immunol-031210-101322] [PMID: 21219177]

[102] Todoric J, Löffler M, Huber J, *et al.* Adipose tissue inflammation induced by high-fat diet in obese diabetic mice is prevented by n-3 polyunsaturated fatty acids. Diabetologia 2006; 49(9): 2109-19.
[http://dx.doi.org/10.1007/s00125-006-0300-x] [PMID: 16783472]

[103] Huber J, Kiefer FW, Zeyda M, *et al.* CC chemokine and CC chemokine receptor profiles in visceral and subcutaneous adipose tissue are altered in human obesity. J Clin Endocrinol Metab 2008; 93(8): 3215-21.
[http://dx.doi.org/10.1210/jc.2007-2630] [PMID: 18492752]

[104] Hotamisligil GS. Inflammation and metabolic disorders. Nature 2006; 444(7121): 860-7.
[http://dx.doi.org/10.1038/nature05485] [PMID: 17167474]

[105] Lumeng CN, Saltiel AR. Inflammatory links between obesity and metabolic disease. J Clin Invest 2011; 121(6): 2111-7.
[http://dx.doi.org/10.1172/JCI57132] [PMID: 21633179]

[106] Kim CS, Park HS, Kawada T, *et al.* Circulating levels of MCP-1 and IL-8 are elevated in human obese subjects and associated with obesity-related parameters. Int J Obes 2006; 30(9): 1347-55.
[http://dx.doi.org/10.1038/sj.ijo.0803259] [PMID: 16534530]

[107] Stienstra R, Tack CJ, Kanneganti TD, Joosten LA, Netea MG. The inflammasome puts obesity in the danger zone. Cell Metab 2012; 15(1): 10-8.
[http://dx.doi.org/10.1016/j.cmet.2011.10.011] [PMID: 22225872]

[108] Poitou C, Viguerie N, Cancello R, *et al.* Serum amyloid A: production by human white adipocyte and regulation by obesity and nutrition. Diabetologia 2005; 48(3): 519-28.
[http://dx.doi.org/10.1007/s00125-004-1654-6] [PMID: 15729583]

[109] Kiefer FW, Zeyda M, Todoric J, *et al.* Osteopontin expression in human and murine obesity: extensive local up-regulation in adipose tissue but minimal systemic alterations. Endocrinology 2008; 149(3): 1350-7.
[http://dx.doi.org/10.1210/en.2007-1312] [PMID: 18048491]

[110] Friedman JM, Halaas JL. Leptin and the regulation of body weight in mammals. Nature 1998; 395(6704): 763-70.
[http://dx.doi.org/10.1038/27376] [PMID: 9796811]

[111] Pradhan AD, Manson JE, Rifai N, Buring JE, Ridker PM. C-reactive protein, interleukin 6, and risk of developing type 2 diabetes mellitus. JAMA 2001; 286(3): 327-34.
[http://dx.doi.org/10.1001/jama.286.3.327] [PMID: 11466099]

[112] Yusuf S, Hawken S, Ounpuu S, *et al.* Effect of potentially modifiable risk factors associated with myocardial infarction in 52 countries (the INTERHEART study): case-control study. Lancet 2004; 364(9438): 937-52.
[http://dx.doi.org/10.1016/S0140-6736(04)17018-9] [PMID: 15364185]

[113] Hashimoto I, Wada J, Hida A, *et al.* Elevated serum monocyte chemoattractant protein-4 and chronic inflammation in overweight subjects. Obesity (Silver Spring) 2006; 14(5): 799-811.
[http://dx.doi.org/10.1038/oby.2006.93] [PMID: 16855189]

[114] Kiefer FW, Zeyda M, Gollinger K, *et al.* Neutralization of osteopontin inhibits obesity-induced inflammation and insulin resistance. Diabetes 2010; 59(4): 935-46.
[http://dx.doi.org/10.2337/db09-0404] [PMID: 20107108]

[115] Pérez LM, Pareja-Galeano H, Sanchis-Gomar F, Emanuele E, Lucia A, Gálvez BG. 'Adipaging': ageing and obesity share biological hallmarks related to a dysfunctional adipose tissue. J Physiol 2016; 594(12): 3187-207.
[http://dx.doi.org/10.1113/JP271691] [PMID: 26926488]

[116] Donato AJ, Henson GD, Hart CR, *et al.* The impact of ageing on adipose structure, function and vasculature in the B6D2F1 mouse: evidence of significant multisystem dysfunction. J Physiol 2014; 592(18): 4083-96.
[PMID: 25038241]

[117] Das M, Gabriely I, Barzilai N. Caloric restriction, body fat and ageing in experimental models. Obes Rev 2004; 5(1): 13-9.
[PMID: 14969503]

[118] Ahima RS, Saper CB, Flier JS, Elmquist JK. Leptin regulation of neuroendocrine systems. Front Neuroendocrinol 2000; 21(3): 263-307.
[PMID: 10882542]

SUBJECT INDEX

A

Activity 13, 14, 35, 44, 45, 46, 47, 49, 56, 84,
    89, 92, 108, 119, 135, 153, 156, 157,
    159, 166, 170, 183, 187, 188, 192
  aerobic 192
  anti-inflammatory 47
  antimicrobial 47
  catalytic 166
  cytokine release 170
  endocrine 84
  endothelial 135
  enzymatic 187
  lipoprotein lipase 14, 35, 108
  metabolic 119
  natural killer cell 49
  neuron 56
  neuronal 44, 45, 153
  phagocytic 159
Adipocyte apoptosis 15, 71, 105
Adipocyte(s) 24, 30, 31, 35, 63, 65, 68, 69, 70,
    71, 81, 83, 84, 85, 86, 105, 108, 111,
    112, 113, 116, 120, 132, 137, 156, 161
  dysfunction 81, 83
    expansion 31, 35
    hyperplasia 85
    hypertrophy 65, 69, 85, 105, 111, 112, 113,
      116, 120
    lipid metabolism 69
    mitochondrial dysfunction in 63, 65
  necrotic 86
  necrotic-like 68
  white adipose tissue 24
Adipocytokines 81, 157
  prothrombotic 81
Adipogenesis 9, 11, 15, 68, 71, 81, 84
Adipokines 23, 31, 32, 35
  anti-inflammatory 23, 32, 35
  proinflammatory 35
  pro-inflammatory 31, 32
Adipokine 23, 31, 32, 35, 81, 169
  secretion pattern 81
  influence 169

secretion 23, 31, 32, 35
Adiponectin 23, 24, 26, 27, 28, 32, 33, 55, 56,
    65, 67, 68, 73, 74, 91, 92, 114, 115, 136,
    159, 170
  circulating 26, 27, 28
  globular 26
  protective 33
  release of 67, 68, 74
    secretion 28
    sensitivity 27
    synthesis 26, 65
Adipose tissue 16, 33, 63, 64, 65, 66, 71, 72,
    86, 95, 111, 112, 113, 116, 117, 134,
    157, 190, 195
  dendritic cells (ATDCs) 64, 72
  dysfunctional 86, 95, 195
  excessive 157
  infiltration of 112, 190
  inflammation 16, 63, 65, 66, 116
    macrophages 33, 66, 71, 111, 117
    meta-inflammation 134
Adipose tissue dysfunction 63, 64, 65, 66, 70,
    71, 72, 86, 88, 152, 163
  features of 65
  hallmarks of 63, 66
Alzheimer disease 131, 132, 182
AMP-activated 27, 170
  kinase 27
  protein kinase, activating 170
AMPK pathways 161
Amyloidogenesis 135, 143, 167
  astrocyte-mediated 167
Amyloid 138, 142, 145, 146, 162, 182
  plaques 138, 142, 146
  precursor protein (APP) 142, 145, 162, 182
Anorexigenic 24, 46, 47, 48, 56
  hormones 24
  neurons 46
  neurotransmitters 48
    proopiomelanocortin 56
    neurotransmitters 47
Anti-inflammatory 33, 64, 66, 67, 68, 69, 70,
    113, 121, 145, 182

www.ingramcontent.com/pod-product-compliance
Lightning Source LLC
Chambersburg PA
CBHW050839220326
41598CB00006B/403